A **WOMAN'S GUIDE** TO

Sexual Health

Mary Jane Minkin, M.D.

Carol V. Wright, Ph.D.

YALE UNIVERSITY PRESS   **NEW HAVEN & LONDON**

First published as *The Yale Guide to Women's Reproductive Health* in 2003 by Yale University Press.

Published with assistance from the Louis Stern Memorial Fund.

Printed in the United States of America.

Library of Congress Control Number: 2002035738
ISBN 0-300-10594-0 (pbk. : alk. paper)

A catalogue record for this book is available from the British Library.

The paper in this book meets the guidelines for permanence and durability of the Committee on Production Guidelines for Book Longevity of the Council on Library Resources.

10 9 8 7 6 5 4 3 2 1

The information and suggestions in this book are not intended to replace the services of your physician or care-giver. Because each person and each medical situation is unique, you should consult your own physician to get answers to your personal questions, to evaluate any symptoms you may have, or to receive suggestions on appropriate medications.

The authors have attempted to make this book as accurate and up-to-date as possible, but it may nevertheless contain errors, omissions, or material that is out of date by the time you read it. Neither the authors nor the publisher has any legal responsibility or liability for errors, omissions, out-of-date material, or the reader's application of the medical information or advice in this book.

Although the case histories have been drawn from Dr. Minkin's medical experience, the names of the patients have been altered to protect their privacy.

▶ CONTENTS

▶ ILLUSTRATIONS

FIGURES

TABLES

BOXES

SOME of the most important choices you must make as a woman are those for which you may be least prepared. Your decisions about sexual activity, contraception, family planning, and reproductive health can affect your life in profound ways. Ideally you should make these choices, sometimes in conjunction with your doctor or health care provider, based on accurate information and thoughtful consideration. The purpose of this book is to provide you with that information and to start you thinking (when you have leisure and are not under pressure) about making these decisions: Is this the right time to become sexually active? What is the right contraception for me? If I'm planning to get pregnant is there anything I should know before I stop using contraception? Can I do anything about my menstrual cramps? How can I protect myself from sexually transmitted diseases? Do I really have PMS (premenstrual syndrome), or do all women feel this way during the second half of their cycles?

Your need for a solid bedrock of knowledge on which to base your decisions has been heightened in recent years by changes, both positive and negative, in the way medicine is practiced. On the one hand, women are beginning to get more attention from a medical community that has not always responded to their needs. While earlier research often focused exclusively on men, the Women's Health Initiative, a fifteen-year study by the National Institutes of Health, is investigating chronic diseases that threaten women. Women physicians now play major roles in the health care system—as policymakers and as practicing doctors.

The year before I entered medical school, there were seven women in a class of one hundred at Yale, a proportion that reflected the numbers at other medical schools throughout the country. When I enrolled in 1971, my class had twenty women, a figure also comparable to national statistics. I found it interesting that all of a sudden 20 percent of the qualified applicants happened to be women, compared to a meager 7 percent the year before. Who said there were no quotas?

In another two years, the ratio of women to men was 30 percent; currently slightly more than half the class are female. Of course, this is a wonderful change. However, I do believe that it partially reflects the changing attitude of Americans about health care and physicians. People used to marvel at female equality in the former Soviet Union—after all, more than 80 percent of the physicians were women. However, in the Soviet Union being a physician was an insignificant job; being an engineer was the pinnacle, and only about 1 percent of the engineers were women. I suspect that part of the reason that women are now welcomed more warmly into the medical profession in this country is that the aura surrounding physicians has markedly diminished, so it is all right to have plenty of women doctors.

Significant changes have also come to my particular specialty. I was the second female resident in obstetrics and gynecology at Yale Medical School; now, nationally, well over half the residents in this specialty are women, and during some days of interviewing prospective residents we see no male applicants at all. Obstetrics used to be a field for the lower-ranking students of the medical school class. But with scientific advances including fetal monitoring and in vitro fertilization, and significant leaps forward in understanding the molecular biology of cancer, gynecology today attracts some very fine students, both male and female. Most important, our clientele—women—have been upgraded in the eyes of the world, so taking care of them has become a worthwhile endeavor. Consequently, we have more qualified "ob-gyns" than ever before.

While the enhanced role of women in medicine has been a positive development, the health care system itself has generally become less responsive to the needs of both men and women. The rise of health maintenance organizations (HMOs), which control the business end of medicine, has meant that you may have less access to your caregiver. It may take longer to get an appointment, and when you do get one, you may find the office a very busy place. Reimbursement by HMOs is ever more limited, so that practitioners need to see more patients to cover their operating expenses. The amount of paperwork has expanded exponentially. Less time per patient is the outcome. Surely most of my colleagues would like to spend more time with their patients, but they cannot if they want to see their own families in the evening.

Thus, the HMO-ization of American health care has undermined what I perceive to be the major advantage offered by women practitioners, increased communication with patients. Your caregiver may not be able to devote as much time to your appointment as either of you would like. You may not have the luxury of time to talk about prevention—the things you can do to maximize your health and ward off possible problems.

In view of all these developments in the health care system, it is crucial for you to educate yourself to participate in your own care. If you know basically how your body works, which problems may arise, and what solutions are available, you can better sift through the available health care choices, preferably with the help of your caregiver. My hope, then, is that this book will augment some of the information you may have received directly from your health care provider. And perhaps it will help you frame the questions you would like to ask in the limited time you have together, so that you can make decisions that in the long run will help you stay healthy. Although this book has two authors, the "I" who answers and discusses the questions is M.J.M., the physician.

As a gynecologist, I do breast examinations on my patients every day, but for the chapter on breast health, I consulted with my friend and colleague, Dr. Kristin Zarfos, assistant professor of surgery at the University of Connecticut Medical School. Since most vasectomies are performed by urologists, another friend and colleague, Dr. Ralph De Vito, associate clinical professor of urology at Yale University School of Medicine, helped with that section. Carol Wright and I thank our agent, Mildred Marmur, for her wisdom and encouragement. We are grateful for Vivian Wheeler's impeccable copy editing. Jean Thomson Black at Yale University Press offered fine editorial advice and shepherded this project along as it assumed larger and larger proportions. Finally, we both acknowledge the many contributions of our families to our lives and work: Steve, Allie, and Max Pincus, and Fred and Catherine Wright.

M.J.M.

A WOMAN'S GUIDE TO SEXUAL HEALTH

1 Your Reproductive System and How It Works

▶ **MYTH** Your sexual response depends on your anatomy. For example, the size of your clitoris determines whether you will have orgasms.

FACT Your mind is more important than your body in determining your sexual response.

THIS chapter describes the basics of your reproductive anatomy, tells you how it works, and explains how to keep your body in good working order throughout your life.

THE FEMALE ANATOMY

The external female genital organs, collectively called the vulva, include the mons pubis, labia majora, labia minora, clitoris, urethral opening, hymen, vaginal opening, and perineum.

The mons pubis, or mons, is a fatty pad that covers the pubic bone. The labia are two pairs of skin folds, one inside the other, that cover and protect the vagina. The outer ones, the labia majora (large lips), are derived from the same embryological tissues that give rise to the scrotum in males. After puberty the mons and labia majora are covered with hair. The inner pair, the labia minora (small lips), are flaps of soft skin. Like the lips of your mouth, they are covered with epithelium and are delicate and pink. At the top or front, the

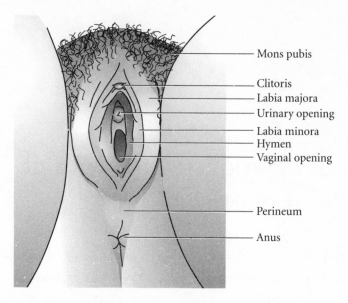

Mons pubis

Clitoris
Labia majora
Urinary opening

Labia minora
Hymen
Vaginal opening

Perineum

Anus

FIGURE 1. The external female reproductive organs.

narrow labia minora come together to form the hood of the clitoris. The labia minora can vary quite a bit in size from one woman to another; they can be hidden by the labia majora or may extend beyond them. The clitoris is a small cylindrical organ made of erectile tissue located where the folds of the labia minora come together toward the front of the body. It is derived from the same embryological tissue as the penis and plays an important role in female sexual pleasure and orgasm.

The opening of the urethra (the tube that carries urine from the bladder to the outside of the body) is located inside the labia minora between the clitoris and the vaginal opening. The vaginal opening is also covered by the labia minora. In virgins it may be partly covered by the hymen, a delicate membrane that usually encircles the opening like a ring or ruffle. The hymeneal tissue narrows the opening but still allows menstrual blood to flow out. In rare instances the hymen is completely closed. Women who have not had sexual intercourse may or may not have an obvious hymen; it can be ruptured by exercise or tampon use. Many women do not have a show of blood on the occasion of their first intercourse.

The perineum is the area of less hairy skin and tissue that lies between the vaginal opening and the anus. It has very little fat, so the skin in this area lies close to the muscle beneath.

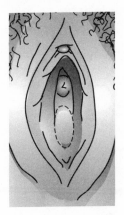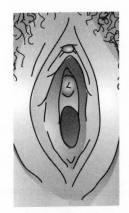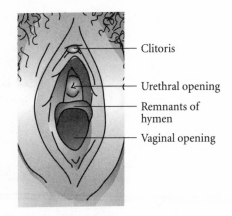

Clitoris

Urethral opening

Remnants of hymen

Vaginal opening

FIGURE 2. The hymen, a membrane that surrounds the opening of the vagina, can vary in shape and thickness. At the left is an imperforate hymen, which completely closes off the vagina. The appearance of the hymen after childbirth is shown at the right.

The most prominent of the inner organs is the vagina. The canal, usually 3.5–4 inches (9–10 cm) long, connects the vulva with the uterus. It is lined with epithelium and surrounded by layers of muscle. The vagina is ridged and expands like the folds of an accordion during intercourse and childbirth. Its muscular walls contract during orgasm, which helps the sperm deposited there ascend to the uterus. (The sperm can readily do so without help; thus it is definitely possible to become pregnant without having an orgasm.)

The cervix, the lower neck of the uterus, extends down into the vagina. If you think of the uterus as a pear sitting, stem end down, on a drinking glass, the cervix is the part inside the glass. Made of elastic and connective tissue and some muscle fibers, it serves as a gateway to the organs above. Looked at from below (as your doctor sees it during a pelvic examination), the cervix looks like a tiny doughnut. If you have not had children, the opening is small and round; once you have had a child, the opening becomes wider and more horizontal.

After intercourse the sperm pass through the cervix and uterus and head upward to the fallopian tubes. Certain glands in the cervix secrete mucus that seems to nourish sperm and definitely kills bacteria, thereby helping to prevent infection. Except around the time of ovulation, this mucus is sticky and opaque, and there is little of it. At the time of ovulation, the glandular cells secrete more mucus. It becomes thin, slippery, and rich in carbohydrates and amino acids, a perfect medium for the upward migration of sperm. During labor and delivery, the cervix thins out and dilates, increasing in size by a factor of about fifty, so that the baby can leave the uterus and enter the birth canal.

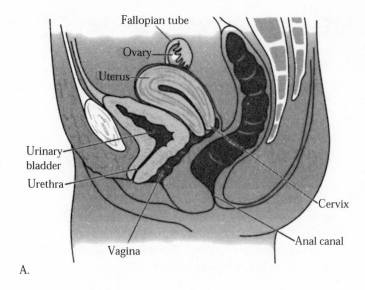

A.

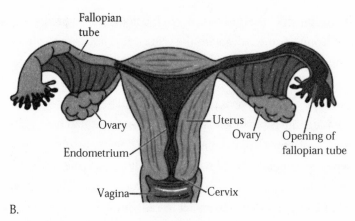

B.

FIGURE 3. The internal female reproductive organs. A, lateral view; B, frontal view.

The uterus, or womb, is a thick-walled, hollow, pear-shaped muscular organ, whose job is to protect and shelter the fetus as it grows. In women who have never been pregnant, the uterus is about the size of a pear: 4 inches (9 cm) long, 2.5 inches (6.5 cm) wide and 1.4 inches (3.5 cm) thick. The main body of the uterus has three layers. The outer layer is a thin peritoneal covering. The myometrium, the middle and thickest layer, is made of muscle that responds to hormonal and other chemical signals. This layer contracts rhythmically at the onset of menstruation and during labor and delivery. The inner layer, the endometrium, is composed of glandular tissue. The endometrium (along with some other fluids and cells) is shed during menstruation.

The fallopian tubes are the passageways through which eggs travel from the ovaries to the uterus. The tubes are attached to the uterus and reach out toward the ovaries without actually touching them. Each tube is just under 5 inches (10–12 cm) long and about 1 inch (2.5 cm) wide at the broad end near the ovary. As they join the uterus, the tubes narrow to the width of thin spaghetti. The ends near the ovaries flare out like the bell of a trumpet and are surrounded by a fringe of specialized cells whose hairlike "fingers" (*fimbriae,* the Latin for "fringe") wave rhythmically, beckoning the egg into the tube. The fimbriae have quite a range of motion and can even drape themselves over the ovary like the tentacles of an octopus, making it easier for an egg to "find" its way into the tube.

The two ovaries, at the ends of the fallopian tubes, are the center of the action; they produce eggs. Each ovary is 1–2 inches (3–5 cm) long, 1 inch (2.5 cm) wide, and 0.75 inch (2 cm) thick, about the size of an almond in its shell, although the ovaries change in shape and size during the menstrual cycle. Each ovary produces, on average, one egg every other month, but if one ovary is lost through surgery or some other cause, the surviving ovary can usually manage double duty. The ovaries also produce hormones that serve the process of reproduction—mainly estrogen and progesterone, and a few others.

Many teenage girls and some women worry about whether their anatomy is "normal." If something about your reproductive anatomy worries you, don't hesitate to ask your caregiver, who will probably be able to set your concerns to rest. There is a wide range of what is normal in sex characteristics—patterns of hair growth and breast size and symmetry, for example—just as there are wide ranges of height and weight, hair color, and skin shade. The various parts of the female reproductive anatomy come in different sizes and shapes. Women can have short or long labia minora; sometimes the inner lips can be so long that they get in the way of underclothing, which is unusual but certainly normal.

> Amy is a fine athlete. In high school she played soccer and in college she rows competitively, training every day on one of the local rivers. Amy has long labia that keep getting caught in her workout clothes. While this is not dangerous, it is annoying. Amy decides to have minor surgery, to trim back her labia and make her more comfortable when she works out.

Generally the clitoris is large enough to be seen externally between the folds of the labia minora, but sometimes it is not. In rare instances an abnormality that causes too much testosterone production (all women produce a little of this male hormone) may result in an enlarged clitoris.

There is also considerable normal variation in breast size and appearance. The colored area around the nipple (the areola) can be large or small, dark or light, ranging from pink to dark brown. Many women have one breast that is larger or slightly higher than the other.

Facial and body hair is another issue for some women. In general, your genes determine how much hair you have and where it grows. Almost a third of women between the ages of 15 and 44 have some upper-lip hair. Of this group maybe 6–9 percent have some hair on the sides of the face or the chin as well. If you are of Mediterranean descent, you may well have more facial hair than someone whose background is Scandinavian. If your hair is dark, it will be more noticeable. Only in rare cases—when a woman makes too much testosterone—can facial hair signal a problem.

Men and women have different distributions of pubic hair, though again there is a wide range of normal for each sex. Women's pubic hair is generally in a triangle with some spread to the inner thighs. Pubic hair also covers the outside of the labia majora between the legs and the area around the opening of the vagina. In men, pubic hair may extend up toward the belly button in the shape of a triangle or diamond. Some women too have a line of hair that reaches toward the belly button; others have hair that extends down inside the thighs. Some women have dark hairs around their nipples.

Chances are that your own pattern of pubic hair will resemble your mother's (though by the time you get around to checking, she may have gone through menopause and have less than she did as a young woman). Or your pattern will follow that of some other female relative, perhaps on your father's side of the family.

When one of my patients worries that she has some anatomical problem that interferes with her sex drive, I am able to reassure her about 99 percent of the time that nothing is physically wrong. There may be a psychological component to these persistent anxieties, and many women find counseling helpful.

If something should prove to be anatomically wrong, it probably will be a relief to know that nowadays gynecologists or surgeons can construct the external female anatomy quite easily. Years ago when I was a medical student, I did a routine checkup on a woman who had had a sex change operation, a total reconstruction of her anatomy. Of course she did not have a uterus or ovaries, and she took estrogen to make sure that she had breasts and the other female secondary sex characteristics, but outwardly—in terms of her genitals and her general appearance—she looked like a perfectly ordinary woman.

THE PHYSIOLOGY OF THE MENSTRUAL CYCLE

Although menstruation usually begins when a girl is between 10 and 16 years of age, the reproductive process actually starts before birth. It continues until menopause, which in this country generally occurs between the ages of 45 and 55.

The ovaries along with the primitive egg cells are among the first structures formed during fetal life. Before a baby girl is born, her ovaries have produced all the eggs she will ever have. By the twentieth week of pregnancy, the future baby girl has some 4 million to 6 million egg cells, which then decrease in number throughout her life. At birth, the number has dwindled to somewhere between 1 million and 2 million. When she reaches puberty, about 300,000 remain. (These figures represent informed guesswork.) During her reproductive life span, fewer than 400 will mature completely and be released into the fallopian tubes to await fertilization. The others deteriorate and are reabsorbed by the body, so that by the time a woman reaches menopause, only a very few remain.

The fact that women do not produce new eggs during their lifetime has an important impact on reproduction. The egg with which a woman becomes pregnant was formed during her prenatal life and if she is in her mid-40s, that egg will be 40-plus years old. Since men *do* produce new sperm as they go through life, this 40-something egg will be fertilized with sperm that was made perhaps two months previously.

By the time a girl reaches puberty, she has lost more than half the eggs she had at birth. The remainder are at rest, enclosed in structures that will form the ovarian follicles. In their simplest state, each follicle consists of an egg cell surrounded by a single layer of cells called granulosa cells. When the ovaries become more active at puberty, the eggs begin to develop.

Like a car engine that sputters a little before the ignition catches and fires, the cycle does not work perfectly at the beginning. Young girls who are just starting to menstruate may have heavy periods, light periods, or irregular periods as their cycles adjust. Once normal cycles begin, they repeat themselves each month, generally without much variation unless pregnancy takes place. Stress, severe weight loss, and certain birth control methods can also disrupt the regular pattern.

Every month some of the follicles start growing. In each growing follicle, the granulosa cells divide and reproduce many times. Instead of a single layer, many layers of cells now surround the egg cell; these granulosa cells produce most of the estrogen in the body. The cells in the ovary surrounding this developing follicle cause the outer layer of the follicle to grow and stimulate its cells to differentiate.

About a week into the menstrual cycle, the biggest follicle of the group that is growing

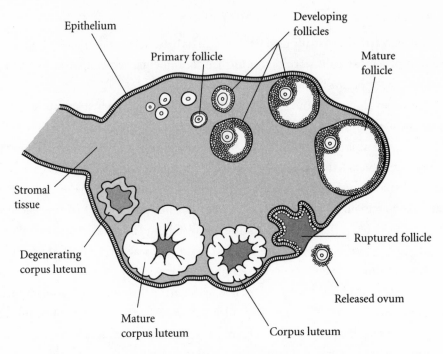

FIGURE 4. The ovary, with follicles developing and degenerating during the menstrual cycle.

and differentiating is chosen to be "follicle of the month"—in scientific terminology, the dominant follicle. It continues to get bigger while the other follicles degenerate and die off. Occasionally more than one follicle continues to develop, creating the possibility of fraternal twins.

When the dominant follicle reaches a certain size, it ruptures. The egg cell and some of the surrounding granulosa cells burst through the wall of the ovary, an event known as ovulation. This happens on about day 14 of a twenty-eight-day menstrual cycle. If all goes well, the egg cell is swept into the fallopian tubes by the specialized fringed cells. Once in the tube, the egg may or may not be fertilized. This first part of the menstrual cycle, which deals with the development of the follicles, is called the follicular phase.

Back in the ovary, what is left of the ruptured follicle becomes active again. It changes into a yellowish glandlike structure called the corpus luteum (Latin for "yellow body"). If the egg cell in the fallopian tube does not meet any sperm and become fertilized, the corpus luteum grows for about ten days (until day 24 of the cycle), then in its turn begins to degenerate. During its short life span (in a nonpregnant woman), the corpus luteum secretes large amounts of the hormones progesterone and estrogen.

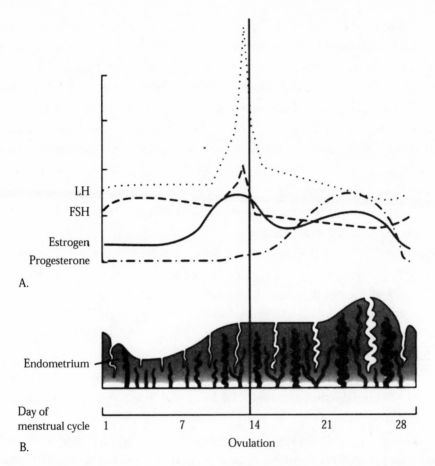

LH
FSH
Estrogen
Progesterone
A.

Endometrium

Day of
menstrual cycle   1   7   14   21   28
B.   Ovulation

FIGURE 5. Hormone levels and changes in the uterine lining during the menstrual cycle. A, levels of pituitary and ovarian hormones in the bloodstream; B, maturation and thickening of the lining of the uterus and its blood supply.

All this hormonal action stimulates changes in the uterine lining (endometrium). As the follicles develop in the ovaries, the lining of the uterus begins to thicken, responding to the estrogen produced in the ovaries. After ovulation takes place, the estrogen level surges again. The additional progesterone produced by the corpus luteum acts on the endometrial tissue to stabilize it and make it hospitable to a fertilized egg, should fertilization occur. Stimulated by progesterone, glandular tissue and blood vessels proliferate in the endometrium, making it thick and spongy. The endometrium itself now begins to produce various chemicals, including prostaglandin, which are responsible for menstrual cramps and other premenstrual symptoms.

If fertilization of the egg does take place, a hormone produced by the placenta, human chorionic gonadotropin (hCG), keeps the corpus luteum active for another six to eight weeks as the embryo develops. If fertilization does not occur and the corpus luteum dissolves, on about day 25 of the cycle a sudden shutdown in the production of both progesterone and estrogen occurs. The endometrium loses its support system and the uterine blood vessels constrict, so that the lining has a diminished supply of oxygen and nutrients. The muscular walls of the uterus begin to contract rhythmically, stimulated by prostaglandin. Soon the uterine lining disintegrates and is sloughed off as menstrual blood. A thin, deep layer of cells remains, from which the endometrium will regenerate for the next cycle. This part of the menstrual cycle, from ovulation on day 14 to the onset of menstruation on day 28, is called the luteal phase.

This routine is as carefully organized as an intricately plotted novel. The organizers and controllers—the agents that start and stop the different actions of the cycle—are hormones. Although the ovaries are the chief producers of the female sex hormones estrogen and progesterone, they do their job as part of a chain of command that begins (to the best of our knowledge) in the brain.

The action starts in the cerebral cortex, the mass of gray matter that plays a role in memory, language acquisition, and motor control. We do not know precisely how the cerebral cortex regulates the hormones of the menstrual cycle, but changes such as the loss of periods during times of stress seem to be influenced by the cortex.

The next player in the sequence is the hypothalamus, a small region of the brain that lies above the pituitary gland and below an area called the thalamus. Though tiny, the hypothalamus has an important role in regulating the body's internal environment: influencing eating behavior, the daily sleep and waking cycle, and the water balance within cells and tissues. The hypothalamus also releases the hormones that trigger menstruation.

After a girl reaches puberty, the hypothalamus begins the ovarian cycle each month by secreting a hormone called GnRH, gonadotropin-releasing hormone. The gonadotropins that get released are luteinizing hormone (LH) and follicle-stimulating hormone (FSH). These gonadotropins control the gonads (the organs that make reproductive cells, eggs or sperm; that is, the ovaries in women and the testes in men).

The chemical messenger GnRH alerts the appropriate region of the pituitary gland, geographically a close neighbor of the hypothalamus, to secrete its hormones, LH and FSH. The hormones from the pituitary will in turn stimulate the ovaries. The FSH does just what its name suggests: it stimulates the follicles to develop. The LH, whose presence in the blood surges at midcycle, causes the dominant follicle to release the egg cell, culminating in ovulation.

This complex regulation is governed by a control system called negative or reciprocal feedback, which works more or less like a thermostat. Once set, the thermostat in a room senses the temperature and turns the furnace off or on to keep the temperature at the pre-set level. Within your body the regulating factors are chemical, rather than thermal, but the principle is the same. A constant adjustment takes place between your brain and your ovaries, as the brain responds to the levels of estrogen it senses. For example, a lack of estrogen in the blood causes the LH and FSH to rise, during the menstrual cycle and also at the time of menopause.

Month after month this sequence repeats itself until you reach menopause, though gradually the cycle changes as you grow older. Women in their late 30s sometimes have shorter menstrual cycles, often less than twenty-eight days, because during the second half of the cycle, the corpus luteum of an older woman produces less progesterone than that of someone in her 20s. Less progesterone means the lining of the uterus may break down and be sloughed off sooner. Eventually the reduced number of follicles and their lowered quality lead to lower estrogen production. When estrogen drops below a certain level, there is not enough to produce the LH surge and ovulation. Older women approaching menopause, like adolescent girls, have irregular periods for a while and do not ovulate during their cycles. Eventually estrogen levels drop so low that menstruation stops altogether.

2 You and Your Gynecologist

▶ **MYTH** If you have a gynecological exam before you are sexually active, you will no longer be a virgin.

FACT Unless there is some special problem, your gynecologist can use a small speculum that will not rupture your hymen.

GYNECOLOGISTS are specialists in women's reproductive health, but internists or family practitioners, trained nurse-practitioners, and physician's assistants are all trained in routine gynecological care. These professionals can do physical exams and tests, write prescriptions (under the supervision of a physician), treat common problems, and answer most of your questions. Gynecologists, unlike these other professionals, are trained in surgery. Throughout this book I speak from my own point of view as a gynecologist, but remember that your family doctor or your nurse-practitioner can also help you.

You may start seeing a gynecologist because you have a problem—perhaps painful, heavy, or irregular menstrual periods, or a vaginal discharge. Or you have started having intercourse and want to discuss your options for contraception. These are excellent reasons for starting a relationship with a gynecologist. Going to a gynecologist for preventive care is also worthwhile, just as you go to your dentist for a semiannual checkup and cleaning to help prevent dental disease.

Like many women, you may want to use your gynecologist as a primary health care provider, especially if you have few common ailments or general aches and pains. When you go for your gynecology appointment, maybe for help with contraception or care during pregnancy, you can ask questions about your general health. However, after age 35 or so, it is advisable to establish a relationship with an internist, who can get baseline readings on factors related to your general health.

YOUR DOCTOR

Gynecologists are trained to deal with problems related to your reproductive system and your sexuality. They can answer questions about menstrual difficulties, sexuality (sexual response, sexual desire, sexual orientation), safe sex and sexual responsibility, contraception and family planning, fertility and infertility, miscarriage and abortion. They can provide a starting point for dealing with the psychological problems surrounding some sexual issues: they can give basic counseling or refer you to a therapist on difficulties involving body image, fear of cancer, or sexual response. If you have been raped or been the victim of incest, your gynecologist can help you or refer you to someone to assist in resolving the issues that surround these traumatizing experiences.

▶ *At what age should you start seeing a gynecologist?*

Many gynecologists believe that age 14 or 15 is appropriate, and current medical training seems to further this view. I disagree; I believe there is no single right answer.

Sexually active teenagers need information about contraception and safe sex. If a girl has a solid relationship with her pediatrician and the pediatrician is skilled in basic gynecology, that doctor can serve as her first gynecologist, especially since many gynecologists who treat adult women are not attuned to teenagers. Very few young girls have anything seriously wrong with them physically, but on the rare chance that something demands more specialized training (diagnosing an ovarian mass, for example) the pediatrician can refer the patient to a gynecologist.

Young women who are not sexually active can wait until their late teens or early 20s to see a gynecologist. There is no point in forcing a young girl to have a pelvic exam until she becomes sexually active or wants to see a gynecologist because she has some problem.

An appropriate time to start is just before college. Many young women who have not been sexually active in high school may become active in college, so it is reasonable to discuss birth control and safe sex. Although many high schools offer sex education, hearing the information from a health care professional outside of school may provide further support. If the college is far from home, the college health care program can serve as a backup in an emergency. Some schools have better programs than others, a factor you might check when looking at colleges.

▶ *Should a teenager with menstrual problems have a gynecological checkup?*

You probably do not need a pelvic exam if you're 14 years old and have irregular periods, since most girls do not have regular periods for about two years. By letting nature take its course, your body will develop its own schedule.

If you have cramps, probably you have just begun to ovulate. Most girls begin having periods before they ovulate; when they do ovulate, perhaps a year later, they produce more prostaglandins and get cramps. Before you consult a gynecologist, try the familiar self-help methods: Continue your exercise program. Try over-the-counter pain remedies, beginning with a little Tylenol. If that does not help, try a little aspirin; if you still do not get relief, try ibuprofen (sold over the counter as Advil) or even naproxen (Aleve), which is stronger than ibuprofen.

If you have heavy bleeding, it may be related to periods in which ovulation has not taken place. One of the usual therapies for heavy bleeding and also for cramps that do not respond to over-the-counter medications is birth control pills, for which you will need a prescription. If the heavy bleeding does not respond to the pill, it might be worth investigating. Sometimes irregular or heavy periods can be caused by blood abnormalities that can be diagnosed with a blood test.

If your menstrual irregularities cause so much emotional anguish that they interfere with school work and social life, perhaps you need to explore these anxieties with a pediatric counselor. In general, if you are losing time from school and other productive activities because of menstrual difficulties, it is worth talking with your pediatrician or with a gynecologist.

Whatever your age, when you are about to undergo your first gynecological exam, you should feel comfortable with your physician. You should be confident that you will receive quality care and satisfied that she (or he) is attentive to you. You will not know this until the two of you meet, but if you do feel uncomfortable, it is quite all right to leave. I know this is not easy, but you can just say something like, "I don't think this is going to work out." You will probably be charged for the visit, since you took up the doctor's time, and you should pay the bill without complaint. It is still much better than going through an examination with someone who makes you feel uneasy.

When you make the appointment, check to see what the routine is. Will there be a discussion with the doctor before the actual examination? On a first visit, your physician should talk to you before you undress for the exam. On later visits it might be all right to chat while you are wearing a hospital gown, but not on the first. If the office manager, receptionist, or nurse says that that doctor does not schedule a talk in an office setting before the exam, it is perfectly reasonable to ask for one. Unless this is a first visit, gynecological exams are usually scheduled as fifteen-minute appointments.

TALKING THINGS OVER

Before you have your actual physical, your doctor will want to learn about your general health and your gynecological health. As an opener, I usually ask my patients what brought them to the office; that gives them a chance to voice their concerns, and I try to chat a little to make them comfortable and create a connection between us.

Jot down questions before you go to your appointment, or you may kick yourself afterward for forgetting to bring up something important. People do get nervous when they go to the doctor. I call it the "white-coat syndrome" and it can cause a spike of twenty or thirty points in blood pressure, as well as a bout of forgetfulness.

After your gynecologist has determined why you came for the visit, she will take your medical history—focusing first, usually, on your gynecological history. How old were you when you had your first period? How frequently were your periods initially? How frequent are they now? Do you have cramps? Do you have problems with heavy flow? How many days do your periods last? Has there been a change in your cycle or your periods?

Then the doctor will ask about your general medical history. Have you had any significant illnesses? Been in the hospital? Had an operation? Next she will go through a review of systems. What about your heart—do you have palpitations or chest pains? Do you have problems with your lungs—for example, asthma? How about your digestion? Constipation or diarrhea? Abdominal pain? And so on, through all your major organ systems.

Since your physician may check your family history, it is probably worthwhile to get this information together before the initial visit. Especially if you are older, your doctor may try to assess your risk for heart disease, osteoporosis, or certain kinds of cancers. Your family history is important in two ways. First, with conditions such as heart disease or osteoporosis, adopting a certain kind of behavior early in life can really help you. If you know your grandmother or mother lost 4 inches of height at the end of her life, you would be smart to start getting plenty of calcium as a young woman and to monitor your intake throughout your adult life. (Actually all women should do that, but awareness of your increased risk might be the "scare factor" needed to keep you on the mark.) Second, when you plan for pregnancy, your doctor should know about genetic diseases in your family (for example, cystic fibrosis, sickle-cell anemia, or Tay-Sachs disease).

Sometimes people who have been adopted (or for other reasons do not know their family medical history) worry that some terrible unknown disease may lurk in their background that they will be unable to avoid. While in the case of Alzheimer's disease or osteoporosis it is helpful to know that you have a family history of that condition, you are not at a tremendous disadvantage in general. Family history counts, but not to the extent that many people imagine. For example, most women with a grandmother who has had breast cancer are concerned about their own risk. In actuality, your grandmother's history means very little. If she died of breast cancer at the age of 85, you have nothing to worry about. Your *maternal* history is what counts. If your grandma died of breast cancer before menopause, say at age 40, and your mother is 55, postmenopausal, and free of breast cancer, then genetically speaking you are in good shape. If some disease in your family history does concern you, bring it up; your doctor may be able to reassure you.

Your doctor may ask about your preferences in matters of health, or you may bring up these issues yourself. Do you prefer a "natural" approach to your health? Do you buy organic food, herbal medicines, and natural cosmetics, utilizing chain supermarkets and drugstores only as a last resort? You accept medical intervention if it is absolutely necessary—for example, insulin for diabetes—but you would rather treat a urinary tract infection with cranberry juice than go to a doctor and get sulfa? Or perhaps you have no objection to "manufactured" medications. You eat a healthy diet, get adequate exercise, and look after your general well-being, but you have no strong feelings against taking antibiotics or other medications.

Let your doctor know how you feel. She may be able to take your preferences into consideration when suggesting medications or other therapy.

Your gynecologist will ask if you are sexually active, because it influences the issues you and she discuss and your treatment if a problem turns up. If you are concerned about confidentiality, ask before you make the office visit. My own policy is to treat what any patient tells me with absolute confidentiality.

I encourage teenagers and younger women to be open with their parents, so that if an issue does arise, parents and children will be able to work together to solve it. We have all heard about terrible consequences resulting from unintended teenage pregnancies, tragedies that could have been prevented if daughters were not afraid to trust their parents.

On the other hand, I have been a doctor long enough to be a realist. I encourage abstinence, and I counsel young women not to rush into sex just because everyone else is doing it or because their current boyfriend is urging it. But I know from experience that many young women do have intercourse and that their mothers would be angry and distressed if they knew. (Ironically, I have treated some of those mothers and know that they too were sexually active before they were married.)

Many doctors don't mind if you bring an advocate to your appointment. Some young girls are frightened and want their mothers with them for comfort. Others would have preferred to come alone and make this opinion clear by subtle or not-so-subtle signals. In this case I talk about whatever issues the daughter and mother want to discuss together during the interview, then I ask some of the important questions again when the daughter and I are alone in the examining room. The mother's main concern may be her daughter's menstrual cramps, whereas the daughter really wants to talk about birth control. If that is the case, the daughter and I can also talk in private about sexually transmitted diseases and safe sex.

Another reason for privacy in the examining room is that one of the markers for sexual abuse and physical violence in a relationship is that the husband, boyfriend, or significant other comes to every appointment.

Anna was pregnant with her second child. Her husband, a resident physician at a nearby hospital, accompanied her on every prenatal visit. My colleagues thought he was really generous, taking time out of his busy schedule to accompany Anna. I felt it was a little strange, but his presence failed to set off any alarms in my mind, especially since he had a fine reputation among his colleagues and patients. Much later I realized he had been physically violent with Anna and did not want her to talk to me alone. She never mentioned abuse and we never saw physical evidence of it on her body. She had plenty of psychological scars, however.

One day, years after her last child was born, Anna arrived in our office unannounced, without an appointment. The abuse had been going on so long that her sense of self-worth had been utterly destroyed. She told me that she had figured out exactly how she was going to kill herself, and I was afraid that she would follow through the minute she left my office. She and I went in my car directly to the psychiatric unit of our hospital, where she received help and support.

Since this experience, I have been more aware of the possibilities of abuse and more likely to view the ever-present spouse with a little suspicion.

Some girls are comfortable going to the doctor who treats their mother. Others are not. Sometimes a mother will see me and the daughter will see one of my partners, keeping them in the same "medical family" but maintaining a little distance. Some young women prefer getting birth control information and prescriptions from Planned Parenthood; others use the health care system at their college.

When I first started practicing, some of the mothers asked if they could bring their preschool daughters into the examining room, where they played with toys in the corner. I used to think this was rather strange, but I have come to believe it is a good idea. Actually I am treating some of those girls now as young adults, and I think the experience gave them a sense of what the exam was like and a greater feeling of comfort.

THE PHYSICAL EXAMINATION

Once you and your doctor have talked over your history, your health care preferences, and your general concerns, you will have the actual physical exam. The nurse (probably) will show you to the examining room to undress. I encourage women to disrobe entirely, because I like to do a breast exam and it is hard to do one through a bra. You may want to leave your socks on, as they will make you more comfortable in the stirrups on the examining table.

After you have undressed, you will put on a gown. In our office we use cloth gowns, which are comfortable, quite modest, and more attractive and ecological than the paper gowns that many offices use for sanitary reasons. The federal Occupational Safety and Health Administration (OSHA), which oversees health and safety issues, has high standards of sanitation, so we send the cloth gowns to an OSHA-approved laundry more than a hundred miles away. Our patients often comment that they like the cloth gowns, so we continue to use them.

WEIGHT, BLOOD PRESSURE, AND OTHER LAB TESTS

The nurse will start by weighing you. You are not alone if you think getting weighed is the worst part of the exam. Our society simultaneously encourages women to be rail thin and bombards us with ads for soft drinks and fatty fast food, so it is not surprising that many women carry a lot of psychological baggage on the subject of body weight. I never force anyone to be weighed, but I think it is worthwhile to know where you are and where you are headed. Realizing that you are gaining every year is an incentive to work at keeping your weight down. If you are staying in the healthy range, it is satisfying to know you are where you should be.

Blood pressure is another indicator worth checking. If you are one of those people with white-coat syndrome, your reading may be high simply because you are nervous. If your blood pressure is still high when taken a second time because you are still nervous, then I might suggest that if your local pharmacist has a cuff, you have your pressure taken there in a less intimidating setting. Other doctors suggest that you stop in one day when you happen to be driving by the office, without an appointment weighing on your mind, and have your blood pressure taken then.

Some doctors ask for a urine sample to test for protein and sugar in the urine. The protein measurement checks kidney function and the sugar test is for diabetes. Because these tests can signal complications of pregnancy, I do them routinely for pregnant women, but not for others. Some doctors routinely do a blood count, which involves a finger prick with a needle.

THE BREAST EXAM

When the doctor comes in to examine you, she will first probably listen to your heart and lungs. Most gynecologists will palpate (feel) your breasts to check for a discharge from the nipple or for lumps, checking also under your armpits, where lumps sometimes appear. Your doctor may also check for enlargement of the liver (by pressing in the right upper quadrant beneath your ribs) or of the spleen (under the left side of the rib cage) and palpate in the groin region, feeling for enlarged lymph nodes.

VAGINAL EXAMINATION

Then comes the part that no one likes. You lie on your back and put your feet into the little footrests, called stirrups, on the examining table. Your knees are bent and apart. This awkward posture, known as the dorsal lithotomy position, offers your doctor the best access to your reproductive organs. You will probably be asked to scoot down so that your buttocks are as close as possible to the edge of the table. This is important, especially if you are a first-timer, because the closer you are to the end of the table, the less discomfort you are likely to experience. Being in stirrups makes us all feel vulnerable. Sometimes women ask me if it is absolutely necessary to use the stirrups; unfortunately, it is.

If you have severe arthritis or other disabilities that prevent you from getting your feet into the stirrups, the office nurses can hold up your legs for you. It is possible to do pelvic exams on women with hip problems and even spinal cord injuries, though achieving the correct position is a little more difficult.

Once you have your feet in the stirrups, you should just let your knees flop apart and relax like a rag doll. If you tense your thigh muscles, you will also tense your vaginal muscles and the exam will be more difficult and uncomfortable than if you are limp.

▶ *Does your first pelvic exam hurt?*

If you have an intact hymen, the exam may be uncomfortable—but it may not. If your hymen is very tight, the doctor may not be able to do a speculum exam. (I have encountered this situation only about three times in my twenty-plus years of practice.) If you have this problem, you and the doctor may talk about surgical removal of the hymen at some later time.

A speculum is a double-sided instrument made of metal or plastic, whose sides can open, expanding the vagina so that the doctor can see your cervix. If the speculum is

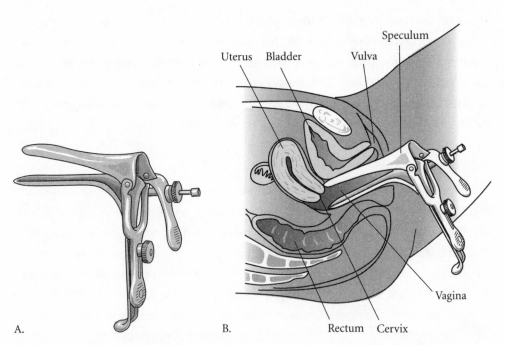

FIGURE 6. A, a speculum; B, the speculum holding open the vaginal walls to make the cervix visible.

metal, your doctor may warm it before insertion into your vagina, using either warm water or an electric heating pad. This is a courtesy and not all doctors do it, but when I teach I encourage residents to do so, especially for a first pelvic exam. Some doctors prefer plastic speculums, which do not get as cold. I prefer the metal ones because they are easier to adjust and they slide better.

Speculums come in different sizes, with narrow ones available for virgins and elderly women, and for special circumstances. If this is your first exam, the doctor will use a small one. If you have had several children, a wider one is appropriate. Your physician will insert the speculum gently into your vagina and encourage you to relax. Try to stay as loose as you can. If you are tense, your doctor will probably give you a little extra time. The cervix is in different locations in different women. Sometimes it just pops into view once the speculum is opened, but sometimes it is wedged high up in the vagina and is difficult to find. Once your doctor has located your cervix, she will perform a Pap test.

THE PAP TEST AND WHAT IT MEANS

This relatively simple test is named after its creator, Dr. George Nicolas Papanicolaou (1883–1962), and since its widespread use, the incidence of cervical cancer has fallen considerably. Dr. Papanicolaou's first published paper on the topic, entitled "New Cancer Diagnosis," was presented at a minor medical meeting in Battle Creek, Michigan, in 1928, but was generally ignored. By the mid-1940s, his idea that early-stage carcinomas not visible to the naked eye could be identified from vaginal smears was finding general acceptance. Today the Pap test, or smear, is one of the nation's most widely used tests and is credited with saving millions of lives and reducing the incidence of cervical cancer by about 70 percent.

A Pap test consists of taking a sample of the cervical cells and checking them microscopically to look for or rule out cervical cancer. Since precancerous changes may occur in the cervix years before the disease actually develops, regular Pap tests can help catch the disease while it is most curable. Most women tell me that the sampling feels "weird" or "strange," but does not actually hurt. Others interpret the feeling as discomfort or pain. Fortunately the process only lasts a few seconds.

There are two tools for collecting the cells. The first is a small plastic brush shaped to fit up close to the cervix; it is used to scrape cells from the outer side of the cervix. Then the second tool, a swab that looks like a tiny pipe cleaner or bottle brush, is rubbed around the inner part of the cervix where precancerous changes are most likely to occur. A generous sampling of cells from this area is desirable, and the brush takes off more cells than a simple Q-tip would.

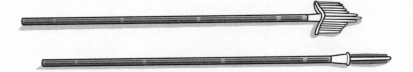

FIGURE 7. Tools for sampling cells from both the outside and the inside of the cervix.

The old-fashioned standard Pap smear involved wiping the swabs onto a glass slide and examining the sample microscopically. Newer techniques call for placing the sample in a liquid solution in a jar. A pathologist centrifuges the solution to gather the cells and puts the concentrated cells onto a glass slide. This is called a thin-prep or autocyte Pap test; its advantage over the older method is that the sample contains more cells for examination. For the last five or six years, insurance companies have been willing to pay for this test, which costs between twenty-five and fifty dollars.

After the Pap test and possible sampling of cervical secretions, your doctor will remove the speculum as gently as possible. If it is plastic, it is discarded. If it is metal, it is put in a receptacle for articles that will be sterilized.

A Pap smear is a guide, not a definitive test. It may indicate that everything is fine—no cells look cancerous or precancerous—or that some cells should be further investigated. The test will not invariably show exactly what cell changes are taking place in the cervix, but it will show that there *are* changes. Most of the changes that show up on Pap smears are benign or precancerous, and almost all can be cured with small interventions.

Although the main purpose of a Pap smear is to reveal abnormal cells that may lead eventually to cervical cancer, a Pap test can also detect about 25 percent of endometrial cancers and, very rarely, show the presence of ovarian cancer. In my twenty-five years of practice, I have seen this happen only once.

Josie, the mother of four children, has a Pap smear that shows odd-looking cells, unlike the kinds of cells commonly associated with cervical cancer. Her pelvic exam is normal and does not turn up any unusual mass within her abdomen.

At first I suspect that the abnormal cells may be from her uterus, so I do a D&C (dilation and curettage), scraping out the lining of her uterus and sending samples for microscopic examination. Although the cells from the D&C show no abnormal endometrial cells, they do show psammona bodies, abnormal cells associated with ovarian cancer.

Since ovarian cancer is now a distinct possibility, Josie and I decide that a hysterectomy is in order. One of my colleagues who specializes in cancer surgery stands by at the operation. We remove Josie's uterus and her ovaries, which are indeed cancerous.

It turns out that the cancer cells from her diseased ovaries have been picked up by her fallopian tubes and have traveled through her tubes and uterus down to her cervix. Josie has no symptoms whatsoever, which is often the case with ovarian cancer. Her abnormal Pap smear has saved her from serious disease.

It is also possible to test for some STDs by looking at your cervical secretions. Often, if someone tells me she does not practice safe sex, I will get her permission and take samples using a long swab like a Q-tip. The samples can be evaluated for gonorrhea or chlamydia by means of sophisticated testing techniques in a laboratory. Since some four million cases of chlamydia occur every year, it is prudent to be checked if you are at high risk.

Your doctor can put samples of any vaginal discharge onto glass slides and check them microscopically for bacteria. Certain bacteria have what are called clue cells (cells from the vaginal surface coated with bacteria) and can be recognized simply by looking through the microscope. Yeast, which is a fungus, and trichomonas, a parasite, can also be detected through a microscope.

▶ *Is something wrong if you bleed after your Pap test?*

Bleeding a bit after a Pap test is not unusual because of the swiping and rubbing of the cervix to sample the cells. Some women have a little spotting, and some even have a little flow. The amount depends on the "friability" or fragility of your cervix, the tendency of its cells to "crumble." Bleeding heavily after a Pap test is unusual; call your doctor if this happens to you.

▶ *What should you do if your Pap test is abnormal?*

If you have an abnormal Pap smear—and many women do at some point in their lives— do not panic. Proceed slowly. Have a repeat Pap test. Have biopsies. You probably do not need a hysterectomy because of one or two abnormal Pap smears unless a biopsy shows that you have invasive cancer. You have time to talk to your doctor and to get another opinion if you want. (See Chapter 9 for a discussion of Pap smear results and a description of treatment choices.)

A while ago, Scandinavian researchers studied a group of more than ten thousand women. Several thousand had carcinoma in situ of the cervix, a precursor stage of cervical cancer in which cells are abnormal but do not shown signs of spreading. The researchers followed these women for ten years but did not intervene medically. One third got well spontaneously and the cells in their cervixes reverted to normal. One third stayed the same. The final third progressed toward cancer. Although I do not advocate not treating carcinoma in situ just because the Scandinavian study said that some women got better spontaneously, remember that the time frame of the study was ten years, not twenty minutes. You have the luxury of time, unless a biopsy says otherwise.

THE BIMANUAL EXAMINATION

The next part of your checkup is the bimanual examination, a physical exam of your internal organs during which your doctor will use her two hands to feel for abnormalities. She will wear surgical gloves, so if you are allergic to latex, mention it; vinyl gloves are available as well as the more common latex ones. People who are sensitive to latex feel itching and burning from just a few moments' exposure. This sensitivity, while not common, seems to be an acquired allergy and increases with exposure. In our office we color-code the charts of women with allergies, but there is no harm in reminding your caregiver before the exam that you are latex sensitive.

Again, as with the earlier part of the exam, try to relax during the bimanual exam and stay as loose as you can. Try Lamaze breathing or other relaxation techniques; think pleasant thoughts of being in the Caribbean, the shoe store, or whatever relaxes you.

Your doctor places one, two, or occasionally three fingers in your vagina, and the other hand on your abdomen. Between her two hands she can check your pelvic organs for position and size. Is your uterus tipped back (which we call retroverted or retroflexed) or is it in the usual position? Is your uterus its normal size or is it enlarged? Are fibroids present?

With experience and under normal circumstances, we can tell a great deal. We can feel significant endometriosis. We can feel large ovarian cysts—or rather we can feel that the ovary has enlarged to three times its normal size. We can feel large fibroids, though not pea-sized ones. We can tell whether the fibroids move around. (Fibroids tend to be mobile; scar tissue from pelvic inflammatory disease and adhesions from endometriosis tend to be stuck in place.) If you have considerable body fat, are very muscular, or simply cannot relax, the bimanual exam may not reveal much.

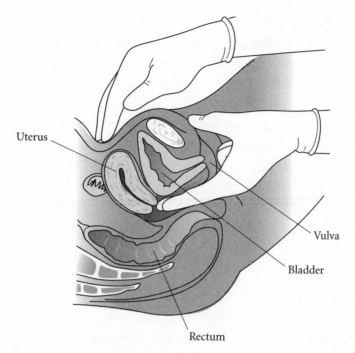

Uterus

Vulva

Bladder

Rectum

FIGURE 8. In a bimanual examination, the examiner presses on your abdomen from the outside with one hand while pushing upward from within your vagina with the other. This helps her feel your cervix, uterus, fallopian tubes, and ovaries.

▶ What if something abnormal turns up during the bimanual exam?

The bimanual exam gives a relatively accurate indication of the size and position of your organs and what is happening in the larger physical sense, but it does not reveal the inner composition of anything unusual. I may feel an enlarged ovary, but I am unable to tell from the physical exam whether it is a cyst filled with fluid, perhaps from endometriosis, or a solid mass that might be a cancerous tumor. To get this kind of information, I might recommend an ultrasound study, because this kind of imaging can distinguish between solid and fluid-filled growths.

THE RECTAL EXAMINATION

Finally, your doctor may perform a rectal exam. I tend to do this exam only on women who are 40 years of age or more, because it is an exam for cancer of the lower bowel and older people, both men and women, are more at risk. The rectal exam also gives the doctor another way to feel your pelvic organs. Your ovaries, for example, are often easier to feel from the rectum than from the vagina. If I suspect endometriosis or pelvic inflammatory disease in a younger woman and need another way to check the uterus, I may decide to do a rectal exam.

Your doctor will insert one well-lubricated finger into your vagina and another into your rectum, then feel between the fingers for any abnormalities. Most women do not find it painful, though it can be a little uncomfortable. Like the other parts of the pelvic exam, it is easier if you relax. And it lasts only thirty seconds or so.

AFTER THE EXAM

If the examination turns up nothing suspicious, your doctor should tell you right away, ask if you have any questions and answer them, and suggest a time for your next appointment—perhaps next year for a routine checkup.

If I find something suspicious, especially if I have an inkling that it could be serious, I will ask you to dress and come back to my office. People seem to listen better with their clothes on. Once there, we will talk about what might be wrong and what might be the next step in diagnosing the problem. Between these two extremes—everything all right and something possibly seriously wrong—we will discuss ways to solve the problem that brought you to the office in the first place. If you have pelvic pain during your periods and the exam has shown no endometriosis, for example, we can talk about therapy with birth control pills. If you are unsure how to take a medication—perhaps you have not taken birth control pills before—ask your doctor or the nurse.

Your doctor may give you a free sample of the medication she is prescribing for you. Samples given out by pharmaceutical companies are identical to the product available at the drugstore. They usually come with a leaflet that contains in very fine print everything anyone could possibly need to know about the medication: how to use it, its chemical structure, its action in the body, reasons for using it (indications) and for not using it (contraindications), and how it interacts with food or other medications. The insert warns about conditions the medication may cause or be statistically associated with. It tells the findings of laboratory tests: for example, whether the medication changes clotting time or the amount of calcium in the blood. It goes into great detail about possible side effects of the drug. These are reported in no particular order, though sometimes the most common ones are listed first, with the others lumped randomly together. The brochure is intended to alert you and your doctor to the effects and possible risks of the medication, but the detailed listing of side effects and possible negative consequences also helps protect the manufacturer from lawsuits. The *Physicians' Desk Reference,* known as the PDR, published yearly, has the same information, as do the Web sites of some pharmaceutical manufacturers.

If the prescribed medication gives you side effects, before you automatically stop taking it, call your physician or your pharmacist. He or she is knowledgeable about side effects associated with the drug and the potential seriousness of what you are describing.

Lauren has just started taking birth control pills. She calls me to say that her breasts are tender, she feels bloated, and she has gained six pounds. I know that these side effects are fairly common and I reassure her that they are not signs of anything seriously wrong. I suggest that perhaps a different dosage or another brand will work better for her.

Megan asked for birth control pills when she went to college as a freshman. She calls to say that the very first day she started taking them, she began to feel achy and feverish, and she wonders whether the pills have caused these symptoms. I can tell her that fever and chills are not recognized side effects of the pill. At college she has been exposed to all sorts of new and unfamiliar germs and perhaps is coming down with an infectious disease.

▶ *How often should you see your gynecologist?*

If things are going well, seeing your gynecologist once a year is usually adequate. If you are starting on birth control pills, your doctor might ask you to come in after six months. If your exam has shown a mass on an ovary or a cyst in your breast, you will probably be asked to come back in two or three months. Ask when you should have your next appointment, if your doctor doesn't tell you.

Since physicians' offices are much busier these days than they used to be, you might bring along your datebook and schedule your next appointment as you leave, or at least ask how far in advance your doctor is scheduling. Many book six months ahead, so if you want an appointment at a specific time, ask early.

Doctors routinely leave slots open in their schedule for emergency problems. If you are taking birth control pills and have chest pain, leg pain, or headaches, call your doctor right away. Although phlebitis (inflammation of the veins) and phlebitis with blood clots in the lungs are extremely rare, they must be attended to quickly.

Women taking the pill often call about bleeding between periods. This is a fairly common side effect of birth control pills, even low-dose pills, and is not usually worrisome. On the other hand, if you have already gone through menopause and have unexpected vaginal bleeding, alert your physician immediately.

TELEPHONE PROTOCOL

I encourage my patients to call if they have questions. If your doctor's office is very busy, you may not get to speak with the doctor, but a specially trained triage nurse, a nurse-practitioner, or, in the case of a gynecologist, a midwife can answer frequently asked questions.

If you have vaginal itching and burning and a discharge that resembles cottage cheese, the nurse will be able to tell you that you probably have a yeast infection. She can look at your chart, see that when this happened before Terazol helped you, and (under the supervision of a physician) call in a prescription for you. If the nurse does not know the answer to your question, she will refer it to the physician.

If, on the other hand, you are in the worst pain you have ever suffered in your life, or if you are hemorrhaging and are unable to get out of bed, you *do* need to talk to the doctor. The triage nurse is trained to make this kind of judgment, and your physician trusts her. Some, but not all, doctors review the decisions of their triage nurses. Most physicians review Pap smears, blood tests done at an outside laboratory, x-ray reports, pregnancy tests, mammograms, urine cultures, and so on. If I see an abnormal Pap smear or a hematocrit (a count of red blood cells) that has dropped dramatically, I will ask my nurse to call you and schedule more tests or another appointment.

All this information, including the questions answered by the triage nurse or the nurse-practitioner, is recorded. So if you call a second time about your yeast infection because it has not improved, your physician can look at your chart, see what treatment you were taking, and recommend something else.

▶ When is the best time to call your doctor?

Unless you are having an emergency, it is advisable to call your doctor during office hours. This is not just a matter of courtesy (though courtesy does help make the world run more smoothly). It helps your doctor make an accurate diagnosis or recommendation because she has access to your chart. People sometimes call with questions like, "What was that medicine you gave me when Judy was born?" Judy is now 15 years old, and I probably will not remember what I prescribed. But if I have the chart, I can say, "Oh yes, it was Methergine," a blood-vessel constrictor given to control bleeding after childbirth.

Late at night while at the hospital, I have gotten calls from patients who want to know when they had their last Pap test. If I am on the delivery floor, I cannot answer that question (though my office nurse can answer it during office hours). Most offices have not yet computerized their charts, although doing so would give physicians easier access to their patients' records.

If you are calling for a prescription refill, again—call during office hours. Your chart will have the prescription information and will also tell when you had your last checkup; perhaps you have run out of pills because it has been more than a year since you were examined.

In the United States, in these days of managed care, medical practice has become more uncomfortable for both doctors and patients. For doctors payments for services have gone down, while paperwork and the expenses of running an office have gone up. Most of us are seeing more patients in the same amount of time. For patients, all of this means longer waits, less access to your doctor, and glitches in the smooth operation of the system (for example, a prescription not called in on time).

Both you and I are often vexed by these problems. When something goes wrong, I feel bad. I apologize, but I know that my staff too is overworked.

Some offices are run more efficiently than others. If you are not happy with the office you are using, consider switching. Be careful about burning your bridges, however, because you may discover that you would like to return to your former physician. So be tactful when you leave.

3 Menstruation: Problems and Possible Solutions

▶ **MYTH** Bleeding between menstrual periods means that you have cancer.

FACT Although this is a possibility, it is a slim one; in young women, the chances are less than 1 percent. In the vast majority of instances, hormonal problems are the cause.

MENSTRUATION is your body's monthly response to not being pregnant. The menstrual cycle starts every month with preparation for the release of an egg from the ovary and continues with the buildup of the uterine lining to nourish that egg if it is fertilized. If fertilization does not take place, the lining sloughs off as the menstrual flow.

Although women differ from one another in their personal patterns of menstruation as much as they differ in other areas, there is nonetheless something called a normal menstrual cycle. While the average cycle (counting from the day bleeding begins one month to the day it begins the next month) is twenty-eight days, a normal cycle is somewhere between twenty-one and thirty-eight days, and the normal menstrual period lasts somewhere between three and seven days. In the United States, the average age of menarche (pronounced MEN-ar-key), the onset of menstruation, is 12.8 years; most girls begin menstruating between the ages of 11 and 14, but the normal range extends from 9 to about 17 years.

The most important factor in determining when you will start menstruating is genetic. Your genes have programmed you to follow the pattern of some female relative,
probably your mother. However, sisters may begin at different ages, so maybe you take after your grandmother or your aunt, and your sister takes after your mother. Other factors
that influence menarche include nutrition, general physical health, and behavioral factors
such as your exercise level.

During the first fifty years of the twentieth century, improved nutrition lowered the
age of menarche in this country until it stabilized in the 1950s. Some researchers believe
that girls must reach a critical weight, about a hundred pounds, for menstruation to begin.
Others think that the proportion of body fat to weight is more significant than total body
weight. Diabetics and moderately obese girls (20–30 percent above normal body weight)
begin menstruating earlier than girls of normal weight. Anorectics and athletes who exercise intensely (including athletes with normal body weight but proportionately more
muscle and less fat) usually begin later.

The menstrual flow is made up of blood, cervical mucus, vaginal secretions, and debris from the cells of the uterine lining that is being shed. When the flow is moderate, anti-
clotting substances within the uterus keep the blood liquid. But when the bleeding is
heavier, clots sometimes form. Although they are not dangerous, they can cause cramping; the uterus perceives them as foreign objects and contracts to get rid of them.

▶ *Should you worry if your cycles are not regular?*

At both the beginning and the end of your reproductive life, you probably will have irregular periods. Teenagers do not usually establish a normal pattern for a year or so, and
women approaching menopause become irregular, often with shorter cycles, before they
stop menstruating altogether.

With those exceptions, you will probably maintain the same pattern once you have established a cycle. Yet no one is completely regular. Stress, anxiety, significant weight loss
(not just a pound or two), travel across a couple of time zones, illness, and some uncommon diseases can cause erratic periods. Contraceptive methods that depend on abstinence
during fertile days can fail, since these factors may alter your cycle.

If you have no periods at all, very short cycles, or heavy bleeding, talk to your doctor.
Hormonal imbalances often cause these difficulties, and most therapies prescribed for
them are also hormonal.

NO MENSTRUAL PERIODS

The technical term for not having periods is amenorrhea. If you have never started to menstruate, you have primary amenorrhea; if you have had periods but they have stopped, then the condition is called secondary amenorrhea. Under the official definition of secondary amenorrhea, you have not had regular menstrual periods for more than six months when you are not pregnant, breast-feeding, or approaching menopause.

PRIMARY AMENORRHEA

I generally consider 16 years the upper cutoff age for menarche. If you are 14 and have not yet had your first period, don't worry. Most often the cause is simply late puberty. Some girls mature faster than others, and as long as you have some signs of puberty—pubic hair and breasts that are beginning to develop—chances are that you are a late bloomer.

A second cause can be heavy athletic training. Occasionally the mother of a young teenager tells me during her own appointment that she is worried because her daughter has not started to menstruate. When I ask what sports the daughter plays, sometimes the mother will say, "Oh, my daughter is extremely athletic. She runs, she plays tennis, she swims." I point out that running, swimming, and playing tennis are wonderful activities for adolescent girls, but all that exercise keeps body weight down, leads to a high propor-tion of muscle to body fat, and often delays menarche. I usually suggest that girl and mother talk to their pediatrician (most girls this age still go to a pediatrician for their gen-eral care). If their pediatrician is not well versed in these matters, he or she can always con-sult with a gynecologist or an endocrinologist.

There are a couple of anatomical causes for primary amenorrhea, but they are quite rare. One is an imperforate hymen, which means that the hymen is completely closed, leaving no way for the menstrual flow to exit the body.

Tracey was sent to me by her pediatrician when she was 14 years old, because she had cramps every month but no menstrual flow. When I checked her, I discov-ered that she had an imperforate hymen. The answer was a simple surgical pro-cedure, performed under anesthesia, during which we cut an X-shaped opening in her hymen. When we did so, we found blood from her previous menstrual pe-riods collecting in her vagina.

The surgery solved her problem, and I didn't see Tracey for about ten years. After college and marriage, she came back for prenatal care and the delivery of her first child, a birth that took place with no problems at all.

A few rare genetic conditions can cause amenorrhea. One of these is androgen insensitivity syndrome (AIS); the other is Turner syndrome.

Androgen Insensitivity Syndrome

This rare condition, also called testicular feminization syndrome, develops in women who have XY chromosomes (like males) rather than XX chromosomes (like females). A woman with this condition is born without a uterus or fallopian tubes. Instead of ovaries, she has incompletely developed testes, which nevertheless can produce testosterone. The testes may be in either her abdomen or her groin area. After puberty these women may have no pubic hair or only a small amount, and their breasts usually do not have much glandular tissue. Women with AIS never menstruate and cannot bear children, but their psychological outlook and behavior are feminine, so they often adopt children. Their bodies are apt to be slender and strong.

The condition is caused by a recessive gene that interferes with proper sexual differentiation. During early fetal life all embryos have the potential to become either males or females, but at the seventh week or so, a gene on the Y chromosome (the one that males have) causes the testes to develop. If the embryo has no Y chromosome, then ovaries develop at about the eleventh week of fetal life.

Once the testes have formed, the fetus responds to male hormones and the other male internal and external structures form. An embryo with an XY genetic makeup that carries the faulty recessive gene will have testes, but the fetal cells do not respond to the masculinizing hormones (androgens) that would continue the process, so the male organs do not develop fully. The condition is diagnosed by a physical exam, blood testing for testosterone levels, and chromosomal testing.

Turner Syndrome

Turner syndrome (also called gonadal dysgenesis) is another rare genetic condition, caused by complete or partial absence of one of the two X chromosomes that women normally have. The cause is not yet known, but Turner syndrome has not been associated with any of the environmental factors that sometimes cause genetic problems. Usually the condition turns up at adolescence, when the girls affected fail to develop adult sex characteristics and do not start menstruating. These girls have a distinctive physical appearance: they are short (the average adult height is 4' 8"); they may have a webbed neck, many moles, no breast development, and childlike genitals. Blood tests can show whether hormonal levels are normal. Turner syndrome can be detected during fetal life through genetic testing. Estrogen replacement therapy can encourage normal breast development and menstruation. Sometimes growth hormone is given to increase height. Most women with Turner syndrome do not ovulate, but modern reproductive techniques such as fertilization with donor eggs can sometimes help these women to become pregnant.

SECONDARY AMENORRHEA

If you are a teenager just starting to menstruate, or in your 40s headed toward menopause, don't worry if you go several months without a period. In adolescents the feedback system that regulates periods is not yet finely tuned. Women approaching menopause have irregular cycles because their ovaries no longer produce enough progesterone to maintain the regular rhythm of the system.

A girl aged 16 or 17 who has established her periods and then developed anorexia nervosa or otherwise lost a great deal of weight may stop having periods. And of course any woman who has been sexually active and ceased menstruating should consider pregnancy as a possibility.

The other day Rose Ann called, worried and upset because her period was five days late. I knew she was involved in a new relationship, so I asked whether she could be pregnant. Not a chance, she said, because she and her boyfriend had not had sex. They were waiting.

She mentioned that she had been suffering from something called irritable bowel syndrome, and that she had had severe diarrhea and had lost ten pounds in less than two months. I guessed that the weight loss had caused her to stop menstruating, and indeed after she got the diarrhea under control, her periods came back.

Changes in diet that bring about significant weight gain can also cause your periods to cease temporarily, as can drastic changes in exercise pattern. If you have been a couch potato and suddenly start running ten miles a day, you may very well stop menstruating for a time.

Tension can interfere with your menstrual cycle in a major way. If you are under heavy stress at school or have recently gone away to college, you may have irregular periods—or no periods for a while. An illness in the family or a death can have the same effect.

Organic causes are possible too, some of them related to the endocrine system and some fairly common. The pituitary gland, which plays a major role in ovulation, produces a hormone called prolactin that acts to start milk production when you give birth. For some reason, the pituitary gland can start producing too much prolactin when you are not pregnant, and elevated levels can interfere with regular periods. Certain medications can raise your prolactin levels, notably Risperdal (risperidone), an antipsychotic drug. Women with thyroid disorders can also lose their periods. It is easy to test for thyroid function and easy to alleviate problems via medication.

Another rather rare cause is premature menopause, which can happen as early as age 35. If you are having hot flashes, sleep problems, and night sweats while you are in your early 30s, your doctor may have you tested for premature menopause. The problem is unlikely if you are in your mid-20s.

▶ Should you be concerned about your general health if your periods stop?

If amenorrhea caused by too little estrogen continues for some time, it can affect your bones. Because you are not ovulating, and thus not producing the estrogen that protects your bones, you are at increased risk for osteoporosis (a disease in which the mineral content of bone is gradually lost). Very thin women (models, runners, ballet dancers, and women with anorexia) have this kind of risk.

Women with a lot of body fat make plenty of estrogen, even if they have no periods, so their bones are not at risk. However, because they are not getting a monthly clean-out bleed, they may develop overgrowth of the uterine lining.

▶ Should you worry if your cycles are longer than thirty-four days?

If you are a teenager who has just started menstruating or an older woman headed for menopause, you may well have widely spaced periods. Chances are that either you are not ovulating frequently or that your hormonal levels at the time of ovulation are not quite high enough.

For women in their 20s and 30s, skipping periods or having very long cycles can cause two problems. If the underlying problem is that you don't ovulate frequently, you may have trouble getting pregnant, but rest assured that there are ways to bring about more frequent ovulation. Very long cycles, with periods that come so far apart that they are not regular at all, can also lead to hyperplasia (overgrowth of the uterine lining). If your body fails to clean out the endometrium every 90 days or so, the uterine lining keeps growing and growing. Hyperplasia can lead to cancer if it is not treated. (See the discussion of how endometrial cancers develop in Chapter 9.)

▶ *What can you do if you have very long or very short cycles?*

To shorten very long cycles, your doctor may prescribe progesterone for five to twelve days every couple of months. When you stop taking the progesterone, you will have a period and thereby clean out the lining of the uterus.

If you have short cycles, say twenty-one or twenty-two days, you have no reason to worry, even though bleeding that often is rather inconvenient. If you bleed both heavily and frequently, there is some risk that you may become anemic. A red blood count will tell you whether this is a problem.

If you are unable to tolerate bleeding every three weeks, you can space your periods further apart by taking birth control pills, which shut down ovulation and then bring on a period by means of progesterone withdrawal.

BLEEDING BETWEEN PERIODS

Bleeding between periods is called breakthrough bleeding, dysfunctional uterine bleeding, or metrorrhagia. It can happen when you ovulate, or just randomly. It can amount to an occasional spot of blood now and again, or it can be heavy bleeding. But it happens when you don't expect it. Sometimes, but not always, bleeding between periods is accompanied by heavy periods.

Bleeding between periods, like irregular periods, is quite common in girls just starting their periods and in older women heading toward menopause. They may not ovulate every single month and when they do, they do not produce enough progesterone to stabilize the uterine lining through the second half of the monthly cycle. But if you bleed between periods once you have established a regular cycle and before you are close to menopause, talk to your doctor. Irregular bleeding can be a sign of endometrial (uterine) cancer or some other medical condition.

▶ *Is it dangerous to spot a couple of days before your period starts?*

Spotting just before your period is quite common and probably nothing to worry about. It probably means that your progesterone levels are dropping before your period, but you should probably mention this to your physician.

▶ *Is it dangerous to spot or bleed a little at the time of ovulation?*

This is fairly common; as long as the bleeding is related to the hormonal changes at the time of ovulation, it is nothing more than a nuisance. When a mature egg is released from the ovary during ovulation, your estrogen level peaks and then falls off rapidly, around day 14 of the cycle. At about the same time, production of LH also peaks. Usually the bleeding caused by these hormonal spikes amounts to a bit of spotting that lasts a day or two. Some women simultaneously feel pain on one side of their abdomen (technically known as mittelschmerz, or middle pain). Your doctor may want to rule out other possibilities by using an endometrial biopsy or an ultrasound scan. For some women mittelschmerz can be very uncomfortable. Once you and your doctor have determined that the bleeding results from normal hormonal changes, you can decide to live with the bleeding or you can try birth control pills, which solve the problem by preventing ovulation.

Among the medical conditions that can cause bleeding between periods are endometriosis, adenomyosis, fibroids, polyps, pelvic inflammatory disease, a tubal or ectopic pregnancy, or an incomplete miscarriage (all of these problems are discussed elsewhere in this book). Another possibility is cancer, particularly cancer of the endometrium (uterine cancer), which is relatively rare among women in general—about six times less common than breast cancer—and extremely rare in young women (see Chapter 9).

HEAVY PERIODS

Heavy bleeding with menstrual periods, officially known as menorrhagia, can mean heavy flow or longer periods or both. Most of the time, heavy menstrual bleeding does not mean that something has gone terribly wrong or that your life is endangered, but you and your doctor will want to figure out the cause, which can be either hormonal or anatomical. Perhaps you have a fibroid, or perhaps for some reason you are not ovulating.

It is difficult to know what is meant by "heavy" bleeding, because what seems like threatening blood loss to one woman does not bother someone else. Almost everyone seems to overestimate her own blood loss, especially women who tend to worry about their health in general, and every day at work I get at least one phone call from someone who says she is bleeding heavily.

A research study that weighed tampons and pads to determine blood loss during periods showed that the heavier bleeders in the group lost about 4.5 fluid ounces (135 ml, or roughly a half cup) of blood each month. Some doctors suggest that you can consider yourself to be bleeding heavily if you have to change a thoroughly soaked super tampon every hour for twenty-four hours; others suggest a standard of every half hour for six hours. Even though this rate of loss could be considered heavy, it is not life threatening.

Your physician can gauge your blood loss by using a hematocrit, a measure of the proportion of red blood cells in the blood. The normal hematocrit in women is somewhere between 37 and 40. (For men it is in the mid to high 40s.) Anything below 30 might be worrisome. If you lose a significant amount of blood, your hematocrit will fall, indicating objectively how much you have lost.

> Courtney comes into the office sure that she is bleeding heavily enough to be in serious trouble. I send her to the lab for a blood count, and her hematocrit turns out to be a very high 43. Courtney was not anxious about her health, but she simply had no basis for comparing her bleeding with "heavy" bleeding.

On the other hand, one of my partners got a call from the emergency room in a local hospital about a patient who had an episode of heavy bleeding during a period and ended up in the hospital with a hematocrit of 16. The hematocrit drops by roughly three points for each unit (pint) of blood lost, so to get to a hematocrit of 16 when she started out with 37, this woman would have lost seven units of blood, well over half her blood volume.

When you call your gynecologist because of heavy bleeding, try to quantify what is happening. If you tell me you are wearing a super tampon plus a pad and have to change them every hour, something has to be done. If you say you are changing a maxipad every two hours, I can see why you are upset, but I can assure you that your bleeding is not dangerous unless it goes on for weeks. Between those extremes I have to make a judgment call.

A small percentage of women bleed heavily enough during their periods to lower their hematocrit slightly, but as long as it stays in the range of 35 or 36, the blood loss will not threaten their health or keep them from their normal activities.

▶ What can you do to maintain your red-blood-cell count during heavy periods?

If you can live with your heavy periods but worry about becoming anemic, you can boost your blood count by taking iron pills, available over the counter at your drugstore. Start with 325 mg of iron sulfate daily, more than is recommended for pregnant women and enough in many cases to maintain a hematocrit of 37–40 despite heavy periods. Have your doctor check your hematocrit again after a month or two. If it is still too low, you probably need more iron. Most women cannot absorb more than three 325-mg tablets of iron sulfate daily.

To optimize the amount you absorb, take iron tablets on an empty stomach, an hour before a meal or several hours afterward. If they upset your stomach, take them with food. Supplementary iron can make you constipated, so drink plenty of fluids, get lots of exercise, and eat fiber-rich foods, including bran, whole-grain breads and cereals, and fresh fruits and vegetables (with their skins).

If you are not afflicted with heavy bleeding, it is fairly easy to get enough iron in your diet, especially if you eat red meat. But if you are trying to avoid anemia in the face of heavy bleeding by increasing dietary iron, you will have to pay careful attention to what you eat. Many foods contain iron, but not all iron is absorbed equally.

There are two kinds of iron. Heme iron, which makes up about 40 percent of the iron in animal tissues, is found in meat (especially liver and red meat), poultry, and, to a lesser extent, fish. Nonheme iron is found in dairy products, egg yolks, dark green vegetables, legumes, and grains, and is used to enrich flour and cereals.

Your body absorbs about 30 percent of the heme iron in your diet, but only 5 percent of the nonheme iron. Cooked broccoli, for example, contains 1.8 mg of iron per cup, of which only 5 percent actually gets absorbed. Therefore, to get 15 mg, the daily requirement for menstruating women who do not have heavy bleeding, you would have to eat more than 160 cups of broccoli to reach the recommended iron level. This silly example shows how carefully you have to plan if you want to get enough iron without eating red meat or taking supplements. A nutritionist may be able to help you reach your goal.

▶ What diseases or medical conditions cause heavy bleeding?

Fibroids, noncancerous muscular growths in the uterus, can cause heavy bleeding and are fairly common in older women. (For more about fibroids, see Chapter 8.) Polyps, estrogen-stimulated growths of the endometrium that stick out into the uterus, can also produce significant bleeding. They tend to be small and may be attached to the uterine wall by means of a pedicle (a small stalk). Sometimes they protrude through the cervix into the vagina. Usually diagnosed via a D&C, they can be removed surgically from the wall of the uterus, often during the D&C. Hypothyroidism (too little thyroid hormone) can cause very heavy menstrual bleeding. Women with hyperthyroidism (too much thyroid hormone), on the other hand, usually have very light periods.

Certain blood diseases, including von Willebrand's disease (an inherited clotting disturbance), can also cause heavy bleeding. This disease is uncommon and generally not much of a problem. But it can be risky during labor and delivery, surgery, or a tooth ex-

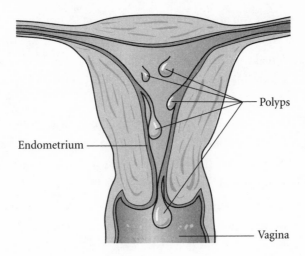

FIGURE 9. Endometrial polyps.

traction, so alert your doctor if you know you have von Willebrand's disease. It is easy to detect, by drawing blood to test for clotting factors.

▶ Can an IUD cause heavy periods?

Women who use an IUD (intrauterine device) for birth control often have heavy menstrual periods, with an increase in both the flow and the length of the period. They may also have premenstrual spotting and bleeding between periods. If you are using an IUD and bleed or spot between periods, tell your doctor so that the two of you can make sure that the IUD is indeed the culprit—not some other condition.

HORMONAL TREATMENTS

Usually hormonal problems are at the root of heavy menstrual bleeding. If you did not ovulate (often the case with young girls and women near menopause), there may not be enough progesterone in the right place at the right time to keep menstrual bleeding in check. You may have heavy bleeding. Occasionally, problems with thyroid, adrenal, or pituitary hormones may result in an imbalance that can cause heavy periods.

▶ *Can you do anything to lighten heavy periods?*

Once you and your doctor have ruled out the possibility of disease, you can try birth control pills, since most women who use them have fairly light periods.

If your heavy periods are caused by ovulatory problems, you can try progesterone therapy , which simply provides "outside" progesterone to make up for what your body is not producing. Doctors often recommend medroxyprogesterone, a synthetic progesterone sold as Provera. The dosage is usually 10 mg daily for ten to twelve days.

> Sarah usually goes about thirty-eight days, more than five weeks, without a period and then bleeds heavily. To get her heavy bleeding under control, we decided that she should take progesterone in pill form beginning on day 16 of her cycle and continuing for ten or twelve days each month. The progesterone stabilizes the lining of her uterus and prevents the tremendous overgrowth during the second half of her cycle that was causing her heavy bleeding. When she stops the progesterone, she gets a clean-out bleed of moderate volume, controlled by the progesterone. The progesterone therapy works for her, because low progesterone was the cause of her heavy bleeding.

This treatment does not always work. Sometimes when I look under the microscope at a sample of endometrial tissue, I see that different parts of the sample look like tissue from different parts of the menstrual cycle. Some parts look as if they come from the first week in the cycle, some from later. So at any one time some of this tissue is bleeding.

If progesterone therapy does not work for you, your doctor may suggest therapy with birth control pills, which contain both progesterone and estrogen, in the hope that adding back some estrogen will "get the cycle together." That is, it will get all the tissue in the endometrium on the same schedule. Here is the "magic" schedule for birth control therapy: four birth control pills a day for three days, then three birth control pills a day for three more days. That comes to twenty-one pills, a whole cycle's worth of pills in six days. After that, you break into your next pack of pills and take two pills a day for three more days, and then one pill a day until the second pack is gone. When you have finished the second pack, you should have a controlled withdrawal bleed, not a flow that resembles Niagara Falls!

SURGICAL TREATMENTS

If hormonal treatments do not work for you, there are several surgical approaches that can help control heavy bleeding. A D&C removes the endometrial tissue that is causing the heavy bleeding, but leaves the underlying layer of cells, which generates a new endometrium every month after your menstrual period. Other procedures—endometrial ablation, cryoablation, and hot-water balloon ablation—aim for a more permanent result: they remove the glandular endometrium and scar the underlying layer so that no new endometrium is produced. Another new treatment for women whose heavy bleeding is caused by fibroids is to deprive the fibroids of their blood supply by injecting particles, something like tiny styrofoam balls, into the arteries that lead to the fibroids. The procedure is done in a hospital setting with the assistance of a radiologist. The surgical procedure of last resort for uncontrollably heavy periods is a hysterectomy.

D&C (Dilation and Curettage)

During this procedure the cervix, the narrow opening to the main body of the uterus, is dilated. Then the lining of the uterus is scraped out with a sharp-edged tool called a curette. The old slang among physicians for a D&C was a "dusting and cleaning." While not quite accurate, the term describes the procedure's purpose, which is to clean out the glandular lining and get back to the underlying muscular layer of the uterus.

One common reason for performing a D&C is diagnostic. Why is there such heavy bleeding? Is the cause a hormone imbalance? Are polyps or fibroids the underlying cause? Or could the bleeding be an early indication of endometrial cancer? Whenever I do a D&C, I send tissue samples to a pathologist for careful examination and a definitive diagnosis. The procedure can also be used to perform an early-term abortion (though today suction aspiration is more common) or to clean placental tissue from the uterus after a miscarriage.

If you have a D&C, you will not be disabled for weeks and weeks; in fact, you will probably feel quite all right the next day. Most women have some cramping the day of the procedure, similar to the cramping of a heavy menstrual period. A mild painkiller such as Tylenol or Advil will probably take care of it. Spotting or staining for up to two weeks after the procedure is not uncommon, nor is it indicative of anything dangerous. You can usually return to your normal activities, including work, in a day or two. Much of the speed of recuperation depends on what type of anesthesia you were given.

Frequently a D&C can be done with local anesthesia in a doctor's office or surgicenter.

The most commonly used technique is a paracervical block, in which Novocain or an equivalent is injected right into the cervix. A D&C with a paracervical block does cause some discomfort. The block anesthetizes the cervix, but it does not act on the inside of the uterus. A biopsy usually involves taking samples from different parts of the uterus to ensure getting representative bits of tissue, and women respond differently. I have had reactions ranging from "This is no big deal; why did you tell me it was going to be uncomfortable?" to "This is the worst thing that has ever happened to me." A middle-of-the-road group responds with "This is not fun, but who wants to go through general anesthesia?"

I tell patients who are about to have any procedure under local anesthesia that if it gets too distressing they can ask me to stop and have it done later under general anesthesia—and sometimes I have abandoned a procedure because the patient is too miserable. If the procedure is being performed in an operating room facility, you can start with a paracervical block and proceed to general anesthesia if necessary.

Fifteen or twenty years ago, a D&C with general anesthesia was a major production. You were admitted to the hospital the night before and stayed a day or two afterward. Nowadays, even with general anesthesia, the vast majority of D&Cs are performed in surgicenters or other outpatient settings. You go in at about seven-thirty in the morning, the procedure is done an hour later, and you go home before lunch.

It makes sense that a D&C will help someone with polyps or fibroids, which can cause heavy bleeding, but sometimes women who have nothing visibly wrong may also improve after a D&C for reasons that are not understood. Usually these women do well for a year or two; then their periods may get heavy again.

Endometrial Ablation

Like a D&C, endometrial ablation removes the glandular lining of the uterus, but it uses the intense heat of a laser beam or an electrocautery instead of a curette. The doctor looks inside the uterus with a hysteroscope (a narrow, lighted viewing tool) and under its guidance focuses the laser beam to "fry" the endometrium. As in a D&C, the goal is to remove the entire endometrium and get back to the underlying muscular layer. Even if some bits of glandular tissue remain, the heavy bleeding is usually relieved. Like any surgical procedure, endometrial ablation should be performed by a skilled practitioner who has done it many times.

While endometrial ablation has its place in the range of available procedures, it is not without risks and potential drawbacks. If the uterus is large, the laser must be used extensively. Through the hysteroscope the physician can see an area about the size of a nickel, so must move the scope and the laser extensively to see and remove all the endometrial tissue. Ablation can also be difficult if the uterus has a lot of nooks and crannies (for example, a fibroid or two pressing inward through the outside of the uterine wall).

Some physicians insist that a woman go on hormonal medication like Lupron or danazol for a month or two before the ablation (see Chapter 8). The medication "flattens out" the uterine lining and makes the procedure easier. The same physicians may also recommend continuing the hormone therapy for a month or two after the ablation, to let the endometrium scar and keep it from growing back.

> Melissa has three children and doesn't want any more. She is seriously over-weight and has high blood pressure. Because of her obesity, she tends to bleed heavily with her periods. She has tried progesterone but it hasn't helped her.

Melissa might consider endometrial ablation. Since she plans to have no more children, she could have a hysterectomy. However, she is not a good surgical risk because of her weight and because other therapies have not helped her. She should choose this procedure with the same seriousness with which she would approach a D&C.

Other Methods

One new technique uses a "roller ball," a little electric ball that rolls around the lining of the uterus and scars the endometrium with electric current—instead of a laser, which scars it with intense heat. It is perhaps safer than laser ablation because there is less risk of burning the bowel, which is close to the uterus in the abdominal cavity.

Another new method, which has been approved by the Food and Drug Administration (FDA), uses a hot-water balloon, a little sack at the end of a long slender tube. The sack is placed in the uterus and filled with very hot water. It remains there for slightly less than ten minutes, while the heat destroys the endometrium.

Cryoablation, recently approved by the FDA, uses cold instead of heat to destroy the endometrium. The physician inserts a probe into the lining of the uterus and freezes the area with refrigerant gas. I helped out during preliminary research for FDA approval of this procedure by checking temperature gauges attached to the surface of the uterus to make sure that nearby organs did not become damaged by the cold.

All methods that destroy the endometrium should be used only if you are certain that you have completed your family. They scar the uterus, which hinders fertility.

Hysterectomy

If you are sure you do not want more children and all other therapies have failed, hysterectomy is your final recourse. It is a major surgical procedure; you should anticipate two or three hours in the operating room and six weeks of recuperation time.

> After Michelle's second child was born when she was 30, she had her tubes tied. Unfortunately, she bleeds heavily every month. Birth control pills control her heavy periods but give her migraine headaches, sometimes as many as five a week. She decided to stop the pills, but started bleeding again and felt bad enough to miss work. We did a D&C with the aid of a hysteroscope, and the procedure confirmed that she does not have cancer or fibroids.
> Michelle did not want to live her life choosing between migraines and heavy bleeding. After weighing her options carefully, she came in one day and said, "I can't take this any more. I'm just going to have a hysterectomy and be done with it." She had the procedure, during which her uterus but not her ovaries were removed; she has been happy with the results and has not missed a day of work since she returned after her postoperative recuperative period.

▶ *Will insurance pay for a hysterectomy to stop heavy bleeding?*

If your heavy bleeding is caused by endometrial cancer, of course your HMO (health maintenance organization) should pay. If it is caused by large (grapefruit-size) fibroids, usually HMOs are willing to cover the costs. If your fibroids are smaller, the company may ask whether you have tried progesterone therapy or birth-control-pill therapy; if you say you have, the company will probably ask why you did not tolerate the pills. If you meet several criteria, you may be able to convince your insurer to pay. You will have to submit a blood count; if it shows that you are anemic your company may cover you because the hysterectomy is for treatment of a recognized disease. You also must submit clotting studies to be sure you do not have some clotting problem that could be life threatening after surgery. In short, you may be able to get your HMO to pay, but you will probably have to jump through hoops to do so. Just be sure to obtain preauthorization before you undertake the surgery, to avoid any nasty financial surprises afterward. Your doctor's office staff will help you, but you will probably have to do some of the work yourself.

PAINFUL PERIODS

Dysmenorrhea is the medical term for painful menstrual periods. Many women feel some pain or discomfort on the first day or two of their periods, but usually the pain subsides once the flow is established. However, at some time in their lives about 50 percent of women experience menstrual pain severe enough to interfere with their normal activities, and 10 percent have cramps that keep them home from work or school one to three days a month.

Menstrual pain can begin a day or two before your period or it may start just as the flow begins. It can vary from mild discomfort that responds to common painkillers to pain that keeps you in bed because even walking around is too uncomfortable. Sometimes menstrual pain feels like sharp cramps in the lower abdomen and sometimes like a dull ache, which may or may not spread to the lower back or upper thighs. Some women also have headaches, nausea, diarrhea, or dizziness. A few vomit or faint.

Primary dysmenorrhea, which I call ordinary garden-variety dysmenorrhea, is the kind for which physicians can find no underlying physical cause. You are perfectly healthy, but you have cramps. In general, primary dysmenorrhea afflicts younger women. Secondary dysmenorrhea is menstrual pain caused by a known medical condition (for example, endometriosis or fibroids) and is more likely to be a problem for older women.

Menstrual pain, which may begin in the midteen years, becomes more common during the mid-20s and then decreases. Unless there is some medical cause, women who have had comfortable periods in the past do not ordinarily begin having cramps in their 30s, though some women continue to have cramps if they have had them before.

Obese women (those at least 20 percent overweight) are more likely to have menstrual cramps than thin women. Athletes are less likely to get them than other women, and highly trained, very thin athletes may stop getting menstrual periods altogether. Women who have regular periods are more apt to have cramps than women who do not. Women with longer periods are more likely to get cramps than women whose periods last fewer than three days.

Most girls just starting to have periods have no cramps at all because they are not yet ovulating. Prostaglandins, hormone-like chemicals that are responsible for ordinary cramps, are not produced until after ovulation begins—usually a year or so after periods start. If you are a teenager and have started getting cramps after a couple of years of comfortable menstrual periods, chances are that you have just begun to ovulate. It is unlikely, though possible, that you have endometriosis or fibroids or some other condition that is causing cramps. If you are worried, talk to your doctor.

PRIMARY DYSMENORRHEA

The main causes of primary dysmenorrhea are prostaglandins, produced by the uterine lining after ovulation toward the time of the menstrual period. These hormones stimulate the contraction of smooth muscle, including the muscular walls of the uterus. Some women produce more prostaglandins than others do, and this overproduction causes not only menstrual cramps but also the headaches, nausea, and other symptoms that sometimes accompany the abdominal pain.

Before the discovery of prostaglandins, researchers offered several theories to explain menstrual pain. One was that menstrual cramps were all in your mind. Another hypothesis suggested that dysmenorrhea was caused by narrowing of the cervix: because the menstrual flow could not easily escape through this constricted opening, the uterus contracted to help get rid of it. For that reason one of the early treatments for menstrual pain was a D&C, during which the cervix was mechanically dilated and the uterine lining scraped out.

Although physicians no longer believe that cramps are imaginary, menstrual cramps like any other pain can have a psychological component. If you expect something to be painful, it may well be so. If a girl sees her mother lying in bed two or three days a month, complaining of "the curse" and its "terrible pain," the daughter may tend to repeat the pattern. Mothers can do their daughters a favor by encouraging a positive attitude toward this normal function.

A few teenagers have psychological issues surrounding menstruation. Counseling can help a young woman who has a phobia about bleeding, an aversion to her developing body, or problems with becoming a woman.

▶ *What can you do to relieve menstrual cramps?*

The best drugs for menstrual cramps are prostaglandin synthetase inhibitors. As the name suggests, these drugs block the body's production of prostaglandins. They are also called nonsteroidal anti-inflammatory drugs (commonly called NSAIDs, pronounced *en-seds*) and are used to treat arthritis, tendonitis, gout, and other inflammatory diseases. We know them in the drugstore as Advil, Aleve, Anaprox, Motrin, and Naprosyn, among others. Aspirin, the first common NSAID, was used even before scientists knew why it worked, but the newer drugs are often more effective. When I was in medical school thirty years ago, Motrin was a relative newcomer, available only by prescription. We considered it a miracle drug, because it relieved menstrual pain so effectively.

The first rule with NSAIDs is, Take them early. Don't be a John Wayne type, strong and silent, until you can't stand the pain any longer. NSAIDs will stop the production of more prostaglandins, but they won't do anything about the prostaglandins currently at work in your pelvis. Once your body produces prostaglandins, you have to wait until the normal metabolic processes break them down to get relief. If you have a regular cycle and can predict when your period will start, you can take prostaglandin inhibitors ahead of time, maybe a day before your period begins, and shut down prostaglandin production before the pain begins. The second important rule is, Take NSAIDs with food or milk. They are hard on the lining of your stomach and may cause nausea or stomach pain.

You are not harming yourself by depriving your body of prostaglandins for a couple of days a month. Their only real use is in starting the contractions of labor. And you need not worry that taking NSAIDs during your periods will keep you from having a normal pattern of labor when or if you start your family. Your body keeps on making prostaglandins, so they are always available when you need them (and sometimes when you do not).

A second line of attack on dysmenorrhea caused by prostaglandins is birth control pills. They suppress ovulation, and in menstrual cycles without ovulation, not much prostaglandin is produced.

Some mothers are concerned that when I prescribe birth control pills for their daughters' cramps, I am giving license for intercourse. That is not my intention at all. The issue of when it is appropriate to become sexually active depends on moral, social, and religious factors as well as physical ones, and these factors are beyond the scope of my role as physician. I am simply treating a young woman for a medical condition, just as I would give her penicillin if she needed an antibiotic. So it is important that there be an open relationship between mother and daughter, or within the family, and a mutual understanding of shared values.

If you are taking birth control pills, remember that while they will prevent pregnancy they will do nothing to protect against sexually transmitted diseases, including herpes, the condyloma virus, and AIDS. If you use birth control pills, you must also practice safe sex, which means using condoms, unless both you and your partner are monogamous.

You can stay on the pill as long as you wish. It is fine if you want to stop in six months or a year and see how you feel. If you then have no pain and do not feel like going back on the pill, that is fine. If you want to resume taking the pill, that is also fine. There is nothing wrong with going off and on the pill, as long as you use other forms of contraception when the pill is not protecting you from pregnancy.

▶ Are NSAIDs safe?

Individuals who must take nonsteroidal anti-inflammatory drugs daily for long periods (for example, people with arthritis) can develop stomach ulcers or kidney problems. Some physicians are so concerned about these potential side effects that they discourage NSAID use for menstrual cramps. But if you take NSAIDs in moderation—for only the first few days of your period—and with food, you should have no trouble. Do not take NSAIDs if aspirin or some other anti-inflammatory has given you asthma.

▶ What is the standard dosage for anti-inflammatories?

Most over-the-counter ibuprofen tablets come as 200-mg tablets, though you can get them in dosages of 400–600 mg. The standard dosage for prescription Motrin is 600 mg (three 200-mg tablets) every six hours. If you are taking one Advil and it does not help, try two or three—but take them with food or milk and use them short term. Some anti-inflammatories, Advil and Naprosyn for example, come in liquid form for those who cannot swallow pills.

Anti-inflammatories come in a range of strengths, the stronger ones available only by prescription. Tylenol and aspirin are probably the mildest. Next in strength I would rate ibuprofen (Advil or Motrin); then come naproxen (Naprosyn, Aleve, and Anaprox), indomethacin (Indocin), and finally ketoralac (Toradol), the most potent of all.

▶ Is it all right to take both anti-inflammatory medications and birth control pills for menstrual pain?

If you get some relief from taking birth control pills but are still uncomfortable, you can try Motrin or some other nonsteroidal anti-inflammatory drug as well. The two medications are totally different and do not interfere with each other.

▶ Does exercise help with menstrual cramps?

Exercise can be very beneficial for menstrual cramps and is in fact one of the most important things you can do to promote your own general physical and mental health. Research has shown that female athletes of whatever weight, not just lean long-distance runners, have less menstrual pain than women who do not exercise. You do not have to become a marathoner, as one of my patients did, to deal with menstrual discomforts, but you do need to get regular exercise—running, walking, aerobics, or whatever appeals to you.

▶ *Are there alternative treatments that help with menstrual pain?*

Some women find that fish-oil supplements help. Fish oil has been shown to be effective in treating rheumatoid arthritis and seems to have anti-inflammatory properties. It does not seem to have adverse effects, and while you must take a great deal of it (eating salmon, mackerel, sardines, or other oily fish three times a week or swallowing 10–18 gm in fish-oil capsules), you are unlikely to overdose.

There are also herbal and folk remedies, most of which have not been tested scientifically. Raspberry tea is one traditional herbal remedy for cramps. While no clinical studies have discovered a chemical agent that relaxes the smooth muscles of the uterus, raspberry-leaf tea has long been considered useful for expectant mothers as well as menstruating women. When you buy raspberry tea, be sure you get the kind made from the leaves of the raspberry plant, not just tea infused with raspberry oil to give it a fragrant aroma. Herbalists sometimes recommend peppermint tea for menstrual cramps, though it is usually used to treat indigestion. Peppermint leaves seem to have an antispasmodic effect, at least in the upper digestive tract, which may account for the popularity of peppermint tea in treating cramps.

Herbal products, like prescriptions you buy at the drugstore, contain chemicals that may have significant side effects; they may cause interactions with other drugs or withdrawal symptoms. If you use these products, tell your doctor what you are taking. Because herbal medicines are not tested for safety by the FDA and are not offered in standard dosages, you may not know how much you are getting or even, in some cases, what you are getting.

Acupuncture, often used to control other kinds of pain, has been found to help women with menstrual cramps. It may be effective in controlling pain through a connection with endorphins, natural narcotic-like substances produced by the brain.

Another home remedy is alcohol. When your grandmother had cramps, she perhaps took a shot of brandy and went to bed. Alcohol works because it is a smooth-muscle relaxant, so effective that in the old days doctors gave alcohol intravenously to stop premature labor. While a little alcohol at bedtime does relax you, you should not take alcohol in the morning if you have to go to work, and you should be sure not to overdo whenever you take it.

▶ *Are narcotic pain relievers useful for menstrual pain?*

Occasionally I prescribe codeine for women who have prostaglandin-caused menstrual pain if they cannot tolerate ibuprofen or other NSAIDs. Some women take two or three codeine pills a month during the first days of their period so that they can sleep at night. Narcotics are very high risk drugs, and like other physicians I am aware of the possibility of addiction or abuse. I try to have the kind of relationships with my patients whereby I know who is vulnerable, and I prescribe them only to patients who are not.

SECONDARY DYSMENORRHEA

Among the medical conditions that can cause menstrual pain are pelvic inflammatory disease, fibroids, endometriosis, and adenomyosis.

Pelvic inflammatory disease (infection of the cervix, uterus, fallopian tubes, and/or ovaries, usually associated with sexually transmitted diseases) may cause no symptoms whatsoever, or it may cause dull, constant pain in the lower abdomen, not only during your period but at other times (see Chapter 7).

Fibroids, which are noncancerous growths of the uterine wall, do not necessarily cause pain during menstruation or at any time, and many women with fibroids do not know they have them. However, fibroids may press on nerves within the pelvis and cause backache or abdominal heaviness not necessarily related to the menstrual cycle. Or sometimes the uterus may "decide" that a fibroid is a foreign body and begin contracting, trying to expel it. Fibroids can, however, cause heavy menstrual bleeding.

Endometriosis, a condition in which the tissue normally lining the uterus somehow migrates to other locations within the body, causes pain during the menstrual period and sometimes at other times of the month (see Chapter 8). This tissue responds to hormones just as if it were in its normal location inside the uterus: it swells and breaks down and bleeds. Since it has no natural exit, it bleeds into the abdominal cavity or surrounding tissues.

Adenomyosis, which used to be called internal endometriosis, is a sort of reverse endometriosis, in which the endometrial tissue turns inward and invades the muscular wall of the uterus beneath the endometrium. Like all endometrial tissue, wherever it may be, adenomyosis responds to hormones and bleeds into the surrounding tissues at the time of the menstrual period. Unlike endometriosis, which is a disease of younger women without children, adenomyosis usually targets women in their 30s and 40s who have already given birth several times. Women who have had a cesarean section or a D&C are also at increased risk. Researchers believe that pregnancy, labor, and the shrinking of the uterus after delivery may damage the uterine wall, allowing small islands of normal endometrial tissue to work their way into the muscular lining of the uterus.

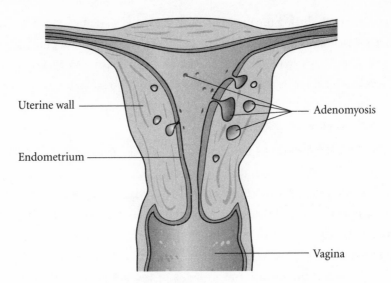

FIGURE 10. Adenomyosis, a condition in which the endometrium grows into the wall of the uterus.

Like fibroids, adenomyosis usually causes no symptoms at all. When symptoms appear, they usually include increasing menstrual flow—periods that become both longer and heavier—and increasing menstrual pain, which may become severe. Some women notice pain on intercourse and pelvic pressure before the menstrual period begins.

▶ *What is the treatment for adenomyosis?*

If you have symptoms that suggest adenomyosis, your doctor will give you a pelvic exam to check your uterus. Sometimes the uterus is enlarged and either hard or soft—different from its usual consistency. To differentiate between a possible pregnancy or fibroids, you may be given a pregnancy test and an ultrasound.

Unfortunately, adenomyosis is difficult to treat. If the symptoms are mild, sometimes NSAIDs take care of the pain. Often adenomyosis will go away by itself after menopause. Hysterectomy is the definitive treatment. If you have have completed your family or do not intend to have one, a hysterectomy need not be a disastrous event.

PREMENSTRUAL HEADACHES

Many women have migraine headaches just before or during the first day or two of their periods. The culprit seems to be the sudden drop in estrogen level that accompanies the beginning of the period. This loss of estrogen causes the blood vessels in the scalp and head to constrict, which in turn causes the headache. If you notice a pattern of headaches associated with the onset of your period, talk to your caregiver about taking estrogen just before your period begins. The hormone causes the blood vessels to dilate again, restoring the blood flow. The therapy is effective for about 50 percent of women. If it does not work for you, you may find relief through working with a neurologist.

TOXIC SHOCK SYNDROME

Toxic shock syndrome (TSS) is a rare disease associated with a common bacterium. Although recorded cases of toxic shock date back many years, in the late 1970s the disease suddenly reappeared and seemed to be reaching epidemic proportions in this country. Physicians identified several hundred cases, first in children and then in young women, including teenagers, who became very sick at the time of their menstrual periods. Their symptoms included high fever, severe nausea and vomiting, massive diarrhea, a dramatic drop in blood pressure, and sometimes kidney or liver failure.

As cases accumulated, the Centers for Disease Control and Prevention (CDC) began tracking this "mystery" disease. In 1978 it was identified as TSS, and in 1980 researchers linked it to tampon use. Approximately 80 percent of those stricken turned out to be menstruating women, and about 3 percent of the reported cases were fatal. The incidence of TSS among teenagers was surprisingly high: in 1981, 44 percent of TSS cases in menstruating women occurred in the age group 10–19 years.

Laboratory tests indicated that the underlying cause was *Staphylococcus aureus,* a bacterium that normally lives fairly harmlessly on the skin, in the mouth, or in the vagina. Tests of the stricken women showed that staphylococcus bacteria were not present in the bloodstream, as might have been expected. Instead, the blood of TSS patients contained exotoxins, poisons secreted by the staph bacteria and somehow transmitted into the bloodstream, where they caused the severe symptoms associated with the disease.

Doctors could not offer their patients anything except supportive therapy. Antibiotics could destroy the staphylococcus bacteria and help prevent recurrences; but since the toxins already released by the bacteria had done the damage, antibiotics did not relieve the symptoms. So physicians continued to treat the symptoms, relieving the dehydration that accompanied the vomiting and diarrhea, offering dialysis to people whose kidneys had shut down, and giving antibiotics to prevent the disease from coming back. Most people did well and eventually recovered.

▶ *How did tampon use contribute to the epidemic of TSS?*

At the time of the epidemic a great deal of research was done on tampons, investigating whether they introduced bacteria to the vagina, changed the vaginal environment so that bacteria could flourish, or in some other way encouraged bacterial growth. Researchers suspected that somehow the tampons changed the environment of the vagina, or themselves provided a place where bacteria could flourish. A new superabsorbent tampon, Rely, had just come on the market. Since a cluster of cases involved Rely, researchers reasoned that the disease might have something to do with the material used in the tampon or the vaginal dryness it created. Maybe this superabsorbent tampon took so much moisture from the vagina that the vaginal tissues were injured by inserting and removing the tampon and became more vulnerable to infection. Or perhaps the tampon itself, with its extrathirsty fibers, provided an oxygen-rich breeding ground for bacteria that produced more and more toxins.

The Rely tampon was taken off the market. Women were warned by the FDA to use the least absorbent tampon that served their needs and to notify their physicians if symptoms of TSS appeared. After Rely was withdrawn, new cases dropped in number but did not disappear, so the Rely tampon could not have been the sole cause.

The epidemic wound down, though occasional cases of TSS still occur: fewer than 1 case per 100,000 menstruating women per year. Not all these cases can be attributed to tampon use. We occasionally see TSS in women and men who have had surgery on their nose or throat and had nasal packing after the operation.

What caused the epidemic? My own explanation for the dramatic appearance of TSS in the 1970s is that the "brand" of *Staphylococcus aureus* that appeared then was a strain (called a phage type) that produced potent exotoxins, unlike some other strains. Research has suggested that certain classic phage types were associated with TSS, but no one knows why we no longer see those phage types. A significant outbreak of TSS occurred in Australia in the 1920s, when tampons had not yet been invented. That suggests that TSS is a cyclical disease; it comes and goes like the flu. If that is the case, it may well come back when a form of *S. aureus* turns up that has toxin-producing capacity.

▶ *What are the symptoms of TSS?*

The CDC has developed a definitive set of symptoms for this syndrome. The most common are high fever (over 102.5 degrees Fahrenheit), vomiting, diarrhea, a sunburn-like rash, a rapid drop in blood pressure, and peeling or sloughing skin, sometimes on the palms of the hands or soles of the feet. Other markers are muscular aches and pains, headaches, sore throat, bloodshot eyes, and confusion. The symptoms can come on rapidly and progress swiftly from discomfort to overwhelming infirmity. Many diseases have some of the symptoms that define TSS, but their severity and appearance in combination leads doctors to think of TSS.

One of the first cases in which I participated as an expert witness was a product liability lawsuit brought against tampon manufacturers.

Mrs. X, the plaintiff, did not feel at all well when she had her period. She ached all over and felt tired. She also had small spots on her index finger that became irritated during her period, for some reason that has never been understood. Her physician, a general practitioner, told her that her problem was "mild recurrent toxic shock."

He did a vaginal culture and it revealed that she did have staphylococcus in her vagina, though not *Staphylococcus aureus.* She had *S. epidermis,* a strain that has never been associated with TSS and has not been shown to produce exotoxins. Her doctor treated her with antistaphylococcal medications.

Mrs. X had none of the symptoms listed by the CDC as defining TSS: no fever, no diarrhea, no vomiting, no drop in blood pressure, no peeling of the skin (though she did have itchy bumps on her index finger). She just did not feel well during her period.

This lawsuit lasted a month in federal court. The jury found the manufacturer innocent and dismissed the case, but not before thousands and thousands of tax dollars had been spent because Mrs. X did not feel well during her menstrual period.

On another occasion, I was reviewing a case that involved a lawsuit brought by the wealthy family of a 15-year-old girl.

Caitlin came into the hospital during her menstrual period, extremely sick, with a high fever and an unusual group of symptoms that included peeling skin on her fingertips. The doctors in the emergency room thought her symptoms did not quite fit the picture for TSS and they were unable to culture staphylococcus from her vagina. They were concerned about TSS because of her age and the fact that she had come in during her period. She was treated and recovered quickly, but her family decided to sue the tampon manufacturer.

However, Caitlin's chart showed that a urine test taken at the time of her admission to the hospital showed a positive result for amphetamines. Her problem was not toxic shock but an amphetamine overdose. Her family dropped the case.

▶ *What is the treatment for TSS?*

Today, as in the 1970s, there is no real cure for TSS. It is treated with antibiotics to decrease the number of bacteria that produce the toxins, and to prevent recurrence. If vomiting and diarrhea have caused severe dehydration, then intravenous fluids are sometimes provided.

▶ *How can you protect against toxic shock syndrome?*

Although, theoretically, anyone is at risk for this disease, women who use high-absorbency tampons, especially teenagers and women in their 20s, seem to be more vulnerable. It makes sense, then, to use the least absorbent tampon that meets your needs. Perhaps you have to use a "super" tampon for the first couple of days of your period, but you can change to a "regular" or even a "junior" size as the flow diminishes.

Second, alternate tampons and pads. If you want to wear tampons during the day, use pads at night or when you are at home. Tampons have real advantages—no odor and no mess—but you may need these advantages more when you are out in the world than when you are at home. Research has shown that it is safe to leave a tampon in place for twelve or thirteen hours, but I recommend that if you do wear a tampon overnight, you start the next day with a pad.

Change your tampons frequently. Don't wear tampons when you're not having your period. Avoid superabsorbent tampons. If you do have some sign of TSS, for example a fever or a rash, remove your tampon immediately, as this may prevent your symptoms from worsening. Call your doctor right away.

▶ *Have manufacturers changed the way tampons are made since the epidemic of TSS?*

Although the Rely tampon, which included materials to increase absorbency, was recalled, tampon manufacture has not changed much. The standard brands are still made from cotton, rayon, or a combination of the two. Both fibers come from plant materials, though rayon fibers are derived from the cellulose obtained from wood pulp. Several companies make all-cotton and organic-cotton tampons, available at health stores and sometimes at supermarkets. Other cotton tampons, whose fibers are processed without chlorine bleach, are also available at health stores.

Since 1990 the Food and Drug Administration has developed uniform standards for absorbency and required tampon manufacturers to print them on the box, so you can judge the relative absorbency of different brands. Before 1990 the "regular" size of one well-known brand was more absorbent that the "super" size of another. Tampon manufacturers must print a warning about TSS and advise you to use the least absorbent tampons that work for you.

▶ *Are all-cotton tampons safer than rayon tampons?*

Higher-absorbency tampons are believed to be riskier than lower-absorbency tampons when the latter will suffice, but no research has suggested that rayon itself is more likely than cotton to foster toxins. Tampon companies, aware of product liability, have tested cotton, rayon, and combinations of the two. They have found that the substance itself is not the problem; the absorbency is what matters.

▶ *Is the bleach used to whiten rayon tampons dangerous?*

Some women are concerned that the chlorine bleach used to whiten rayon tampons may put the tissues of the vagina in contact with harmful chemicals, particularly dioxin. Research by tampon manufacturers shows that currently manufactured tampons do not release measurable amounts of dioxin into the vagina. No research has shown that tampon use heightens the risk of endometriosis, either spontaneously or through the presence of dioxin.

MENSTRUAL HYGIENE

▶ *Can teenagers who have just begun to menstruate use tampons?*

There is no reason why you cannot use tampons if you have just started mensturating, although it takes most girls a while to learn how to insert them. Try different brands; choose "junior" or "slender" tampons, the narrowest ones available. Read the package inserts and follow the directions carefully.

Very occasionally, a young girl who has not been sexually active has come into the office because she could not pull out a tampon that had become stuck on her hymen. I have helped remove it, which I could do without breaking the hymen. If it is impossible for a girl to use a tampon, she and her mother might want to consult a gynecologist about identifying and solving the problem.

▶ Do tampons interfere with virginity?

Today most active young women, who bicycle, ride horses, and take part in other athletic activities, do not reach their first sexual intercourse with a completely intact hymen. These activities usually stretch the hymen enough that tampons can be inserted and removed without further damaging it. If someone's hymen is so tight that she cannot insert a tampon, her first intercourse may be painful.

▶ If you don't want to use tampons or pads, are any other products available?

A few other products are on the market, though none has been widely accepted. One is a little rubber cup that is inserted into the vagina to collect the blood; it can be emptied, washed, and reused. There are also menstrual sponges, made of natural materials, that can be washed and reused; some women really like them.

▶ How about scented or deodorized pads and panty liners?

Scented or deodorized pads are not advisable if you have sensitive skin. The advertisements for feminine hygiene products that speak of "delicate tissues" are right: the perineal tissue is probably the most sensitive skin on the body. If you cannot tolerate perfume on your neck, you may end up with irritation from scented pads.

Judy thinks she has vaginitis and comes in for an appointment. She has previously had a number of yeast infections, which cleared up with Monistat. This time she is very uncomfortable and the Monistat is not helping. Her examination shows inflamed perineal tissue but no evidence of infection and no vaginal discharge. A culture of her vaginal secretions does not reveal yeast or unwanted bacteria. It turns out that Judy tried a new brand of deodorized pads and developed a severe inflammatory reaction after using them for a while.

Some women can wear a panty liner thirty days out of thirty with no problem, but if you have sensitive skin, you may develop perineal irritation. Cotton panties or panties with a cotton crotch are "breathable," gentle to your skin, and do not provide the kind of environment in which yeast infections flourish. If your underwear becomes stained, wash it as soon as possible. (But it is better to have a few pairs of stained panties than a chronically inflamed perineum.)

▶ *Which are the best soaps and detergents?*

My dermatologist friends tell me that white Dove soap is the least irritating of the brands commonly available. Though the advertisements for Ivory show babies, suggesting that the soap is gentle enough for their tender skin, it is very alkaline and can be irritating. Be gentle when you wash your perineal area; don't scrub vigorously with a washcloth. If you have sensitive skin, don't take bubble baths, as the perfumes and other chemicals in bubble products can affect your skin.

As for laundry detergent, find what works for you and stay with it. Some women prefer to wash their underwear separately and to use a product like Ivory Snow or Woolite. If you find those products nonirritating, then don't change. Women have come into my office with what they thought was a yeast infection, and it turned out to be inflamed genital tissue. We check out the possibilities: Has the patient changed soaps or purchased a new brand of toilet paper? Sometimes I learn that her supermarket had a special on generic laundry detergent, which irritated her skin after she washed her underwear with it.

4 Premenstrual Syndrome

▶ **MYTH** PMS is all in your mind, a "disease" that exists only because women are ruled by their emotions.

FACT PMS is real, the effect of hormonal changes that take place in the weeks before your period. The symptoms may be emotional or psychological (irritability or depression), but the causes are physical.

THE term "premenstrual syndrome" (PMS) describes a disease that is not entirely understood by the medical profession in general, by psychiatrists, even by women who have it. All sorts of symptoms and disorders can be lumped together under that name. The symptoms can be emotional—irritability, tearfulness, or mood swings—or physical—headaches, pelvic pain, breast tenderness, or bloating.

Any of these symptoms can be caused by other conditions or can appear in milder form in women who do not have PMS. Many women experience sore, tender breasts. Many women get headaches from tension, hormone swings, or other causes. Many women notice that they are tearful, irritable, and have mood swings during the second half of their cycle. But two factors set PMS apart: timing and severity. With PMS, some or all of these symptoms occur during the last week or so before the menstrual period begins. And while many women have discomfort just before their menstrual periods, women with PMS often find that they can carry on their usual activities only with difficulty or not at all.

Who gets PMS? Previous depression, including postpartum depression, seems to be one risk factor. Women who are depressed or anxious at other times of the month understandably worry that these feelings will worsen during the premenstrual days. A family history of PMS seems to increase risk, as does a family history of depression or migraine headaches. Some researchers believe that consuming large amounts of chocolate or alcohol also increases risk. Others note that PMS can become more severe around the time of menopause.

The two most frequently reported symptoms of PMS are bloating and irritability, with sleeplessness a close third. Some women with PMS have breast discomfort, though some do not. Others report mental changes like lapses in memory and shortened attention span or difficulty concentrating; others experience depression as well as irritability. Some women have cravings for certain kinds of food, especially sweets (the chocolate-bar phenomenon is well known), salty snacks like potato chips, and caffeine.

How much anxiety and emotional distress a woman feels when she has PMS depends to some extent on what I call her baseline level of agitation. Some women feel pretty calm most of the time; if they have mild PMS, they feel agitated or anxious just before their pe-

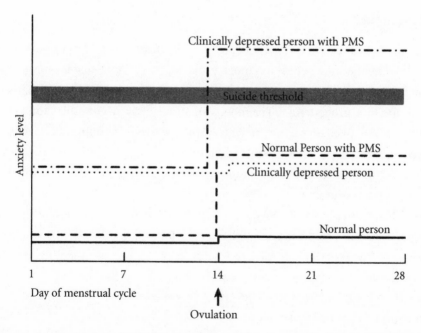

FIGURE 11. Anxiety levels and PMS. Everyone has some baseline anxiety, but the level differs from one woman to another. Most women experience some increase in their baseline level just before their periods; a few women have a very significant increase.

riods arrive. Other women are always fairly volatile and often perturbed, so when their baseline level of anxiety gets worse premenstrually, they feel really bad. These are the women who truly need help with their PMS. But there are also women normally calm and serene, who spike wildly before their periods. For some of these women the emotional effects of PMS are intolerable.

Nowadays, fortunately, PMS is a recognized disease and is no longer considered simply a figment of the irresponsible female imagination. The American Psychiatric Association has developed a list of symptoms for diagnosing and categorizing different kinds of mental illness, one of which is called premenstrual dysphoric disorder (PMDD), formerly known as late luteal phase dysphoric disorder. It seems more or less equivalent to what most people call severe PMS, though the diagnostic handbook issued by the American Psychiatric Association understandably emphasizes psychological symptoms: anger or irritability, mood swings, depression, anxiety or tension, fatigue, difficulty in concentration, loss of sleep, appetite changes; and some physical symptoms: headaches and breast tenderness. To be diagnosed with PMDD, you must have at least five of the symptoms on the list, and they must recur cyclically.

▶ What causes PMS?

No one knows what causes PMS. There are many theories, but no real proof that any is correct. Leading theories include too much prolactin (a hormone that is often produced in greater amounts during stress), too little progesterone, and too much estrogen accompanied by too little progesterone. The most widely accepted current explanation involves levels of serotonin (a chemical messenger used by nerve cells to communicate with other nerve cells or their targets). It is possible, given the wide range of symptoms and the number of competing theories about the cause, that there may be more than one form of PMS and more than one cause.

Since there is no accepted theory as to what chemical imbalance causes PMS, there is no laboratory test for PMS. If someone tells you that for four hundred dollars you can have a blood test that will tell whether you have PMS, just say no. Use the money to buy a membership in a gym or something great to wear.

▶ How can you control PMS symptoms?

Since PMS is so complex and so difficult to treat, you can start at the most basic level by doing things that may help you and certainly won't hurt you.

Many women are helped merely by charting their lives and recognizing patterns in the way they feel. If you have the luxury of organizing your own time and activities, set up your schedule so that on the days you know you are going to feel irritable or bloated, you won't be doing things to raise your stress level. If you know you are not going to be the most delightful person starting Tuesday the 23rd, don't plan to have a college interview, an aggravating meeting with an incompetent employee, or a birthday party with your 8-year-old son's dozen best buddies.

Charting can also be diagnostic. Suppose after a couple of months of monitoring yourself and looking for cyclical patterns, you notice that you feel depressed, irritable, and anxious every day. Because PMS is in the media and therefore on everyone's mind, you have automatically assumed that your bad moods are cyclical. When you start charting, you may discover that they are not. In fact, you may have depression—which is less acceptable socially than PMS and not usually helped by PMS therapies. We are fortunate that today there are good medications for depression. If you do chart your symptoms and find that you are depressed more than half the month, you and your doctor should try to get the correct diagnosis and treat you for that. An antidepressant will work a lot better than treating your depression as PMS. Therapy may help as well.

Another major step in helping yourself through PMS is to eat so that you get close to your ideal body weight; the closer you get, the better you will feel in terms of general health, whatever time of the month and whatever your age. If you need to lose weight (and it's a lot easier to *talk* about ideal body weight than to get there and stay there), try to stick to a relatively low-fat, general-weight-loss diet. Keep your calorie intake high enough to maintain your health, and try to lose weight gradually.

I encourage women who have PMS symptoms to avoid concentrated carbohydrates (like cookies), stay away from chocolate bars if you can manage to suppress the cravings, keep fat intake low, and cut down on salt and caffeine. Decreasing salt intake reduces the bloating associated with fluid retention, and limiting caffeine helps both with breast discomfort and with the caffeine-induced jitters. My standard line is that if your body, like Audrey, the carnivorous plant in the *Little Shop of Horrors*, shouts "Feed me! Feed me!," you have to respond negatively. If you eat the candy bar, you will feel worse with the extra sugar on board. If you eat the salty potato chips, you will increase your tendency to bloat.

Regular exercise is another key. It is good for you even if it turns out not to help your PMS. Researchers have discovered substances called endorphins, natural opiates produced by your brain, which make you feel better just as antidepressant drugs do. Endorphins are produced in greater amounts during exercise and account for the phenomenon known as a runner's high. Since premenstrual depression is an issue for many who have PMS, the endorphins generated through exercise will probably help these women feel better. The goal is a half hour of aerobic exercise (getting your heart rate to about 75 percent of its maximum capacity) three times a week. This is a goal, not a limit; if you feel like exercising more frequently, so much the better.

> Lucy feels out of sorts every month before her period. She decides to start running to see if it will help her to control her negative feelings. She begins with short distances but finds that the more she runs, the better she feels. Eventually she becomes a marathoner and completes the New York marathon several times. With her newfound energy, she later takes up karate. She is now extremely fit and generally serene all month long.

Not every woman who takes up exercise to control PMS will end up as a marathoner or earn a black belt, but Lucy's example shows very clearly that exercise can have a real effect on PMS.

▶ What about vitamins or dietary supplements?

Even though the value of vitamins and supplements in treating PMS is controversial, many women find that vitamin B_6 helps. I recommend 100–200 mg daily, which is a safe dosage despite being much higher than the normal daily requirement (about 2 mg) or even the amount in prenatal vitamins (10 mg a day). However, B_6 taken in huge dosages, let's say 1,500–2,000 mg daily, can be toxic to your nerves and produce symptoms like tingling in the fingers; with any vitamin supplement it is crucial to realize that more is not necessarily better. Just because your symptoms improve with vitamin B_6, don't take more than 100–200 mg daily.

How does vitamin B_6 work? For one thing, it is a natural diuretic and therefore helps with bloating. Furthermore, B_6 seems to antagonize a couple of brain hormones, particularly prolactin, which may be involved in PMS. Researchers have noted that vitamin B_6 plays a role in serotonin metabolism and sometimes helps with the depression linked to oral contraceptives. Maybe 60–70 percent of the women I treat for PMS get some relief when they take B_6, which is much higher than the placebo effect. That is, in any drug trial a placebo (a pill without active ingredients) helps about 30 percent of the people who try it. Thus, to show that a medication actually relieves symptoms, you have to demonstrate an effect greater than 30 percent. And since B$_6$ often helps with breast discomfort, is readily available, and will not harm you if you take moderate amounts, it is worth trying.

A second vitamin useful in treating the breast discomfort that often accompanies PMS is vitamin E. Try supplementation at about 400–600 units a day. Be careful not to overdose on it, for vitamin E is fat soluble and can be stored in the body's fatty tissues. Fat-soluble vitamins can readily accumulate to undesirable levels, whereas water-soluble vitamins are more easily excreted. Vitamin E currently has a reputation as perhaps preventing cancer and promoting cardiac health.

Some physicians recommend calcium supplements (1,000–1,200 mg daily) or magnesium (200 mg daily during the last half of the menstrual cycle). Recent research suggests that calcium can be quite effective; of course, all women should be getting calcium regularly to protect their bones.

▶ What about herbal remedies?

Therapies beyond diet, exercise, and vitamins B$_6$ and E get even more controversial. Many of my patients find that evening primrose oil helps them. Evening primrose is a garden plant rich in an essential fatty acid called gammalinolenic acid—GLA as it is known in the health food business. The theory behind GLA or evening primrose oil is that some women develop a deficiency in their fatty-acid metabolism, a deficiency involving an enzyme called delta 6 desaturase. According to the theory, the women who develop this defect cannot metabolize linoleic acid to gammalinolenic acid. By taking the gammalinolenic acid, they bypass the "deficient enzyme" and improve their fatty-acid metabolism. What this has to do with PMS, no one is quite sure. But 50–60 percent of the women I treat for PMS feel better with evening primrose oil.

The oil is costly, more expensive than vitamin E or vitamin B$_6$. You can buy it at health food stores, where it costs about twenty-six dollars for a two-month supply. Standard dosage is 500 units per capsule; I recommend two capsules a day to women just starting out, though many practitioners who recommend evening primrose oil suggest up to six capsules a day. It has no negative side effects.

▶ Are hormones useful in treating PMS?

If you still feel bad after trying dietary changes, exercise, vitamin B$_6$, vitamin E, calcium, and evening primrose oil, maybe you should consider hormonal intervention. Among the possibilities are progesterone and birth control pills.

The idea of using progesterone to treat PMS came from Katharina Dalton, an English general practitioner who published her findings in the 1940s and early 1950s. Dalton believed that PMS was a progesterone deficiency disorder, an idea that makes sense, especially with older, premenopausal women who often have PMS as well as heavy periods. As women approach menopause, their progesterone production frequently falls before estrogen production does. Since progesterone is important in controlling the heaviness of the menstrual flow, Dalton's idea was to give extra progesterone to replace what a woman was not producing on her own. She treated thousands of women with PMS by giving them supplements of natural progesterone for ten days or two weeks before their periods. According to her published results, her patients improved.

Progesterone must be specially processed, broken down into very tiny particles, to be well absorbed by the digestive system. When Dr. Dalton first started using natural progesterone, this process had not yet been invented. She recommended vaginal suppositories, because natural progesterone can be easily absorbed across the mucous membranes. Although researchers in the United States have tried to duplicate her work, most of the studies show no significant difference between placebo and progesterone.

Even though American research does not corroborate Dalton's work, gynecologists here do use progesterone supplements as PMS therapy. In appropriate doses this supplementation is completely safe, and it does seem to help some women. Some respond well to synthetic progesterones such as Provera, which are readily accessible, but some feel better with natural progesterone.

Progesterone as a therapy for PMS is also available in long-lasting injections, as Depo-Provera, usually used as a contraceptive. The drawback of injected progesterone (aside from the inconvenience of having the shots) is that it is deposited in body fat and once on board, it remains there for three months. Some women experience unpleasant side effects, including breakthrough bleeding, spotting, or staining; depression; and weight gain. Other women, however, respond well to it. Women on Depo do not get periods and are happy with this situation. Because progesterone can act as a sedative, it calms many women who suffer anxiety premenstrually. Nevertheless, injected progesterone is not something to rush into lightly, nor should it be used without supervision.

Sometimes birth control pills are effective. If PMS is a disorder of ovulation, shutting down ovulation (which is what birth control pills do) should help. If you have symptoms of PMS, need contraception, and perhaps have bad cramps, your doctor may suggest that you try the pill for a month or so to see how you feel. You may find that the pill works well for you, but you may also find (for reasons no one understands) that oral contraceptives make your PMS worse. If that is the case, stop taking them and talk to your doctor about trying something else.

If neither progesterone nor birth control pills relieve your PMS, there are certain hormonal medications that will close down your ovaries altogether, making you chemically menopausal for as long as you take them. Lupron, one of the major drugs used to treat endometriosis, does this. Many physicians use Lupron as a diagnostic tool for PMS.

Suppose you are feeling really irritable and depressed. Is your problem PMS or is it clinical depression caused by something else? In order to distinguish between the two, we can shut down your ovaries altogether for a month or two, give you a little estrogen to prevent hot flashes and other discomforts that will result from the shutdown, and see whether your PMS goes away. If it doesn't, then clearly your problem is not PMS; if the symptoms disappear, then at least you know what you are dealing with. Some physicians use Lupron plus estrogen, long term, to treat PMS. However, this add-back therapy is very expensive, costing more than three hundred dollars a month.

Katie's husband, a policeman, is both mentally and physically abusive to her. She is obviously depressed about her personal situation, but she seems to have severe PMS as well. In order to find out whether her problems really do include PMS, we tried Lupron with estrogen add-back therapy. This treatment showed me clearly that she does indeed have PMS. When she is taking the Lupron and her ovaries are temporarily shut down, she feels much better; when we stop the therapy, she again feels depressed.

▶ *What can I do to reduce bloating?*

Some women gain ten pounds during their menstrual cycles. Some even own one set of clothes for the first half of their cycle and another for the second half. Vitamin B$_6$ and evening primrose oil help with bloating, but women who need something more can take a diuretic for a week or two before their periods. The diuretic recommended is spironolactone, sold under the trade name Aldactone. It seems to have some other effects on the symptoms of PMS, perhaps lessening irritability. Aldactone is quite safe: it is relatively mild and will not lower your blood pressure so much that you pass out; it is potassium sparing, which means it does not deplete your body of potassium as certain other diuretics do. However, as with all diurectics, the danger of becoming addicted exists.

If you take a diuretic regularly for mild bloating and then suddenly stop taking it, severe bloating may result. These medications will take care of mild high blood pressure and bloating, but you cannot stop and start them whenever you like; you have to continue taking your diuretic every day for long periods. Diuretics are not intended as weight-control pills. Their use has to be carefully monitored.

Susanna, a very attractive woman in her early 40s, was deeply concerned about her appearance, particularly her weight. Her story is a very sad one and a dramatic example of how not to approach weight control.

She came to me as a patient needing a hysterectomy for fibroids and pain, something totally unrelated to the reasons I subsequently took care of her. One day, years after she had recovered from the hysterectomy, she called me complaining of belly pain. I happened to be at the hospital and saw her in the emergency room. Since she no longer had a uterus, she was not really having a gynecological emergency, but she had no other physician. I examined her and found nothing, though her abdomen was certainly sore. Although I might not normally do so under these circumstances, I asked for a round of blood tests. When requested from the emergency room blood tests often include measurement of the amount of sodium and potassium. Susanna's potassium, which should have been in the 3.5–5.5 range, came back at an exceptionally low 1.8. Certainly that level could give her plenty of belly pain. It also could give her significantly irregular heartbeats, which she was experiencing as well.

We admitted her immediately to the intensive care unit and put her on a heart monitor. Initially we thought Susanna had a rare metabolic illness, because her potassium level was so low. I had never prescribed diuretics for her, so she had no way of purchasing them. Still, someone on the staff did ask whether she was taking diuretics and she said no, that she knew that was wrong and could be dangerous. In fact, she was lying. We sent off a blood screen and urine screen on her again, and the urine test turned out positive for Lasix, a potent diuretic that had been prescribed for her mother, who was taking it for a heart condition.

Susanna had apparently been taking the Lasix for a fairly long time, though of course we couldn't tell exactly how long. (You only have to take it for a few weeks to bring your potassium way down.) Susanna had it in her handbag and was taking it even in the hospital. When she was confronted with the fact, she angrily denied it and signed out of the hospital against medical advice.

She did come back to me several years later for a routine checkup. As we were chatting, I asked who she was seeing as an internist. She mentioned a friend of mine who works in a town nearby. Although it is wrong to gossip about patients, I felt that in this case the internist should know that she had done something that could possibly kill her, so I called and informed him.

When I told him about the episode in the hospital, he replied, "Oh no! She's doing it again. I haven't been able to figure out why she has these very abnormal thyroid function tests." She was getting thyroid extract somewhere, and taking it to try to get thin. She even had tremors. While thyroid is available only on prescription, she had somehow found a source.

A while ago, I read her obituary in one of the local papers. The obituary wasn't specific about the cause of death, but she was a woman in her late 40s, without any life-threatening medical problems. I assume that she died of some medication that she was surreptitiously taking. Whether she got back on Lasix and managed to kill herself with that, or whether she put herself into a toxic condition by taking extra thyroid medication, I don't know. The sad part of it is that she wasn't obese; she was slender.

So while diuretic therapy may be helpful in controlling bloating and the breast discomfort related to bloating, it should not be regarded lightly. It is not a magic bullet for instant weight loss.

▶ Can PMS be treated with antidepressants?

Antidepressant drugs such as Prozac can sometimes help women with PMS, even those who are not ordinarily depressed. Prozac, which belongs to a class of drugs called selective serotonin reuptake inhibitors (SSRIs), has faced allegations that it increases the likelihood of committing suicide or violence against others, but most psychiatrists of my acquaintance believe that Prozac is safe. They believe its bad reputation arose from poorly designed studies and excessive media attention. Individuals who take Prozac are depressed or disturbed in the first place. So a study that compares suicidal or aggressive behavior in one group of generally depressed and disturbed people who are not being treated with another group of depressed and disturbed people who *are* being treated may find little or no difference. In fact, large-scale studies show that those being treated with Prozac commit fewer violent acts against themselves and others. It is their baseline illness, not the Prozac, that makes them violent. The worst that can be said about Prozac is that it does not cure these people of their underlying illness.

As an antidepressant, Prozac is safe when its use is monitored by a physician. Some older antidepressants can have cardiac side effects, but Prozac does not. It is not addictive. It may temporarily depress sexual desire, but when you stop taking it, your libido will return to its pre-Prozac level.

Recent studies have shown the effectiveness of SSRIs for PMS. These drugs can be taken daily for a week or two before your menstrual period. They do not seem to have serious side effects, and they work quickly in relieving PMS symptoms. SSRIs taken for clinical depression take perhaps three weeks to have an effect; but for PMDD, the severe form of PMS, they work in one or two days. In 2000 the FDA approved Sarafem for PMDD; it is basically the same drug as Prozac.

Nancy has had serious PMS for years and recently started taking Sarafem, which made her feel much better. When her teenage daughter, Nina, began having PMS symptoms, Nancy asked whether Sarafem would be all right for Nina too. I checked with Nina's pediatrician, who thought it would be fine as long as Nina used the medication only a few days a month. Last week on a camping field trip from middle school, Nina mentioned to my daughter (whom of course I hadn't told about Nina) that her new medicine was making her feel better.

▶ Are other treatments for PMS available?

Bright-light therapy, which can help with seasonal affective disorder, the depression some people feel when deprived of adequate light, can also help with PMS depression. If anxiety is a major issue with PMS, an antianxiety medication such as Xanax can be very helpful. It is safe for short-term use but does have an addictive potential. You should not take Xanax long term unless the medication has been prescribed by a mental health professional for a severe anxiety disorder. A few pills for a few days before your period are fine. If one of the main issues is migraine headaches, then the beta-blocker atenolol can be helpful. If you have a problem with depression, however, beta-blockers are not advisable at any time.

5   Contraceptive Choices and Responsibilities

▶ **MYTH** You can't get pregnant if you stand up after you have intercourse. Or if your partner ejaculates outside you. Or if you douche with Coca-Cola right after intercourse.

FACT None of these methods will keep you from getting pregnant.

SAFE, legal contraception has given women control over their lives as never before. If you have grown up since the 1960s, in an era when contraception has been largely a matter of personal choice, you may not realize that this freedom is relatively new and was won only after years of struggle.

Margaret Sanger, an obstetrical nurse, saddened by the physical and social consequences of unwanted pregnancies, botched illegal abortions, and widespread sexually transmitted disease, started her crusade for birth control in the early 1900s. Defying existing laws against distributing information about birth control, she was reviled for her work, arrested, and put in a workhouse for a month. Popular opinion was strongly opposed to letting women have access to contraception.

Eventually Sanger and her allies prevailed. In the mid-1930s the government was legally prevented from seizing contraceptives that were sold across state lines. In 1965 in *Griswold* v. *Connecticut,* the Supreme Court declared unconstitutional a state law that made it illegal for physicians to give out contraceptive information. In that landmark decision, the court developed the notion of a "zone of privacy" where individual citizens were protected from government intrusion, a concept that has been the basis of many subsequent reproductive decisions.

CHOOSING A CONTRACEPTIVE

Contraception is something you should think about carefully. It should not be a decision left to your sexual partner, to a frantic last-minute trip to the drugstore, or, even worse, to superstition and luck. Finding the right contraceptive is a personal choice. A contraceptive that is fine for someone else can be absolutely wrong for you, and a contraceptive that is right for you when you are 20 years old may no longer suit your needs when you are 40.

Unfortunately, there is no perfect contraceptive—one that would never fail, would be so easy to use you would not have to think about it, and would have no unpleasant side effects or negative health consequences. But we have come a long way in the thirty-plus years since birth control became legal in this country. Many kinds of contraceptives are available. Some are safer than others, some are less bother, some are more affordable.

So how do you choose? The first guideline is your level of personal comfort. If a contraceptive method makes you physically or emotionally uncomfortable, you probably will not use it faithfully each and every time you have intercourse. If birth control pills upset your stomach or depress you, or if you feel that spermicidal foams or jellies are messy and unaesthetic, choose a different contraceptive.

A second guideline is your reaction to contraceptive failure. How would you feel if you did become pregnant by accident, even though you were using your contraception conscientiously? If you have already had several children and do not want to get pregnant again, no matter what, you will want a different contraceptive from the woman who would like to have a child maybe next year or the year after. While making the right choice balances personal, emotional, and (sometimes) religious factors, there are a couple of ground rules that every heterosexually active woman should follow.

Some contraceptive methods protect you against both pregnancy and disease; most protect only against pregnancy. The combination of a condom and contraceptive foam is probably the best all-around double-duty prevention against sexually transmitted diseases (STDs) and also against pregnancy.

BOX 1. Two Absolutely Basic Ground Rules for Protecting Yourself
Against Pregnancy and Sexually Transmitted Diseases

RULE 1: If you do not wish to get pregnant, you must use some kind of contraception *every time* you have intercourse.

RULE 2: If both you and your sexual partner are not entirely and permanently monogamous, you must protect yourself against disease as well as against pregnancy. Many women have learned that a relationship they thought was mutually monogamous was only monogamous on their side.

▶ *What are the chances of getting pregnant if you have intercourse without using contraception?*

You may believe that the likelihood of becoming pregnant from a single act of unprotected intercourse is close to 100 percent, but that is not true. On the other hand, many women have learned to their dismay or surprise that the percentage is not zero, either. If you have unprotected intercourse once right around the time of ovulation, your chances of getting pregnant are about 10 percent, to the best of our statistical knowledge. That rate will drop to the range of 2–3 percent if the unprotected intercourse occurs a day or two after your period.

You can become pregnant early in your cycle because sperm can remain potent for a day or two, maybe even longer, after ejaculation and because you may ovulate earlier than usual. If you have a twenty-eight-day cycle, you will probably ovulate on the fourteenth day after the beginning of your menstrual period, but you cannot rely on being perfectly regular each and every cycle of your life. Since ovulation is more variable at the beginning and end of your reproductive life, young women—teenagers, in particular—are at increased risk of getting pregnant. Women older than 40, whose fertility is declining, may also ovulate unpredictably, though they may also ovulate less frequently than younger women.

Your chances of getting pregnant during any one complete menstrual cycle if you have unprotected intercourse every other night all month are about 15–20 percent. On a longer-term basis, about 80–85 percent of couples will become pregnant after a year of unprotected intercourse every other night, and 90 percent will be pregnant after two years.

CONTRACEPTIVE RELIABILITY

Contraceptive reliability depends on two things: the reliability of the method and the inconstancies of human nature. Some unintended pregnancies come about because of method failure. Despite your best efforts and those of your partner, condoms can break, diaphragms and cervical caps can be dislodged during intercourse, and intrauterine devices can be expelled or fail to prevent implantation of the fertilized egg. These mishaps are built into the contraceptive method and are the fault of the method or product. All you can do is consistently use your contraceptive as directed. Other unintended pregnancies result from human failure: you forget to take your birth control pills for a couple of days; you leave your diaphragm in the drawer.

Statistics refer to "optimum use" or "best-expected effectiveness" to describe method failure and "typical use" or "estimated actual use" to include both method failure and human failure, or the relative success of the contraceptive in a real-world situation. These data are usually based on a year's use and derive from interviews of couples who say that they are using a particular method of contraception as directed. It is difficult to come up with absolutely accurate numbers: people sometimes forget that they have used their birth control carelessly or not at all, so the statistics that supposedly describe method failure sometimes describe human failure.

▶ *Which contraceptives are the most reliable and the least reliable?*

Starting with the most reliable and working down, the ones that you think about least work best: long-lasting hormonal contraceptives like Norplant and its successors and Depo-Provera, and surgical sterilization (either vasectomy or tubal ligation) are 99 percent reliable, in terms of both expected effectiveness and on-the-job effectiveness. This means that if 100 couples use these methods 100 percent of the time, only one of those couples will become pregnant by the end of the year. Next on the list of reliability are contraceptives that you don't have to think about every time you need contraception: the pill and IUDs. These are followed by condoms and diaphragms.

The least reliable form of contraception is no contraception at all. Also on the list of failure-prone methods are a couple of "folk" methods, which may have a reputation for effectiveness but in fact do not work. These methods include withdrawal (the man re-

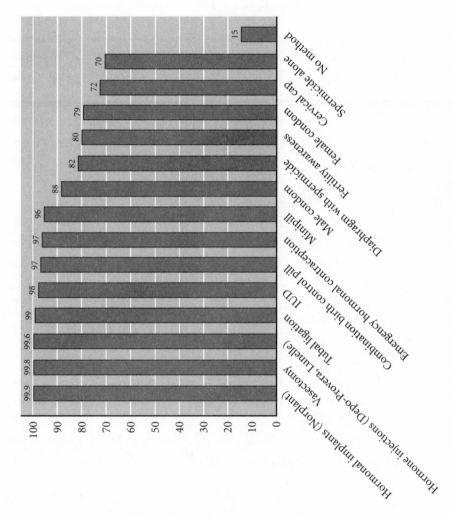

FIGURE 12. The effectiveness of various contraceptive methods during a year of actual use.

moves his penis from the woman's vagina before ejaculating), douching, and breast-feeding. Other rumors falsely assert that you cannot get pregnant if you are having intercourse for the first time, or if the woman fails to have an orgasm.

▶ *Can you get pregnant if your partner withdraws before he ejaculates?*

Withdrawal is one of the most commonly practiced "natural" methods of contraception, but it is risky. If your partner ejaculates only one drop of sperm before he withdraws, you can still become pregnant. Since that first drop is the most concentrated and contains the most vigorous sperm, your risk is substantial. Sperm can migrate upward even if they are not deposited in the vagina, so there is still a possibility of pregnancy even if the man ejaculates entirely outside the woman. Women have gotten pregnant from sperm on their thighs. And of course, in the passion of the moment, the man may not withdraw. On the other hand, if you and your partner suddenly have an attack of conscience in the midst of the sex act, withdrawal is better than nothing at all.

▶ *Why is douching with a spermicide after intercourse ineffective as a method of contraception?*

The sperm en route to fertilizing the egg make their way past the cervix in about a minute, and continue into the uterus beyond the range of the spermicide in the douche within 20 minutes of intercourse. Even if you douche immediately after the act, you still have a chance of getting pregnant; as we have seen, the first sperm to reach the cervix are not only the fastest but the most potent and vigorous. One persistent rumor is that douching with cola kills sperm; this procedure may work in a test tube, but it is not an effective means of contraception.

▶ *Can you get pregnant when you are breast-feeding?*

Although breast-feeding offers some protection for some women, it is unreliable. It may delay the return of fertility after pregnancy, but there is no way to know when ovulation will start again.

> Heather, a midwife, likes to point out that midwives are very successful at breast-feeding. They know all the tricks and techniques, and they are very committed to it. Then she points to her two sons, Tim and Nick, who are ten months apart. Nick is living proof that breast-feeding does not prevent ovulation.

REVERSIBLE CONTRACEPTIVES

Basically, there are three kinds of reversible contraceptives: (1) barrier types, which keep sperm out of the upper reproductive tract where fertilization can take place, (2) hormonal contraceptives, which interfere with ovulation or deny sperm access to the egg, and (3) nonbarrier mechanical devices, which inhibit fertilization or implantation.

Given these three approaches, you have several either/or choices. To begin with one of life's basic natural divisions, there are contraceptives for men and contraceptives for women. Then there are long-term and "per-need" contraceptives. Of the long-term contraceptives, the ones you do not need to think about each time you have intercourse, some (birth control pills or IUDs, Depo-Provera, Norplant) are reversible. Of the short-term or per-need contraceptives, most provide a barrier that prevents sperm from meeting egg; some of these barriers are physical (condoms) and others are chemical (spermicidal jellies and creams). Also in the short-term category are "before" and "after" contraceptives, those you take to prevent conception and those you take when you and your partner have "made a mistake."

BARRIER METHODS

Male Condoms

A condom is a sheath, usually latex, that fits snugly over the erect penis and prevents sperm from entering the vagina. Male condoms are an ancient method of contraception. The

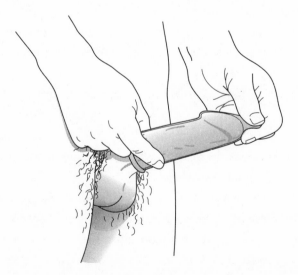

FIGURE 13. Male condoms offer the best protection against STDs including HIV. When used correctly together with a spermicide, they are also an effective means of contraception.

earliest ones, made of animal skin, gave some protection, although they probably did not fit well and must have leaked. Condoms got a big technological boost in 1839 when Charles Goodyear invented vulcanization, a process that made rubber stronger and more resilient. Today they come in all sorts of sizes, shapes, and colors, some with little dots, ticklers, or other devices to enhance sexual pleasure. Some are coated with spermicides, which may offer extra protection, though it is safer to use an additional spermicide in the vagina. Some are prelubricated. However, a basic plain latex condom will certainly suffice.

Certain condoms are still made of animal skin (usually lamb membrane), but these are less effective and more expensive (around four dollars apiece) than the latex ones. Buy latex condoms that are labeled disease protectant. If you are allergic to latex, polyurethane condoms, which cost one to two dollars apiece, are available.

▶ How do you use a male condom properly?

Use a new condom for each act of intercourse, whether oral, anal, or vaginal. Be careful when opening the package, so that you do not tear the condom inside.

Unroll the condom approximately one-half inch, then place the open end over the erect penis. This extra half inch should hang loosely past the head of the penis to catch the semen. Many condoms have reservoir tips that serve the same purpose. Squeeze the end to make sure no air is trapped inside. Then unroll the condom all the way down to the base of the penis, being careful that your fingernails do not puncture or tear the latex. The rolled rim should be on the outside. If the condom is not prelubricated, or if you want additional lubrication, choose a water-based lubricant such as Aqualube or Astroglide, available at many pharmacies. Oil-based lubricants (petroleum jelly, cold cream, hand lotion, cooking oil, or baby oil) can weaken the latex and cause condom failure.

The man should withdraw his penis from his partner while it is still erect (to keep the condom from leaking), holding the condom firmly to keep it from slipping off. Throw away the used condom, preferably wrapping it first in a tissue so that others do not need to handle it; do not flush it down the toilet. Never reuse a condom. And do not use a condom after the expiration date or if it is damaged.

Store condoms in a cool place away from direct sunlight (which also causes the latex to deteriorate). Extreme temperatures—especially heat—can make latex brittle or gummy (like an old balloon). Don't keep them in a hot glove compartment in the car. If you want to keep one with you, put it in a loose pocket, wallet, or purse.

▶ *What should I do if a condom breaks or comes off during intercourse?*

Insert spermicide into your vagina as soon as possible. If you are at midcycle, near ovulation, talk with your caregiver about morning-after contraception.

▶ *How reliable are condoms?*

In theory, male condoms used along with a spermicidal jelly or foam are 98 percent reliable. Condoms used alone, without a spermicide, are said in published studies to have a reliability of about 88 percent, although my medical experience suggests that they are more reliable, perhaps 96 percent.

▶ *What are their advantages and disadvantages?*

Latex condoms have one very important attribute that many other forms of birth control lack: they protect against sexually transmitted diseases as well as pregnancy. Since the active ingredient in many spermicides, nonoxynol-9, is thought to reduce your chance of contracting an STD, condoms plus spermicide give you the best available protection (except, of course, for abstinence) against STDs. Other advantages include reliability, availability (you don't need a prescription), and low cost. Depending on where you buy them, how many you buy at once, and how plain or fancy they are, condoms can cost from less than forty cents to more than a dollar apiece. Spermicides cost seven to ten dollars for a 3.8-ounce tube.

On the negative side, your partner needs to use a condom for each and every occasion of intercourse. Condoms do interfere with spontaneity, but some couples deal with this by having the woman put the condom on the man. Some men dislike them and complain that they dull sensation, but as I say to my patients, if he won't wear a condom to protect you (and himself) against disease, you don't need him.

Female Condoms

Female condoms are a relatively new invention, available in this country since 1993. Currently two brands are on the market: Reality and Femidom, both available without a prescription at some drugstores. You can also buy them over the Internet and sometimes in feminist bookstores. Though not widely accepted in this country, they have some advantages.

The female condom is a loose-fitting, soft polyurethane pouch that lines the vagina

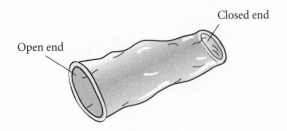

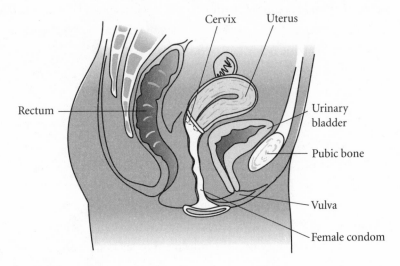

FIGURE 14. The female condom.

and closes off the cervix, preventing sperm from entering the uterus. It has two soft rings, one at each end. The smaller, closed ring is covered with the polyurethane and fits over the cervix, acting as an anchor. The larger open ring stays outside the vagina, covering part of the labia.

▶ How do you use a female condom properly?

Use a new condom for each separate act of intercourse. The condom can be inserted up to eight hours beforehand, unless you have your period, in which case you should insert it shortly before intercourse.

Inspect the condom and make sure it is completely lubricated on the outside and the inside. While holding the sheath at the closed end, grasp the soft, flexible inner ring and squeeze it with your thumb and middle finger so it becomes long and narrow. With the other hand, separate the outer lips of your vagina and gently insert the inner ring. You should feel it go up and move into place.

Next, place your index finger on the inside of the condom, and push the inner ring up as far as it will go. Be sure the sheath is not twisted. The outer ring should remain outside the labia. The sheath adheres to the vaginal wall. The Reality female condom is prelubricated with a nonspermicidal lubricant. If you wish more lubrication, you can use any kind, since the polyurethane sheath is not affected by oil-based lubricants.

During intercourse, gently guide the penis with your hand, to be sure that it enters the sheath and not the space between the sheath and the vaginal wall. It is important to use enough lubricant so that the condom stays in place during sex. If the condom is pulled out or pushed in, there is not enough lubricant. Add more to either the inside of the condom or the outside of the penis.

To remove the condom, twist the outer ring and gently pull the condom out. To avoid spilling, remove it before standing up. Again, wrap it in a tissue and throw it in the trash.

▶ *Can you and your partner use a male condom and a female condom at the same time?*

No, neither will work properly. The material used in condoms is meant to work against skin. If the two condoms rub together, friction could pull off the male condom or push the female condom into the vagina.

▶ *Can you use spermicide with a female condom?*

You can use a spermicidal foam, gel, or film. Put the spermicide inside the vagina before you insert the condom or cover the outside of the condom with the spermicide. No studies have been done to show whether a spermicide increases condom reliability.

▶ *How reliable are female condoms?*

Studies by the manufacturer showed that when used correctly every time, the female condom's failure rate in a six-month study was 3 percent. Its actual failure rate was 12 percent. Based on these results, the annual failure rate is 5 percent for correct, consistent use, and 79 percent for typical use, higher than the failure rate for male condoms.

▶ *What are their advantages and disadvantages?*

Female condoms, like the male ones, protect against AIDS and other STDs. Because their use is controlled by women, they have been endorsed by international AIDS programs, including those sponsored by the United Nations. Female condoms are not made of latex, so they can be used with oil-based lubricants and will not deteriorate. They can be inserted well before intercourse. Female condoms, though more costly than male condoms, are not expensive—about $2.50 apiece.

Some women are put off by the appearance of the female condom and others by the need to insert it into the vagina. Some couples complain that it squeaks during intercourse, though the noise can be reduced by adding extra lubrication. The failure rate is higher than for male condoms; and female condoms are more expensive and somewhat more difficult to insert.

Spermicides

Spermicides do what their name implies: they kill sperm. These chemicals are put into the vagina just before intercourse to prevent pregnancy. Most have nonoxynol-9 as their active ingredient. They come as creams, jellies, foams, and suppositories (Semicid, Intercept, and the Encare Oval) and are packaged in tubes or aerosol cans with special plastic applicators. Spermicides are also available as films (VCF), which are inserted directly into the vagina.

▶ *How do you use a spermicide?*

Insert spermicidal creams, jellies, and foams into your vagina no more than fifteen minutes before intercourse. Suppositories and films can be inserted as long as half an hour before (though it is always best to read the product instructions), but they remain effective for only about an hour. A new suppository or film should be used for each separate act of intercourse.

If the cream or jelly comes in a tube, screw the plastic applicator onto the end of the tube, and squeeze the tube until the applicator is full. Some brands require two tubefuls for each separate act of intercourse, so read the directions. If you are using a foam, shake the can, put the applicator on top of the can, and press down until the foam fills the applicator, pushing the plunger all the way out.

To use a suppository, simply push it into the vagina. Allow the recommended time for the suppository to melt or foam up before you have intercourse. To use a contraceptive film, wrap it around a finger and push it all the way into the vagina to cover the cervix. Do not remove the suppository or film for at least six hours.

If you are using a spermicide with a diaphragm or cervical cap, apply a teaspoonful inside the diaphragm and insert the diaphragm as usual (see the section on diaphragms), then squirt more spermicide into the vagina outside the diaphragm. If you are using it with a male or female condom, or without any mechanical barrier, use the plastic plunger that comes with the product to squirt it up into the vagina.

For any of these methods, you may find it preferable to sit on the toilet, lie in bed with your knees bent, or squat. Remember that you have to reapply the spermicide for each separate act of intercourse. Leave the spermicide in place for at least six hours before washing the vagina.

▶ *How reliable are spermicides?*

Used alone, in theory they are 80–90 percent effective. But combined with other barrier methods (condoms, diaphragms, or cervical caps) contraceptive foams, creams, and jellies are extremely effective and are appropriate if you need a very high rate of reliability.

▶ *Do spermicides protect against STDs?*

Although we have no solid data, there is evidence that spermicides do help prevent infection. However, if you are using a spermicide with a cervical cap or a diaphragm and you put the spermicide only inside the cup, it does not protect against AIDS, herpes, or genital warts. If you put the spermicide into the vagina outside the cervix, then it may protect you.

▶ *What are the differences between brands of contraceptive creams, foams, and jellies?*

All these products rely on nonoxynol-9 to kill sperm, but they have different bases and perfumes. Unless you are allergic to the perfume or the base in which the spermicide is dissolved, the choice is a matter of aesthetics—of color, smell, consistency, and taste. Try different brands, buying only a small quantity until you find one you like. If you do have an allergic reaction (for example, itching, burning, or an unpleasant odor), the culprit is probably the perfume or the base, not the nonoxynol-9, which is rarely allergenic. Ortho makes an unscented product, a good choice if you have allergies.

▶ *What are the advantages and disadvantages of spermicides?*

Spermicidal products are easy to use, either with or without another barrier method. They are available at your local pharmacy without a prescription; they are not expensive (seven to ten dollars for a 3.8-ounce tube with applicator, less for refills). They have no side effects (unless you have an allergic reaction). They do not interfere with later fertility. On the down side, you must use a spermicide for each and every act of intercourse. Used alone, they have a relatively high rate of failure. They can be messy; after intercourse, they can drip out onto your underwear. Occasionally they cause allergic reactions.

▶ *Is a spermicide right for you?*

> Judy is 45 years old, married, and monogamous. She has two children and does not intend to have any more. She uses a contraceptive foam for protection against pregnancy. The 80–90 percent effectiveness rate of a spermicide used alone is probably adequate for Judy, since she is in her mid-40s and her fertility has been reduced by time. She has only one sexual partner; if her husband is also monogamous, she has no need for protection against STDs.

The effectiveness rate that suits Judy would not be adequate for a young, fertile woman who wants to avoid pregnancy. Teenage women whose partners refuse to wear condoms sometimes rely on spermicides alone because these products are easy to get and easy to use. Doing so is risky, in terms of both preventing pregnancy and protecting against STDs.

Diaphragms

A diaphragm is a little rubber cup, between 2 and 3.5 inches in diameter, whose rim is stiffened with a metal spring. The various models on the market differ according to the kind of spring used in the rim. Some come with a special applicator for insertion.

The diaphragm fits across the upper end of the vagina and covers the cervix. It works by preventing sperm from entering the uterus and by holding a spermicidal cream or jelly in place close to the cervix. Before the advent of oral contraceptives, diaphragms were a major form of contraception; for some women they are still a reasonable way to prevent pregnancy.

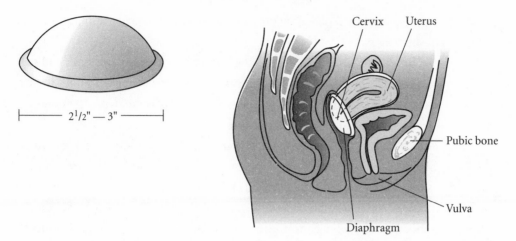

FIGURE 15. When inserted correctly, the diaphragm completely covers the cervix and rests behind the pubic bone.

▶ *How do you use a diaphragm?*

Diaphragms come in different sizes, so your caregiver must fit you and give you a prescription for your personal size, which you can fill at your pharmacy. If you gain or lose more than twenty pounds or have a pregnancy, you will need to have the diaphragm refitted. You can use it during your period (it catches the menstrual blood). Before inserting your diaphragm, be sure it has no rips, tears, or pinholes. If it does, use another method of contraception until you get a new diaphragm.

Inserting a diaphragm takes a little practice, but most women learn without much difficulty. Squeeze about a teaspoon of spermicidal cream or jelly into the dome of the diaphragm and smear a little more just inside or around the outside of the rim. Then pinch the rim together and slide the diaphragm into your vagina, making sure that the cup entirely covers the cervix. When you let go of the rim, the diaphragm springs open. It is easiest to insert lying on your back with your knees bent, sitting on the toilet, or squatting. When the diaphragm is in place, it should fit snugly against your cervix. The front rim should be anchored under your pubic bone. Properly positioned, the diaphragm cannot fall out. Neither you nor your partner should be aware of the diaphragm once it is in place; if it slips around or feels uncomfortable, your caregiver should check and possibly refit it.

You can insert your diaphragm as long as two hours before intercourse, and you must leave it in place six to eight hours afterward, giving the spermicide a chance to work. Do not leave it longer than twenty-four hours. If you have intercourse more than once, you should leave the diaphragm in place but add more spermicide, using the applicator to insert it high in your vagina.

To remove the diaphragm, simply hook your index finger over the front rim and pull the diaphragm out. The positions that made it easier to insert also make it easier to take out. After you have removed the diaphragm, wash it in soapy water, rinse it, and put it safely away in its case. Exposure to light can shorten the life of the rubber.

Some women have difficulty keeping a diaphragm in place. These include women who have certain anatomical problems—for example, a severely prolapsed uterus, which sometimes is the case after the birth of several children. Women who have frequent urinary tract infections might be better off with another form of contraception, since the diaphragm's front edge can press against the urethra and make it difficult for the bladder to empty.

▶ What happens if you forget to take out your diaphragm, or if it gets stuck?

Although you should not leave a diaphragm in place for more than twenty-four hours, nothing dire will happen if you do. There are no documented cases of toxic shock caused by a diaphragm left in too long. However, you may notice a strong or unpleasant odor when you do remove it.

If your diaphragm gets stuck (which happens rarely), ask your partner to help you remove it. If that doesn't work, wait an hour and try again; sometimes waiting helps. Don't be embarrassed to call your caregiver if necessary and ask to have it removed.

▶ How reliable is a diaphragm?

If used faithfully and correctly along with a spermicidal cream or jelly, a diaphragm has a failure rate of about 4 percent. With actual use, which includes women who use the method incorrectly or inconsistently, the failure rate is probably around 18 percent. Diaphragms fail because sperm manage to sneak around the edge and enter the uterus, perhaps because the diaphragm gets dislodged or was incorrectly inserted or fitted, or because additional spermicide was not used for a subsequent intercourse. I have had patients who were themselves gynecologists who became pregnant while wearing a diaphragm, and I assume they inserted it correctly.

▶ *What are its advantages and disadvantages?*

Properly inserted, a diaphragm has a relatively high effectiveness rate. It is quite easy to use. It has no significant side effects. It is under the woman's control, though it certainly helps to have a partner committed to the method. Once it is in place, most couples are unaware of its presence. The spermicide used along with the diaphragm may lower (but not cancel) the risk of being infected with an STD during vaginal intercourse.

On the negative side, diaphragms with their accompanying spermicides are messy. Some people object to the feel or taste of the spermicide. You have to insert your diaphragm each time you have intercourse and remove it after the appropriate interval. You cannot rely on it to protect you absolutely against STDs or vaginal infections. Using a diaphragm may predispose you to urinary tract infections, though you can minimize this risk by using a soft-ring diaphragm in the smallest size that adequately covers the top of your vagina.

The up-front cost of a diaphragm is fairly high—around twenty-five dollars plus the cost of the visit to your doctor. If you get measured for a diaphragm at your annual visit, you do not incur the costs of an extra appointment. Spermicidal creams and jellies cost somewhere between seven and ten dollars for a 3.8-ounce tube, about twelve applications.

▶ *Is a diaphragm the right contraceptive for you?*

Mary is 26, married with one child. She had trouble with blood clots in her legs during her pregnancy, so birth control pills are not appropriate for her. She wants another baby in a year or so, but certainly would not mind if she got pregnant sooner.

A diaphragm might be a reasonable choice for Mary; she and her husband feel comfortable with its effectiveness rate and the need to insert it each time before intercourse.

Carly is 21, a senior in college. Her boyfriend graduated last year and has taken a job in a city hundreds of miles away from her school. Oral contraceptives make Carly queasy, but she is very conscientious about using contraception.

Since she and her boyfriend see each other only occasionally and she is willing to put up with its inconveniences, a diaphragm used along with spermicide might be an acceptable option for her.

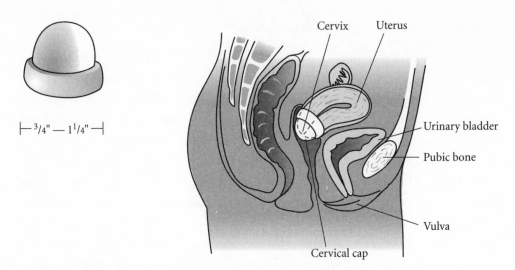

FIGURE 16. A cervical cap in place snugly covers the cervix.

Cervical Cap

A cervical cap is a rubber device something like a diaphragm, but only about an inch in diameter, held in place by suction rather than by the surrounding anatomical structures. While a cervical cap covers the cervix and closes off the entrance to the uterus, it does not block off the entire width of the vagina. For this reason, and also because it is used with less spermicide, a cervical cap is less reliable than a diaphragm, though it is more convenient. Caps are prescribed less frequently than diaphragms, but some women's clinics and university health services do offer them. The woman who might choose a diaphragm might also find a cervical cap suitable.

▶ How do you use a cervical cap?

Cervical caps come in different sizes, so you must be fitted by your caregiver, who will give you a prescription. Some women, especially those who have had several children, are difficult to fit because of the size or shape of the cervix.

You may insert the cap as much as twenty-four hours before intercourse. Fill it about one-third full with a spermicide and insert it into your vagina—directly against the cervix, where it should attach by suction. You need not apply extra spermicide outside the cap, and you can use it for more than one act of intercourse.

After intercourse you should leave the cap in place for six to eight hours to let the spermicide do its work. Some manufacturers say that you can leave it in place as long as a week, but the cap can develop an odor if left that long. It is probably better to remove it at least every other day. You should not use a cervical cap for contraception during your menstrual period, as the flow may break the seal and displace the cap.

▶ *How reliable is a cervical cap?*

Some studies have suggested that a cervical cap has a method failure rate of 6 percent and an actual failure rate of about 18 percent, but my experience with patients suggests that these estimates are optimistic. I estimate the highest possible effectiveness to be somewhere in the range of 92 percent, maybe a little less.

▶ *What are its advantages and disadvantages?*

A cervical cap has the advantages of a diaphragm, plus it can stay in place much longer and is less messy. You can use it for more than one act of intercourse without additional spermicide. On the down side, it does not protect you against disease and is less reliable than other barrier methods. A cervical cap has no known side effects, though occasional women complain of urinary tract infections; these are less likely than with a diaphragm, because the cervical cap does not rest against the urethra.

As with a diaphragm, the initial cost is fairly high. The cap itself costs something more than thirty dollars, but you also pay for the office visit to your caregiver. Since a cervical cap takes more time to fit, your doctor might suggest a special appointment for the fitting rather than doing it during your regular checkup. Spermicides cost about seven to ten dollars per tube.

Contraceptive Sponge

Contraceptive sponges are small, circular sponges impregnated with spermicide that fit into the vagina and cover the cervix. They were withdrawn from the market in this country in 1995, but are available in Canada and may in the future return to the U.S. market.

HORMONAL CONTRACEPTION

Although birth control pills are by far the most popular form of hormonal contraception in the United States and Europe, other available forms include injections (Depo-Provera), hormonal implants, and morning-after contraception (Preven, or special dosages of oral contraceptives). All hormonal contraception is reversible; you can stop taking it and get pregnant, but implants and shots remain effective for months and years, requiring less attention than birth control pills. The hormones used in these methods can cause side effects, generally those associated with the normal menstrual cycle (breakthrough bleeding, queasiness, breast tenderness, acne, headaches, weight gain, and mood changes), but all have been tested for long-term safety. Before you begin to use any of these methods, you should have a checkup and alert your doctor if you have certain medical conditions—for example, a history of problems with blood clots.

Birth Control Pills

Oral contraceptives are the most popular reversible form of birth control today, used by about 30 percent of American women. Introduced in the late 1950s, they found widespread acceptance during the 1960s as a relatively safe and inexpensive form of contraception. For the first time, women had a means of effective contraception they did not need to think about on each and every occasion of intercourse. Some people worried that convenient, reliable contraception would make women promiscuous, and it is certainly true that the availability of the pill did change patterns of sexual behavior.

The pills as first developed contained large doses of estrogen, about 100 μg per pill. Although these high-dose pills often caused bloating, breast tenderness, and depression, many women used them. During the 1970s, high-dose pills were linked to increased risk of blood clots in the veins, as well as heart attacks or strokes, especially for women older than 35 who smoked. Over the years, the estrogen content of birth control pills has gradually been reduced: from 100 to 80 to 50, and now to 30 or 35 μg; a few modern pills contain only 20 μg of estrogen.

Today there are basically two kinds of oral contraceptives: combination pills which contain both synthetic estrogen and synthetic progesterone (progestin) and progestin-only pills, also called minipills.

Combination pills work by blocking ovulation. During the normal menstrual cycle, the rise and fall of estrogen and progesterone levels trigger the monthly release of the egg from the ovary, the thickening of the uterine lining to prepare for a fertilized egg, and the midcycle changes in the cervical mucus that make it easy for sperm to swim toward the egg. During pregnancy both estrogen and progesterone are produced in larger amounts than at other times. Birth control pills that contain these hormones artificially elevate their levels and trick the body into thinking that it is pregnant. The constant high level of estrogen blocks ovulation; the constant high level of progestin inhibits the thickening of the endometrial lining (hindering implantation of a fertilized egg) and keeps the cervical mucus in a state hostile to sperm.

Most pills prescribed today are combination pills. There are several different chemical forms of each hormone, which can be used in different amounts during the month. Ortho-Novum 1/35, for example, has 1 mg of progestin and 35 μg of estrogen. Ortho-Novum 7/7/7 has 0.5 mg of progestin for the first seven days, 0.75 mg for the second seven days, and 1.0 mg for the final seven days.

Brands differ in the kind and amount of progestin they contain, and in the kind and amount of synthetic estrogen. The most frequently used form of the latter is ethinyl estradiol. Older pills contained a different synthetic estrogen called mestranol, which is still used in a few brands—for example, Ortho-Novum 1/50. Oral contraceptives differ also in their progestin content. Among the synthetic forms of progesterone developed early in the history of oral contraception are norethindrone and norgestrel. The second and third generations of progestins include levonorgestrel, desogestrel, norgestimate and, in Europe, gestodene. They are all slightly different chemically, and the newer forms seem to have fewer side effects. Although many women notice no difference whatsoever between the varieties, some women respond differently to the various combinations. You may have to experiment to find the best pill for you.

About twenty years ago researchers began looking at the amount of progesterone in oral contraceptives and trying to achieve an ideal balance. If there is too little progesterone in the pill, women may have bleeding or spotting between periods. If there is too much, there may be undesirable side effects, including a lowering of HDL ("good" cholesterol) and an elevation of LDL ("bad" cholesterol).

Monophasic pills use the same amount of synthetic estrogen and progestin all month long. Biphasic pills have two different formulations, and triphasic pills utilize three different proportions of estrogen and progestin during the month. The changing levels of the two hormones more closely mimic their proportions during the menstrual cycle than do the monophasic pills. Some women believe that triphasic pills have fewer side effects, but otherwise one type does not seem to have advantages over another.

Progestin-only pills (minipills), which contain only progestin, are not quite as effective as combination pills, because they do not block ovulation as well. However, women who cannot tolerate estrogen can use them successfully. They inhibit the thickening of the uterine lining, maintain the cervical mucus in a sperm-unfriendly state, and possibly slow the progress of the egg through the fallopian tube.

TABLE 1. Some Monophasic, Biphasic, and Triphasic Oral Contraceptives

MONOPHASIC	BIPHASIC	TRIPHASIC
Brevicon	Estrostep	Ortho-Novum 7/7/7
Lo/Ovral	Ortho-Novum 10/11	Tri-Levlen
Loestrin	Mircette	Tri-Norinyl
Modicon	Necon 10/11	Triphasil
Nordette		
Norinyl 1 + 35		
Ortho-Novum 1/35		
Ovcon/35		
Yasmin		

▶ *What is the reliability of combination birth control pills?*

The theoretical success rate of combination birth control pills when taken consistently and conscientiously is 99 percent. The success rate with typical use is also quite high, about 97 percent. The progestin-only minipill has a theoretical effectiveness rate of 98 percent and an actual rate of 96 percent. Some people believe that low-dose pills are more likely to fail than the old-fashioned pills with more estrogen, but one of my patients who was taking a 50-μg pill (a high-dose pill for this day and age) did become pregnant, so estrogen dose level is no guarantee of success.

▶ *Do you need to have any tests in order to get birth control pills?*

Your health care professional will want to do a physical exam, including a pelvic exam, a Pap test, and a breast exam. Your caregiver will check your blood pressure and ask whether you have had clotting problems, heart disease, stroke, breast cancer, or diabetes. You will be reminded that oral contraceptives do not protect you from sexually transmitted diseases. You may be asked to have a follow-up appointment several months after you start taking oral contraceptives, to monitor your blood pressure and check for side effects.

▶ *Do other medications interfere with the effectiveness of birth control pills?*

While it is always worth telling the doctor who is treating you for some other problem that you are taking oral contraceptives, most other medications do not interfere with the action of birth control pills. Even a week's worth of an ordinary antibiotic will probably not decrease their effectiveness, though it is worth checking with your doctor about backup contraception (some manufacturers warn about reduced effectiveness with ampicillin and tetracycline). Rifampin, an antibiotic prescribed to treat tuberculosis, interferes with oral contraceptives, so tell your gynecologist of the possible conflict. If you are taking something like Dilantin or phenobarbital for seizures, you might need a higher-dose pill.

Although there is not much scientific evidence one way or the other, it is reasonable to assume that since most medications manufactured by pharmaceutical companies do not interfere with the action of oral contraceptives, most herbal medications will not do so either. Recently, however, some researchers have questioned whether Saint John's-wort reduces the effectiveness of oral contraceptives; check with your doctor.

▶ *Are there reasons not to take birth control pills?*

If you are over 35 and smoke, you seriously increase your risk for heart attack and stroke by taking oral contraceptives. Smokers of any age have higher rates of heart attack and stroke than nonsmokers; smokers who take birth control pills are at greater risk than smokers who use other contraceptives. Many physicians feel that heavy smokers should not use oral contraceptives at any age; others believe that moderate smokers younger than 35 can safely use them. Since oral contraceptives are so safe and effective for nonsmokers, being able to use them throughout your reproductive life is one of the many excellent reasons for not smoking.

If you have had clotting disorders (for example, thrombophlebitis), breast or uterine cancer, severe liver disease, heart disease, stroke, or high cholesterol, your doctor probably will not recommend oral contraceptives. If you have sickle-cell disease, you should consider alternative forms of birth control. If you have migraine headaches, high blood pressure, or depression, tell your caregiver when discussing contraception.

▶ *Can you take birth control pills if you are diabetic?*

Because the progestins in birth control pills can change the way the body processes glucose, oral contraceptives may cause problems for women with diabetes. Some forms of progestin (for example, norethindrone) seem to have less effect than others. Diabetic women may have to adjust their insulin while taking oral contraceptives, and they should be carefully monitored by their physicians. Diabetic women are at increased risk for cardiovascular disease, and progestin is associated with such complications as high blood pressure, lowered HDL and elevated LDL. Pregnancy can cause special problems for diabetic women, and birth control pills are one of the most reliable methods of avoiding accidental pregnancies.

▶ *Can you take birth control pills while you are nursing?*

The American Academy of Pediatrics does approve of their use, but consult your pediatrician. Possible side effects include decreased milk production. Many pediatricians prefer that mothers use a progestin-only pill until they finish nursing.

▶ *Can you take birth control pills to relieve hot flashes and other symptoms if you are approaching menopause?*

Birth control pills can effectively ease the symptoms surrounding the onset of menopause, including hot flashes, irregular periods, and heavy bleeding, while also providing contraception. HMOs will often pay for estrogen replacement therapy; but if the pills are being used for birth control, there is less hope for reimbursement. When one of my patients has had her tubes tied, I send a note documenting the surgery and point out that there is no possibility that she is using the pills for contraception.

▶ *What is the schedule for taking birth control pills?*

Since oral contraceptives only work if you take them, the best schedule for you is the one that helps you remember. For this reason and to keep the dosage consistent, try to take your pill at the same time every day. It does not really matter whether this time is morning or night, unless the estrogen in the pills makes you queasy, in which case it is probably better to take the pill with dinner or at night before you go to bed.

Combination pills come in packets of either twenty-one pills or twenty-eight pills. The twenty-eight-pill packs contain twenty-one pills with estrogen and progestin and seven placebos; you take one pill every day, all month long. The twenty-one-pill packets contain twenty-one hormone pills; you take them until they are gone, then wait seven days and start again, even if you are still bleeding. In either case you get twenty-one days of combined hormones and seven days without hormones.

Some brands are designed so that you take the first pill on the first day of your period. With other brands you begin the Sunday after your period starts. The exact date does not matter, as long as it is close to the time of your period.

The progestin-only pills are taken thirty days out of thirty, even during your period.

▶ *Are you protected from pregnancy during the week you are not taking birth control pills (if your brand comes in the twenty-one-day packs)?*

Yes, because the twenty-one pills you've already taken have blocked ovulation for that month. However, if you fail to start the pills again for an extra week after your "week off," your ovaries may have gotten back on schedule and be ready to send forth an egg.

▶ *Are generic birth control pills safe?*

I prescribe generic drugs whenever I can. By law, the compounds in generic drugs must be as pure as those in brand-name drugs, but the amount in each generic pill may vary a little more from one pill to another. For example, Premarin, a type of estrogen used in hormone replacement therapy for postmenopausal women, was originally marketed by the Wyeth-Ayerst Company, which prided itself that the amount of hormone varied no more than 3 percent from pill to pill. Today there is a generic contraceptive containing the same type of estrogen, but the quantity can vary plus or minus 10 percent from pill to pill, a 20 percent change overall. This amount of variation does not interfere with the pill's effectiveness.

▶ *Will birth control pills protect against pregnancy the first month you take them?*

Although pills are probably effective the first month if you start them on the first day of your period, it is easy to forget to take a pill or two before you establish the habit. Therefore, you would be wise to use a backup method of birth control the first month.

▶ *Can you take oral contraceptives if you are younger than 16 or older than 35?*

Adolescents should wait until they have stopped growing before starting oral contraceptives, perhaps six months after their initial period. It used to be a firm, fast rule that women over age 35 could not use birth control pills, whether they smoked or not. Now many gynecologists have relaxed that view and allow (or even encourage) older women to use oral contraceptives, as long as they do not smoke or have a history of heart disease or stroke, high blood pressure, or liver disease.

▶ *How long can you stay on the pill?*

You can stay on the pill as long as you feel comfortable with it. Speaking for myself, I have been taking birth control pills for more than twenty-five years, because I like knowing when my period will come and I like having no cramps. I see no reason not to continue on them until menopause.

▶ Do birth control pills pose long-term health risks?

Physicians and researchers have studied this problem extensively; so far there are no indications of widespread danger (unless you smoke), despite the fact that in the early 1970s some feminists accused researchers of using women's bodies as "living laboratories" to test the pill's safety.

Early in its history, when the pill contained much higher levels of hormones, oral contraceptives were linked to blood clots, which can cause strokes, heart attacks, or other circulatory problems. Now that the estrogen content has been reduced to 35 μg or less, oral contraceptives do not seem to increase the risk of these diseases, except for smokers.

▶ Do birth control pills offer any long-term health benefits?

Aside from preventing unwanted pregnancies and their related health problems, birth control pills partially protect women from pelvic inflammatory disease (PID), which can cause severe abdominal pain and later infertility; they reduce heavy menstrual bleeding and cramps; and they protect against ovarian and uterine cancer and endometriosis. Usually birth control pills help with PMS; they seldom make it worse.

Photographs taken through the electron microscope have shown that bacteria can attach themselves to sperm and ride up into the female reproductive tract on their "backs." The good news is that oral contraceptives can prevent the sperm and their hostile passengers from making this journey by keeping the cervical mucus hostile to sperm. This ability of bacteria to come along as unwelcome fellow travelers explains why women are most likely to get PID during their menstrual periods. Because the mucus barrier is broken and blood itself is not hostile to bacteria, the bacteria can multiply and move through the cervix into the uterus and beyond.

Although oral contraceptives prevent sperm and their associated bacteria from ascending to the upper part of the reproductive tract where they can infect the fallopian tubes, they do not protect against gonorrhea or chlamydia or other STDs. Chances are, though, that if you are infected, these bacteria will remain localized in your vagina or cervix. A localized infection is easier to treat than one where bacteria have started reproducing inside your pelvis. Nevertheless, you are still infected and can pass on the disease to another partner. Taking oral contraceptives is no substitute for using some kind of protection against disease as well.

▶ Do oral contraceptives increase the risk for breast or cervical cancer?

There is no solid evidence that oral contraceptives raise the risk of breast cancer, even among women who took high-dose pills in the 1960s. Some studies in the early days of oral contraceptives did link the pill to a higher incidence of cervical cancer, but other factors may be at work. First, barrier methods do lower the risk of cervical cancer, but women who take the pill are less likely to use barrier methods also. Second, women who use oral contraceptives may begin sexual activity at an earlier age or have more sexual partners than women who do not (both factors increase risk). Later studies designed to take into account these other factors did not show that oral contraceptives increase risk.

▶ Do oral contraceptives cause high blood pressure?

About 5 percent of women who did not previously have high blood pressure (hypertension) develop it after several months of taking birth control pills. Some of the more recently developed pills seem to have less of an impact on blood pressure than the earlier ones did. The small possibility of developing hypertension is one of the reasons you should have regular checkups if you take birth control pills. If you are unfortunate enough to develop high blood pressure from taking the pill, you will probably have to choose a different method of contraception.

▶ What are the side effects of oral contraceptives?

Nausea or queasiness is probably the most common one. Bloating and weight gain is another. Taking oral contraceptives is not going to make you put on fifteen or twenty pounds (unless you change your eating or exercise habits), but some women gain two or three pounds of fluid weight when they start taking birth control pills, just as women sometimes do on estrogen replacement therapy. If you become bloated when you start taking oral contraceptives, try a different brand or a pill with a different combination of hormones. A new pill called Yasmin has a type of progestin that actually acts as a diuretic as well, decreasing fluid retention for women who have this problem. Other side effects include breast tenderness, skin problems, including rashes or eczema, and brown patches on the face.

BOX 2. Birth Control Pills: Risks and Benefits

1. Birth control pills and thrombophlebitis.
   If you are a nonsmoker or do not have a history of clotting disorders, your risks are slight.
2. Birth control pills and gallbladder disease.
   Birth control pills may increase your risk minimally.
3. Birth control pills and breast cancer.
   A few studies have shown that women who started taking the pill when they were younger than 15 and continued to use it for more than thirty years might have a slightly increased risk. Other studies did not bear this out.
4. Birth control pills and ovarian cancer.
   Women who take the pill have a 50 percent lower rate of ovarian cancer than women who do not.
5. Birth control pills and uterine cancer.
   Women who take birth control pills have a 30 percent lower rate of uterine cancer than women who do not.
6. Birth control pills and benign breast cysts (fibrocystic breast disease).
   Birth control pills have a protective effect.
7. Birth control pills and painful or heavy menstrual periods.
   Oral contraceptives reduce heavy bleeding and cramps.

▶ *Do birth control pills reduce sex drive?*

Some women think that birth control pills do lower their libido; some notice no difference; still others find that freedom from the fear of pregnancy increases their sexual desire. If depressed libido is a problem, try a pill that contains either norgestrel or levonorgestrel for its progestin. These pills may boost your sex drive because the progestin they contain is a little more androgenic—that is, a little more like male sex hormones—than other progestins. But while some women report increased sex drive with these pills, others do not notice any difference.

TABLE 2. Birth Control Pills and Sex Drive

MORE ANDROGENIC (may increase sex drive)	LESS ANDROGENIC (may decrease sex drive)
Levlen (levonorgestrel)	Desogen (desogestrel)
Lo Ovral (norgestrel)	Ortho-Cept (desogestrel)
Nordette (levonorgestrel)	Ortho-Cyclen (norgestimate)
Ovral (norgestrel)	OrthoTri-Cyclen (norgestimate)
	Yasmin (drosipirenone)

▶ Do birth control pills cause migraines?

If you have had migraines around the time of your periods, you may get more frequent or more severe headaches when you take birth control pills. You may also get migraines even though you have never had them before. Or you may find that your headaches are less intense when you are on the pill. If you do get headaches, experiment with different brands of pills and different combinations of hormones. Some women with migraines cannot tolerate any type of oral contraceptive. Occasionally, women who have headaches during their week off the pill benefit by taking a small amount of estrogen during that week. A new pill called Mircette has a small amount of estrogen in the placebo taken the last week of the month.

▶ Do birth control pills cause acne?

Some women find that oral contraceptives, especially those with high levels of progestins, do cause pimples, while other women find that their skin clears up when they start taking birth control pills. Certain progestins, especially ethynodiol diacetate, desogestrel, and norgestimate, are thought to be friendly to your skin. They include pills sold under the brand names Demulen, Zovia, Ortho-Cyclen, Ortho-Cept, and Desogen.

▶ How do birth control pills affect menstrual periods?

In general, women who use combination-type birth control pills have lighter, less painful periods than women who do not. Combination pills make your periods entirely predictable.

Women who use progestin-only pills may have irregular periods and start bleeding anytime during the month. Some bleed quite heavily, others continue to have normal cycles, and some do not bleed at all.

▶ *What should you do if you forget to take a pill?*

If you miss one pill, take two the next day; you should still be protected. If you forget more than one pill, use a backup method of contraception.

▶ *If you bleed between periods while you're taking oral contraceptives, does it mean that the pills aren't working?*

Spotting or bleeding when you do not have your period (breakthrough bleeding) is fairly common for women taking the pill. Even if it happens, the pills are still working. If you take your low-dose pills at significantly different times of day (one in the morning and the next one late at night the following day), you may have breakthrough bleeding. If the bleeding continues even when you take your pill at the same time every day, call your physician. Another brand or another formulation of the pill may solve the problem, but some women find breakthrough bleeding so annoying that they change contraceptive methods.

▶ *How much do birth control pills cost?*

Most birth control pills cost between twenty and twenty-five dollars monthly, plus the cost of an annual checkup visit to your caregiver. Some HMOs will pay for oral contraceptives, just as they pay for other prescriptions, but many do not. If your health plan does not pay, check prices of the pharmacies in your town, because there is some variation from one drugstore to the next. Or try calling femScript (1-800-511-1314), an organization that provides discount birth control pills. After a $9.95 sign-up fee, all products offered by femScript are significantly discounted. Women's advocacy groups are currently pushing for legislation that will cover contraceptives, though their efforts have not yet succeeded in all states.

▶ *Do birth control pills make it more difficult to become pregnant when you stop taking them?*

Although some scientific studies have suggested there might be a delay of several months before ovulation begins, particularly for older women, other studies show no such evidence. By protecting you against pelvic inflammatory disease and possibly endometriosis, the pill may even enhance your fertility.

I always tell my patients to use another method of birth control after they stop the pill unless they want to become pregnant immediately. When I tried to get pregnant with my first child, I had been using birth control pills for about fifteen years. I stopped the pill for three months, then got pregnant my second month of trying.

▶ *Do your menstrual periods return immediately after you stop taking birth control pills?*

Some women have a delay of two or three months before ovulation and menstrual periods begin again. Others begin ovulating right away. Some women, whether they have been taking oral contraceptives or not, spontaneously stop having periods, so it is difficult to tell whether the cause is the pill or something else.

Many physicians recommend a three-month wait after stopping the pill before trying to become pregnant. Some studies have suggested that there may be a higher rate of twins conceived in the first one or two cycles after going off the pill.

▶ *Do birth control pills preserve fertility by preventing ovulation and thus "saving" eggs for later use?*

The ovaries are formed during fetal life, as are the eggs inside them. The future baby girl carries within her immature ovaries about a million eggs. This number drops to about four hundred thousand at birth, and only a fraction of these are destined to reach maturity—maybe about four hundred. So in the reduction from four hundred thousand to four hundred, the ovulations that are suppressed by birth control pills make little difference.

Depo-Provera

Depo-Provera is a reversible, long-lasting contraceptive injected into the muscles of the upper arm or buttocks and slowly released into the body over a period of three months. It contains medroxyprogesterone acetate, a synthetic form of progesterone similar to the progesterone your body produces during the second half of your menstrual cycle. Depo-Provera prevents the eggs in your ovaries from maturing and thus inhibits ovulation. It keeps the lining of the uterus thin (unreceptive to a fertilized egg) and the cervical mucus thick (so sperm cannot penetrate it).

▶ *How effective is Depo-Provera?*

Depo-Provera is more than 99 percent effective, both in theory and in practice when used as directed. It is easy to be consistent and conscientious, since you only have to remember to get a shot four times yearly.

▶ *Are there reasons for not taking Depo-Provera?*

You should not take Depo-Provera if there is even a remote chance you might be pregnant. Tell your doctor if you have had unexplained vaginal bleeding, breast cancer, an abnormal mammogram, stroke, blood clots, or liver disease. Also mention any family or personal history of kidney disease, high blood pressure, migraine headaches, asthma, diabetes, epilepsy, or depression.

Nursing mothers can use Depo-Provera. It does appear in the breast milk, but does not affect its quantity or quality. Long-term studies that followed children through adolescence have shown no adverse effects on babies nursed by mothers who took Depo-Provera. In fact, sometimes the first shot is given in the hospital before the mother goes home.

▶ *At what time of the month should you get your first shot?*

You should get your first shot within five days after a regular menstrual period begins, to be sure you are not already pregnant. Before you get your first shot, your doctor will give you a physical exam; at this time bring up any conditions that might make Depo-Provera a poor choice for you. Most women say that the shot is not painful, though the site of the injection may be sore for a day or so.

If you get your first injection during the first five days after you have begun a normal menstrual period, you are protected from pregnancy immediately: you have not yet ovulated that month, and the hormone will have time to block ovulation before it happens.

▶ *What if you forget your three-month injection or can't come at the scheduled time?*

It is safe to have your injection a week or so early if your three-month date is not convenient, but if you wait longer than three months, you must use another reliable kind of birth control (condoms or spermicides) until you get your injection. Try scheduling your next injection when you get your present one and mark the date on your calendar.

▶ *Does Depo-Provera protect against STDs?*

Because it contains progesterone, Depo-Provera does help protect you from pelvic inflammatory disease, that is, from the spread of disease upward into your uterus and fallopian tubes. But it does not protect you from infection in the first place. You can get HIV, chlamydia, gonorrhea, or any other sexually transmitted disease while you are on Depo-Provera.

▶ *Does Depo-Provera increase the risk of breast cancer? Of osteoporosis?*

Depo-Provera has been available throughout the world for more than thirty years and has been used by more than 9 million women. It was introduced into the United States twenty-five years ago but withdrawn from the market when studies showed that beagle dogs given massive doses of Depo-Provera had an increase in breast cancer. However, beagles were chosen as test animals because of their susceptibility to cancer, and long-term studies on women taking normal doses of Depo-Provera have not shown significantly increased risk. A study undertaken by the World Health Organization in Switzerland reviewed previous research and concluded that Depo-Provera does not increase the risk of breast cancer.

Since Depo-Provera suppresses the natural production of estrogen (which protects against osteoporosis), theoretically it could increase the risk of osteoporosis, a disease in which bones lose their calcium and become weak and porous. One study showed that women who used Depo-Provera longer than five years did show decreased bone density. Other research has shown that bone loss on Depo-Provera is only a problem for smokers, who have increased risk anyhow. Women who have several risk factors for osteoporosis (slender build, fair skin, low calcium intake, lack of weight-bearing exercise) might discuss the matter with their caregivers before deciding on Depo-Provera.

▶ *How does Depo-Provera affect menstrual periods?*

Most women who use Depo-Provera notice some change in their normal menstrual pattern, because Depo-Provera prevents ovulation and the usual cyclical buildup and shedding of the uterine lining. This disruption can be in the form of breakthrough bleeding, usually just spotting or staining. Or the disruption can mean no periods at all, or periods that are regular but lighter than usual. The longer you use Depo-Provera, the less likely you are to have irregular bleeding or any menstrual periods at all. After one year of using

Depo-Provera, 57 percent of women stop having menstrual periods; after two years, the figure is 68 percent.

Unfortunately, some women have long-term irregular bleeding, which means that they can never be sure when they are going to start bleeding. Some women have light bleeding every day for three months; these women usually stop using Depo-Provera because of the nuisance and inconvenience. If you do have heavy or continuous bleeding or a persistent abnormal pattern of bleeding, let your caregiver know so that disease can be ruled out.

▶ *What are the side effects of Depo-Provera?*

Depo-Provera can cause irritability. If it does, you may remain irritable for three months until the effects of the shot wear off—which can be unpleasant for you and those around you. Most women do not have these negative feelings, and in fact Depo-Provera is sometimes used as a treatment for PMS, which has increased irritability as one of its symptoms. Occasionally women become depressed while taking Depo-Provera.

One of Depo-Provera's drawbacks is that it makes some women feel bloated and causes them to gain weight. Studies by the manufacturer show that women who do gain weight on Depo-Provera put on slightly more than five pounds during the first year and keep on gaining. After six years the women who put on weight gained an average of sixteen and a half pounds. This only happens to a few women, but it is distressing for those who do not want to gain weight.

In my medical practice, I have found weight gain on birth control pills to be different from that on Depo-Provera. Women who complain that oral contraceptives have made them put on an extra ten pounds sometimes have gained the weight simply because they have eaten too much. When they change contraceptives, the weight fails to disappear.

▶ *What does Depo-Provera cost?*

The four yearly shots cost in the range of sixty to seventy-five dollars apiece, in addition to the cost of the office appointments, so the annual total is about the same as for birth control pills. Currently many HMOs do not cover contraceptive protection, so you may have to pay these expenses out of pocket.

▶ *Does using Depo-Provera make it difficult to get pregnant later?*

Depo-Provera does not interfere with fertility once the effects of the most recent shot have worn off. Sixty-eight percent of women who become pregnant after quitting Depo-Provera do so within the first year; 93 percent, within a year and a half. The length of time you have been using Depo-Provera bears no relation to how long it takes to get pregnant when you discontinue usage.

▶ *What are its advantages and disadvantages?*

Depo-Provera is convenient and effective. You do not have to think about it. If you have had heavy, painful periods, it may offer relief. It may help with PMS. It gives some protection against pelvic inflammatory disease, and it may decrease the risk of endometrial cancer.

On the negative side, it is long-lasting, so if you decide you would like to become pregnant, you might have to wait for your last shot to wear off. It does not protect against STDs. It can have unpleasant side effects, including weight gain.

Lunelle

Lunelle, long widely used in Latin America, was cleared for use in the United States in 2000. Like oral contraceptives, it combines estrogen and progesterone but is given as a monthly injection. You still have menstrual periods but you do not conceive. The product is almost 100 percent effective and has minimal side effects. Unlike Depo-Provera, which may take months to wear off, Lunelle is easily reversible. The major drawback is that you need to get a shot every four weeks. In many states, pharmacists can give injections, so you need not necessarily go to your doctor's office for the shot. While Lunelle was being developed, researchers discovered that many women would rather have a monthly shot than take a daily pill.

Hormonal implants

A new form of hormonal contraception, Norplant, was introduced in 1990. Developed by the Population Council, a research foundation that works primarily in developing countries, Norplant offered a new option for convenient, long-acting, and reversible contraception. Norplant prevented conception by blocking ovulation and thickening the cervical mucus, thus discouraging sperm on its journey to fertilize the egg.

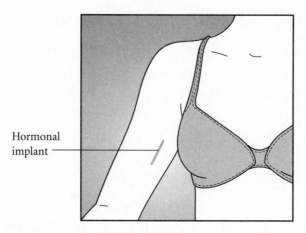

FIGURE 17. Hormonal implants release a small, continuous dose of the hormone progestin, which provides contraceptive protection for about three years.

Norplant came as a set of six flexible silicone capsules, like tiny matchsticks, which were inserted surgically under the skin of the upper arm. The capsules contained levonorgestrel, a synthetic form of progesterone, the hormone produced during the second half of the menstrual cycle. The progestin was released gradually, preventing pregnancy for as long as five years, though the length of effectiveness varied according to body weight and metabolism. The capsules could remain in place for five years and then be removed and either replaced or discontinued. Norplant delivered a very low dosage of progestin and contained no estrogen.

Hailed as a great innovation, Norplant became embroiled in controversy. In 2002, the manufacturer took it off the market because of unpleasant side effects—mainly unpredictable bleeding—and occasional difficulties with removal. A new implant, Implanon, is being developed and will probably be available soon in the United States. It consists of a single soft plastic rod about the size of a matchstick and will be effective for three years instead of five.

▶ How are hormonal implants put in?

Any physician, nurse-practitioner, or other health care professional who has been trained can do the insertion and removal. Be sure your caregiver has received the proper training before you have the procedure. Because you want to be certain you are not pregnant, you should have the insertion within the first week of the start of a normal menstrual period.

The procedure can be done in an office setting and takes only a few minutes. Your caregiver will anesthetize your upper arm with a local anesthetic, make a small incision through the skin, and place the implant beneath the skin using a disposable inserter. The incision will be closed with tape (stitches usually aren't necessary) and covered with a bandage.

The implant site may be sore for a day or so and may swell or look bruised. If the swelling or bruising persists, inform your caregiver. Once the initial soreness has disappeared, you may be unaware of the implant or you may feel a bump or ridge above it. The implant will stay put under your skin and will not move around. It is flexible and won't break if bumped or if pressure is put on it during normal activities.

▶ How are hormonal implants removed?

While removing Norplant usually took less than half an hour and rarely left a scar, sometimes the capsules became embedded in scar tissue under the skin. I had to take one woman to the operating room and remove the implants under general anesthesia because she was just too uncomfortable otherwise. This was a rare complication, but it was a concern with Norplant. Preliminary studies suggest that the design of Implanon will make insertion and removal quicker and easier.

▶ Can the implants be removed before or after the designated time period?

You can have the capsules removed any time you wish if you are unhappy with them or their side effects. While they should be removed at the time the manufacturer advises, nothing dangerous will happen if you delay for a few months. However, hormonal implants gradually lose effectiveness, so your risk of pregnancy increases. A study of Chinese women with an average weight of about 120 pounds showed a cumulative pregnancy rate of 2.3 per 100 women at the end of seven (instead of the recommended five) years of Norplant use.

▶ Is the implanted plastic rod dangerous?

The furor over the safety of silicone breast implants has made many women worry about implants of any kind. The Implanon rod is made of ethylene vinyl acetate, not silicone. But if the notion of having a foreign substance implanted in your body makes you anxious, you should probably try a different form of contraception.

▶ *Will you get menstrual periods with hormonal implants?*

Many women didn't get periods with Norplant and were very happy with the situation. However, as with other progestin-only contraceptives including the minipill and Depo-Provera, women varied in their responses. Some women had so much bleeding that after six months they had the capsules removed.

▶ *What are the side effects?*

The new hormonal implants can be expected to have the same side effects as Norplant, Depo-Provera, and other progestin-only contraceptives. These include changes in menstrual bleeding patterns, lack of periods, or spotting and staining between periods. Twenty-seven percent of women using Norplant reported frequent bleeding or prolonged periods, with an average of one hundred days of bleeding during the first year. A smaller number of women had headaches, skin problems, nausea and appetite changes, weight gain, and nervousness or irritability.

▶ *Do hormonal implants impair fertility once they are removed?*

One advantage of hormonal implants is their quick reversibility. With Norplant, the contraceptive action stopped within two or three days after the implants were removed. More than 75 percent of women who wanted to become pregnant did so within the first year after removal. This rate is higher than the fertility rate in the general population.

▶ *Are there reasons for not using hormonal implants?*

If you have active liver disease and possibly phlebitis (blood clots in the veins), you should not use this form of contraception. Other conditions you should mention to your caregiver are unexplained vaginal bleeding and a history of breast cancer. You should not have the capsules inserted if there is a possibility you are pregnant.

▶ *How much do hormonal implants cost?*

The new implants will soon be on the market in the United States. Norplant had a high upfront cost in this country—between five hundred and six hundred dollars for the implantation procedure—though it was considerably less expensive elsewhere. Many insurers do not cover contraception, so women may have to pay out of pocket. If the cost of implants is spread over their effective life, it is less than the cost of birth control pills.

▶ *How reliable are hormonal implants?*

Hormonal implants are among the most reliable contraceptives available, more than 99 percent effective in terms of both best-expected effectiveness and typical use. Once the implant has been inserted, you do not have to think about it; there is no chance for human error. It becomes effective within twenty-four hours, so you may have intercourse without backup contraception a day later.

Statisticians collecting data on contraceptive effectiveness usually look only at the first year of use. For Norplant, statistically speaking, the failure rate in the first year was only one in five hundred. The failure rate went up slightly during the five years Norplant remained in place, rising to two in five hundred by the fifth year of use, with overweight women having greater risk of pregnancy than thin women.

▶ *Are hormonal implants right for you?*

Because implants are so long-lasting, they are ideal for women who do not want more children, or do not want them for several years. Women who are looking for reversible contraception but do not want or cannot use an IUD might choose implants. There are other, sadder reasons for using this contraceptive as well.

> Nicole, one of my middle-aged patients, has a teenage daughter, Angela, who runs away regularly and is sexually promiscuous. Angela sees a therapist and receives psychological counseling and other supportive treatment, but continues her risky behavior. Nicole worries that Angela may become pregnant or infected with an STD. When she finally realizes that she cannot change Angela's behavior, she urges Angela to have a Norplant and Angela agrees. While the Norplant does not guard against STDs, Angela is at least protected against pregnancy.

NONBARRIER METHODS

Intrauterine Devices

An IUD (intrauterine device) is a small object placed in the uterus to prevent pregnancy. It must be inserted by a health care professional, but once in place it can remain there for months or years. Despite a history filled with accusations and legal actions, IUDs (with certain restrictions) are still a safe and viable means of contraception for many women.

The *Dalkon Shield* (on the market 1970–1974) looked rather like a beetle, with an "eye" at one end, five little "legs" on each side, and a "tail" made of many filaments twisted together. It came in two sizes, a larger one for women who had given birth and a smaller one for women who had not. The Dalkon Shield quickly headed to the top of the sales charts. In its first year, it accounted for about two thirds of all IUD sales, and by 1974 sales had reached 2.8 million.

In the preceding four years, twelve women who became pregnant while wearing an IUD had died of infections after miscarrying. Ten of these women were using the large Dalkon Shields; the other two had another type of IUD. In early 1974 the FDA advised physicians to remove any IUD immediately if its wearer became pregnant. A few months later the manufacturer suspended sales of the Dalkon Shield altogether.

Because of its shape, the Dalkon Shield was slightly more difficult to insert than some other designs and therefore had a higher failure rate; that is, more women became pregnant while wearing one because the device had been inserted incorrectly. Some of these women carried their pregnancies into the second trimester with the IUD still in place and developed infections, which spread beyond the uterus into the pelvis and resulted in miscarriage. In these cases the Dalkon Shield was at fault. We now know that there is an association between IUD use during pregnancy and pelvic inflammatory disease (PID). Indeed, after physicians began following FDA advice and removing IUDs immediately if women accidentally became pregnant, deaths from septic miscarriages stopped being problematic. However, the reputation of IUDs was sorely damaged, since people confused IUD use in general with the problems associated with pregnancy.

Furthermore, some studies at the time showed that women who used IUDs had a higher risk of PID than women who chose another method of birth control. In thinking about the validity of these studies, remember that this era, the late 1960s and early 1970s, was also the time of the so-called sexual revolution, when gonorrhea was increasing dramatically and chlamydia was introduced into the United States.

Many women, attracted by the long-term contraception made possible by the IUD, abandoned their diaphragms (which protect the cervix) and their spermicides (which kill germs as well as sperm). Women also abandoned birth control pills, which do not prevent infectious organisms from being deposited in the vagina, but do offer some protection against the upward spread of sexually transmitted diseases to the uterus and fallopian tubes. Men abandoned condoms (which prevent infection from reaching the female reproductive tract). Therefore, many women who used IUDs and had intercourse with an infected partner did get sexually transmitted diseases that did migrate upward and did indeed destroy their fertility. But it was not the IUD itself that caused the infection.

The problem with these studies on PID was that the researchers designing them compared women who used IUDs to women who used diaphragms or spermicides or birth control pills or condoms, all of which offer certain kinds of protection. The control group (to whom the women with IUDs were being compared) should have been women using no contraception at all.

In the United States today, three IUDs are available: the Progestasert and the Mirena, which contain progestin (synthetic progesterone), and the ParaGard, also known as the copper-T. Other types of IUDs are available in Canada and Europe, and women sometimes go abroad to have these inserted.

The *ParaGard* is a T-shaped plastic device about 1.5 inches long and 1 inch wide. The long vertical arm is wrapped with copper wire and the two horizontal arms have copper collars. At the tail end of the T is a bulb through which a piece of polyethylene thread is inserted so that its two ends hang down to help remove the IUD. The ParaGard can remain in place as long as ten years and is impregnated with barium sulfate so that it will show up on x-rays.

The *Progestasert* and the *Mirena* are also plastic T-shaped devices of the same size as the ParaGard, with two-threaded tails for removal. Each has a reservoir in the vertical stem of the T, which contains a small amount of progesterone; each uses barium sulfate to make it show up on x-rays. Mirena can remain in place for five years, and Progestasert, an older version, for one year, after which the progesterone is used up.

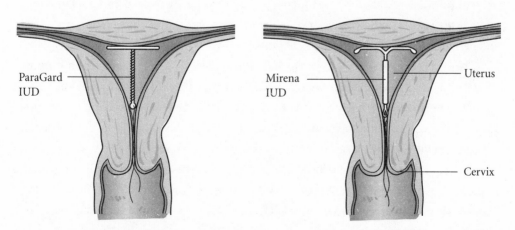

FIGURE 18. Intrauterine devices: A, the ParaGard is wrapped with copper wire; B, the Mirena has a reservoir containing progesterone. It is believed that these devices work by inactivating or killing sperm before they reach the egg.

▶ *How does an IUD prevent pregnancy?*

No one knows exactly how an IUD works. Researchers first suggested that an IUD acted like a foreign body in the uterus, making the uterine lining hostile to the fertilized egg, perhaps through an inflammatory response. Another theory proposed that the presence of the IUD hurried the egg through the fallopian tube, reducing chances for fertilization. If the IUD worked by preventing implantation of a fertilized egg, then researchers would expect to find fertilized eggs in the fallopian tubes of IUD users, but they have instead found inactivated sperm in the uterus.

Nowadays the consensus is that the sperm are inactivated before they even reach the egg. Researchers believe that the progesterone in the Progestasert and Mirena IUDs changes the cervical mucus so that sperm cannot swim upstream to meet the ovum; similarly, it is believed that the copper in the ParaGard makes sperm less vigorous and less able to swim. If IUDs do indeed work by killing or inactivating sperm before they reach the egg, then fertilization never happens. Women who hesitate to use an IUD because they do not want to abort a fertilized egg might reconsider their decision.

▶ *What is involved in using an IUD?*

Before your IUD is inserted, you should have a physical examination that includes a pelvic exam to see whether you have any anatomical problems (such as a severely tipped uterus) that would make an IUD a bad choice for you. Your doctor will make sure you are not pregnant and will take a history to find out whether you have a monogamous relationship and whether you have had STDs or pelvic inflammatory disease. You will have a Pap test and perhaps tests for gonorrhea and chlamydia.

Then your caregiver will insert the IUD through your cervix and position it in the uterus using a narrow tube that presses down the arms of the T into a straight line. Once the IUD is positioned within the uterus, the insertion tube is removed and the arms spring back. The two ends of the string, which is used to remove the IUD and to check its position, remain outside the uterus in the upper part of the vagina against the cervix.

I prefer to insert an IUD during a menstrual period—first, because you are unlikely to be pregnant, and second, because your cervix may be a little dilated, making insertion less painful. Some doctors prefer to insert the IUD at midcycle, believing that infection is more likely during the menstrual period.

IUDs are designed to be easily inserted, but the process can be painful, especially for women who have not had children. Take a little Motrin or Aleve or another anti-inflammatory before you go to your appointment. If one of my patients is extremely anxious or has a sensitive cervix, I may put a little Novocain into her cervix. IUDs are a lot easier to remove than to insert; only rarely does that procedure hurt.

Some women notice cramping or low backache for a day or so after insertion. Others have spotting or staining for a few days as well. Occasionally women faint during the insertion, which is frightening for both the woman and her physician. These women have what is known as a strong vasovagal reflex; they are reacting to the stretching of the cervix, which is touched by the vagus nerve.

Theoretically, IUDs are 98–99 percent effective and rank among the most reliable forms of contraception. In practice, the failure rate is about 3 percent overall, with most failures happening in the first year of use. Among women using this method for seven years, the failure rate is only 1 percent. If your IUD fails and you do become pregnant with your IUD in place, call your doctor and have the IUD removed immediately.

▶ Can an IUD fall out or move around in the uterus?

An IUD cannot fall out, but occasionally one moves around or is expelled by the muscular contractions of the uterus, usually during the first few months after insertion. Sometimes this happens during a menstrual period, and occasionally it happens without being noticed. So it is important to inspect the strings regularly, just after your menstrual period perhaps, to be sure that your IUD is still in place.

To check your IUD, reach into your vagina and feel up toward the cervix. The strings are quite thin, about the size of dental floss. They do not hang down like the string of a tampon, but are wedged up against the cervix. If you cannot feel the strings, call your doctor, who can determine the exact location of your IUD with ultrasound imaging or an x-ray. Chances are that the strings have just migrated inside the cervix, but sometimes the IUD has moved. Usually it turns up somewhere inside the uterus, but occasionally one works its way through the wall of the uterus and into the abdominal cavity. This perforation of the uterus is a rare but potentially serious complication, and it can happen without the user's being aware of it. Surgery may be necessary to remove the IUD. So check the strings frequently.

▶ Does an IUD increase the risk of a tubal pregnancy?

There is no evidence that women who have used an IUD in the past and then become pregnant later have a higher rate of tubal pregnancy than women who used other contraceptives. In fact, some data suggest that women who have used the copper-T before becoming pregnant actually have a lower rate of tubal pregnancy than the general population. However, if you become pregnant with the IUD in place, then you do have a higher-than-average chance of an ectopic (out of the uterus) pregnancy. If you are using an IUD and miss a period, or have a late period with light, scanty bleeding, call your doctor immediately; there is a possibility that you might be pregnant.

▶ *Do IUDs interfere with later fertility?*

There is no evidence that an IUD impairs fertility unless you have had complications, for example, infection or uterine perforation. Often, though, IUDs are prescribed for women who do not want more children.

▶ *How much does an IUD cost?*

IUDs are expensive in the United States. The device itself can cost more than two hundred dollars, plus the expense of an office visit to have it inserted and a follow-up visit six weeks later to check that the strings are in place. Some doctors require two visits at the time of insertion: one to do cultures checking for chlamydia and gonorrhea, and a second visit a week later, when the cultures have been completed, to do a pelvic exam and install the device. The total up-front cost for an IUD can run about three hundred dollars, but there are no ongoing costs. Clinics such as Planned Parenthood usually offer IUDs on a sliding price scale. If the IUD remains in place for a year, the cost is similar to that of birth control pills. If it remains in place longer, it becomes less expensive per year than birth control pills. Abroad, an IUD costs only about forty dollars.

The manufacturers of the leading IUDs in this country claim that the high cost results from passing on to the consumer the expense of carrying malpractice insurance against possible lawsuits. Given the many past lawsuits, the assumption of future lawsuits is realistic. The company that makes ParaGard asks women to sign a consent form stating that they are familiar with the product's possible side effects and risks.

▶ *What are advantages and disadvantages of an IUD?*

Although the Progestasert and Mirena actually seem to decrease flow during menstrual periods, other IUDs including the ParaGard can cause long and heavy menstrual periods. These symptoms are usually most noticeable during the first year of IUD use and often decrease with time. The initial cost of an IUD is high and the insertion process can be uncomfortable. Some researchers believe that women who use an IUD, especially those who have more than one sexual partner, have a higher rate of pelvic inflammatory disease than those who choose other contraception. The rate is highest just after insertion and up to four months afterward. If you use an IUD and have any of the symptoms of PID (abdominal pain, pain during intercourse, a foul-smelling vaginal discharge, nausea, or vomiting), call your doctor immediately. An IUD will not protect against STDs.

The advantages are that, once in place, an IUD continues its work without your thinking about contraception at all. IUDs are reliable and effective. They are long-lasting: eight to ten years with the ParaGard, one year with Progestasert, five with Mirena.

▶ Is an IUD the right contraceptive for you?

Maureen is 37 years old. She has two children and doesn't want any more, but emotionally she is unwilling to consider sterilization. She is also unable to stop smoking. She and her husband have an active sex life and neither wants to bother with barrier methods.

An IUD would be perfect for Maureen. She and her husband are monogamous, so she doesn't need protection from STDs. Because she smokes and is older than 35, she cannot use oral contraceptives.

Although sometimes IUDs are prescribed for a woman who may want children later, they are most often given to women who have completed their families. Mutual monogamy is a must for IUD users, since the IUD gives absolutely no protection against HIV or any STD. Women with multiple sexual partners and women whose partners have multiple partners should use barrier methods of contraception.

You should not use an IUD if you have had pelvic inflammatory disease or an ectopic pregnancy. If you have vaginal bleeding of unknown cause or a vaginal infection, you should wait until these conditions have been investigated and cured before getting an IUD. Choose another form of contraception if you have a condition like leukemia or HIV that makes you susceptible to infection, or rheumatic heart disease that makes your heart vulnerable to infection. You should not use an IUD containing copper if you are allergic to copper.

If you have a strong vasovagal reflex, you probably should not choose an IUD, because of problems with insertion and removal. Once the IUD is in place, however, you probably will not have difficulties. If you have never had a child, your doctor may find it difficult or be unable to insert an IUD.

MORNING-AFTER CONTRACEPTION

If for some reason your contraceptive fails, or you do not use one, you still have the option of morning-after contraception. This is not the same as a nonsurgical abortion, which uses the antiprogesterone RU-486 (mifepristone) seven to nine weeks into the pregnancy.

The concept of morning-after contraception, also called emergency contraception, has been around for some thirty years, though it has been rather a well-kept secret. In the 1960s emergency contraception was used to help victims of sexual assault reduce their risk of pregnancy, and even in the 1990s one third of the prescriptions written for emergency contraception were for rape victims.

Morning-after contraception was "discovered" by two physicians at Yale University: Gertrude van Wagenen, who was a primate researcher, and Dr. John Morris, a gynecologist best known for his work on cancer. Van Wagenen and Morris reasoned that if you administer a heavy dose of estrogen at the time the embryo is about to implant, you can effectively prevent implantation. At first researchers employed the drug diethylstilbestrol (DES). This synthetic estrogen had been used as early as the 1940s to prevent complications of pregnancy, but since the 1960s had been associated with birth defects and, later, disorders of the reproductive organs in the daughters of women who had taken the drug during pregnancy.

As morning-after contraception, DES was prescribed in very high doses for five days after the unprotected intercourse. While DES did prevent pregnancy, it also caused severe nausea and vomiting, which limited its usefulness. Then, twenty-five years ago, researchers discovered that large doses of birth control pills could also prevent pregnancy. In 1974 Dr. Albert Yuzpe, a Canadian researcher, published studies showing emergency contraception using oral contraceptives to be safe and effective, and suggesting the regimen most frequently used today.

Until very recently, emergency contraception was an "off-label" use of oral contraceptives, not one of the uses authorized by the FDA when the drug was approved for marketing. Public health and women's advocacy groups worked with the FDA and with pharmaceutical companies to develop and market an emergency-contraception kit. In 1998 the FDA approved the first one, known as Preven; in 1999 Plan B, an emergency contraceptive containing levonorgestrel, was approved. Generic versions are now available.

▶ *Can you use birth control pills for emergency contraception?*

If you cannot get emergency contraception especially formulated with the correct dosage, you can still use birth control pills.

> About twenty-five years ago Ava, a graduate student in her 20s, came to the rape crisis center after a sexual assault. Along with her other fears and anxieties, she was worried that she might be pregnant. We explained that we could give her DES and prevent a possible pregnancy, but that she would probably be nauseated and vomit off and on for the next five days. At the time we did not know that birth control pills could achieve the same result with less nausea. Because she was studying for her comprehensive exams, a requirement for a degree she had been working on for several years, Ava elected not to take the DES but to wait and then terminate the pregnancy, if necessary. Fortunately it turned out that she was not pregnant. She did pass her exams, despite having many nonacademic worries at the time.

The availability of safe emergency contraception, free of severe side effects, came too late to help Ava, but will benefit other women who share her plight.

Morning-after contraception is not strictly limited to the morning after; it works any time within seventy-two hours of the unprotected intercourse. The required dosage is about 200 μg of estrogen, taken in two equal doses. So you need to take two tablets of a 50-μg pill such as Ovral, or four tablets of a 30-μg pill such as Lo/Ovral, within the first seventy-two hours after unprotected intercourse. Then twelve hours later you take another two 50-μg pills (or another four 30-μg pills).

▶ *How do you know that morning-after contraception has worked?*

About two weeks after the emergency contraception, you should have a menstrual period, as you normally would. The additional hormones you took to avoid pregnancy may make your period heavier or cause more cramping than usual.

▶ *How effective is morning-after contraception?*

While its effectiveness is difficult to assess, since no one knows for sure whether conception has actually taken place, current estimates rate its success at about 98 percent. Statistically, if one hundred women have unprotected sex during the second or third week of their menstrual cycles, an average of eight will become pregnant; but if they correctly use emergency contraception, only two of those hundred will get pregnant. I have never personally seen morning-after contraception fail if used correctly.

▶ *What are the side effects of emergency contraception?*

An estimated 30–50 percent of women feel nauseated after taking such a big dose of estrogen, just as women often felt queasy with high-dose birth control pills in the 1960s, which contained almost as much estrogen as the dose for emergency contraception. Some 15–25 percent vomit, but over-the-counter (Bendaryl or Dramamine) or prescribed antinausea medications, preferably taken one hour before the emergency contraception, can reduce this discomfort. If you are nauseated and have no medication, call your caregiver; even taken after the nausea begins, antinausea medications can help.

Other potential side effects can include headaches, breast tenderness, and irregular bleeding. Because morning-after contraception lasts for only one day, the side effects taper off a day or so after you take the second dose.

▶ *Can you get birth control pills to use for emergency contraception if they are not your regular method of contraception?*

If you usually use a barrier method, you might ask your doctor for a packet of birth control pills when you are discussing contraception in general. Some doctors routinely prescribe a packet to women who use barrier methods, to keep in the drawer in case of an emergency. You can also go to Planned Parenthood or a women's clinic and get a prescription for the Preven kit.

To locate the nearest Planned Parenthood chapter for emergency contraception, call 1-800-230-PLAN. The Reproductive Health Technologies Project hotline, at 1-888-NOT-2-LATE, has a list of the other emergency contraception providers closest to where you live.

▶ *How does the Preven kit work?*

The kit, which includes a pregnancy test, works the same way as birth control pills for morning-after contraception. The instructions suggest taking the pregnancy test first and then the emergency contraceptive pills, but some Planned Parenthood chapters suggest taking the pills and waiting two weeks, then using the pregnancy test to confirm that the pills have worked.

▶ *How much does emergency contraception cost?*

At Planned Parenthood, it costs about fifteen dollars; at a pharmacy the kits are about twenty dollars. The prices are similar for Plan B. A pack of combination pills costs twenty dollars to thirty five dollars; two packs of progestin-only pills cost about fifty dollars; a visit to your doctor or health care provider can run from thirty-five dollars to one hundred fifty dollars.

▶ *What if you are already pregnant but don't know it, and use morning-after contraception to prevent a pregnancy?*

This problem arises sometimes after sexual assaults. Suppose someone has just conceived, and a week later is assaulted by a stranger. She receives morning-after conception because of the assault. Two weeks after the morning-after contraception, she does not have a menstrual period. It is impossible to know at this stage whether the fetus that has been conceived is the child of the rapist or the child of the husband. If it is the child of the husband, and morning-after contraception has been given, then the fetus has been subjected to a big dose of hormones. If it is the child of the rapist, then morning-after contraception simply has not worked. Was it method failure? Or was the woman already pregnant?

Many gynecologists in this situation will recommend terminating the pregnancy because of the exposure of the fetus to such a high dose of hormones. The risk is uncertain—we do not really know much about the effects of exposure.

▶ *Should you have morning-after contraception if you are unwilling to terminate a pregnancy?*

The possibility of morning-after contraception raises other issues. Suppose Jane Smith comes in to a rape crisis center because she was sexually assaulted, and she asks for morning-after contraception. Jane says that if the method does not work and she becomes pregnant, she will not terminate the pregnancy because of religious scruples. Should the physicians at the center give her the morning-after contraception, knowing that it may cause problems for the fetus?

I am asked this question occasionally when working at our local rape crisis center. I do not have the answer and, frankly, I do not believe that even professional bioethicists have it. The chance that the emergency contraception will cause a problem with the fetus is minimal, and the chance that the method will work is very high. Still the decision depends on the conscience and beliefs of the woman who has become pregnant under such unfortunate circumstances. I do think that every woman who asks her physician for morning-after contraception should first ask herself what she would do if the method failed, especially if she might be a week pregnant from a previous act of intercourse.

When discussing morning-after contraception with my patients, I do mention that 3 percent of children born in this country have abnormalities. Most are minor, but there is a small chance, independent of the hormones administered to prevent conception, that your child will be included in the 3 percent. If you will forever blame yourself for taking the hormones and say, "I am responsible for my child's malformation because I wanted morning-after contraception and would not terminate the pregnancy when the contraception failed," think long and hard before you ask for emergency contraception.

▶ *Are there other methods of morning-after contraception?*

Sometimes an IUD is inserted within three days of unprotected intercourse to prevent implantation of a fertilized egg.

> Betty, the mother of two children, calls the office on an emergency basis because she and her husband have had unprotected intercourse and she fears she may be pregnant. She has been planning to get an IUD, but keeps putting it off. Now she is sure she does not want to take any more chances with an accidental pregnancy. Betty comes in the next day and has her IUD inserted.

Women who know they are already pregnant should not use an IUD for any reason. Neither should women who have a sexually transmitted infection or a history of pelvic inflammatory disease. Since the IUD must be inserted by a physician, you can ask whether it is appropriate for you.

▶ *How effective is the IUD as a means of emergency contraception?*

As with any emergency contraceptive measure, time factors are crucial; both the amount of time that has elapsed since the unprotected intercourse and the time in a woman's cycle when the unprotected sex took place. The sooner after intercourse that she receives the emergency contraception, the more effective it will be. The closer a woman is to ovulation, the less likely it is that the method will succeed. However, one study found that since 1976 more than eighty-four hundred copper-bearing IUDs have been inserted for emergency contraception, and only eight pregnancies have occurred, a failure rate of fewer than one in a thousand, or less than 0.1 percent.

RU-486 (mifepristone), the "French abortion pill," may in the future be accepted for emergency contraception, although it is currently approved only as a drug for use in medical abortion. Studies have shown that it is very effective in preventing pregnancy when used as a morning-after pill, and that it has fewer side effects than the present methods.

Also available is a progestin-only emergency contraceptive, called Plan B, containing the hormone levonorgestrel. A British study found that levonorgestrel is more effective than the present birth control pill method (which uses both estrogen and progesterone) and has fewer side effects.

PERMANENT CONTRACEPTION

Both men and women can be sterilized surgically so that they cannot produce more children. The procedure in women, tubal ligation, involves tying, cutting, cauterizing, or otherwise interrupting the fallopian tubes so that sperm cannot reach the egg. In men the procedure, called vasectomy, blocks off the vas deferens, the tube through which sperm exit the body when they are ejaculated.

▶ *Which is better, a tubal ligation or a vasectomy?*

When a patient asks for a tubal ligation, we always discuss whether it is better for her to have a tubal or for her husband to have a vasectomy. Because of the possible consequences of tubal ligation, I urge husbands and wives to think about vasectomy as a safer alternative.

For several reasons vasectomy is the better choice. First, consider what happens if the procedure fails. Vasectomy and tubal ligation have roughly the same failure rate, about one in three hundred. If your partner's vasectomy fails, then you will probably get pregnant. But if your tubal ligation fails, you will probably get pregnant—and very likely have an ectopic pregnancy. About 40 percent of pregnancies that result from failed tubal ligations are ectopic. Such a pregnancy requires invasive surgery; if untreated, it can be fatal.

Second, vasectomy is a less invasive surgical procedure than tubal ligation. It can be performed in a doctor's office with local anesthesia. Men have "outdoor plumbing"; their anatomy is easier to work with because the vas deferens lies just under the skin away from any important organs or large blood vessels. Women have "indoor plumbing": the fallopian tubes are buried deep in the pelvis and lie close to the bowel, the bladder, and major blood vessels.

▶ Are there instances when tubal ligation is a better choice?

Couples may well consider the future: what will happen if one of them dies. Some women have said that, should they die, they would like their husbands to be able to remarry and have more children. If you feel this way and are willing to undergo the risks, tubal ligation is the correct choice.

For women who do not want children (or have completed their family) and have more than one sexual partner, tubal ligation is also a good choice.

> Jennifer, who has three children, comes in for her yearly checkup and requests a
> tubal ligation. I ask her whether she has discussed the matter with her husband.
> No, she says, because she has three sexual partners. Whether or not her husband
> has a vasectomy is not the issue, but I do point out that a tubal ligation will not
> protect her against sexually transmitted diseases.

Although vasectomy does not interfere with testosterone production or erections, some men refuse it because they believe the procedure will diminish their manhood. In this case tubal ligation may be the only choice.

TUBAL LIGATION

Tubal ligation ("getting your tubes tied") literally means tying the fallopian tubes so that sperm cannot meet the egg. In practice, the tubes are usually cauterized with electrical current and cut, but they may be cut and tied or clamped to achieve the same objective.

Sterilization of women has been performed for centuries, and at one time or another the ovaries, uterus, and fallopian tubes have all been surgically altered or removed to control fertility. Nowadays tubal ligation is the preferred technique. It has even been used in Catholic hospitals, where sterilization is not permitted, to "isolate" the uterus and help avoid the spread of pelvic inflammatory disease.

In the past, tubal ligation was almost always performed in a hospital under general anesthesia. Today, newer tools and techniques have made the procedure shorter, so that it is often done in a surgicenter or the outpatient surgical unit of a hospital.

▶ *Is tubal ligation right for you?*

If you do not wish to bear any children, or any more children, at any future time, and you do not want to put up with the inconveniences of other birth control methods, you might consider this procedure. However, when you chose tubal ligation, you should consider it irreversible. If you are not totally sure about never wanting another biological child, and in the back of your mind are thinking that you can always have the procedure reversed, you should *not* have a tubal ligation. Try long-term reversible contraception instead, perhaps Depo-Provera or Norplant. In my experience, women who choose tubal ligation because they do not want any children at all seldom seek to have the procedure reversed.

> Rebecca is the eldest of eight children. She took care of her brothers and sisters from the time she was old enough to help her mother until she left home. When she got married, she already had many nieces and nephews whom she dearly loved, and she was sure she did not want to care for children of her own. Nor did her husband particularly want children. Rebecca had a tubal ligation after several years of marriage and remained content with that decision throughout her life.

If you already have children, you should ask yourself two important questions before going ahead with a tubal ligation. First, if you should lose a child, would you want to have another baby? Second, if something were to happen to your present marriage and you married again, would you want to have a child with your new husband? If you can without hesitation answer no to these questions, then a tubal ligation may well be appropriate for you. Some women are sure they do not want more children because they cannot face the discomforts of pregnancy again.

> Emily has a daughter who is now 5 years old. Throughout her pregnancy she was miserable, so nauseated for so long that the thought of being pregnant again is simply more than she can bear. She has a tubal ligation and is happy with her choice.

You should also consider your surgical risks. You are at higher risk for complications during tubal ligation if you are obese or have scar tissue from previous abdominal surgery (for example, ovarian cysts) or a pelvic inflammation.

▶ *How is a tubal ligation performed?*

There are two surgical approaches: a minilaparotomy and a laparoscopic procedure. Until about twenty-five years ago, minilaparotomy under general or spinal anesthesia was the standard way of performing a tubal ligation. The surgeon makes an incision about 1.5–2 inches wide in the abdomen, works down through the layers of skin, fat, and muscle, enters the pelvic cavity, picks up each fallopian tube, cuts a piece out of each, and ties off the ends. This procedure is still done today, though there are modern variations.

A different time-honored way to approach tubal ligation was through the vagina, a method not often used nowadays. In this procedure the surgeon made the incision in the vagina, reached upward, and drew each tube back down through the vaginal incision. The tubes were then cut and tied off. This procedure had a slightly higher rate of infection than the abdominal method, but women who absolutely did not want an abdominal scar chose this method anyway.

About twenty-five years ago the "belly button" or "band-aid" operation came into favor in this country and has since become the most commonly performed technique of tubal ligation. The surgeon makes a very small incision, maybe half an inch long, just under the belly button, through the abdominal wall. Through the incision the surgeon fills the belly with carbon dioxide, which moves the intestines out of the way, making it easier

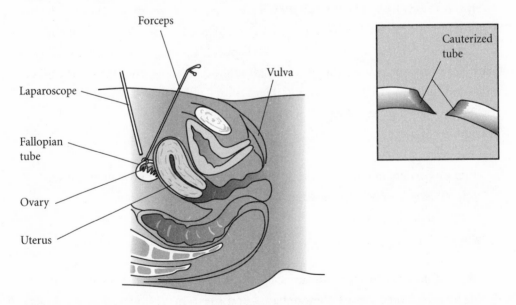

FIGURE 19. In tubal ligation, the sperm cannot meet the egg when the tubes are interrupted by cauterizing or some other method.

to find the fallopian tubes and less likely that the bowel or other organs will be injured during the procedure. Using a laparoscope, a long lighted fiber-optic tube, the surgeon looks inside the pelvis, moving the scope around until the fallopian tubes come into view. (In the old days we looked directly through the tube, but now we hook it up to a video camera, which projects the view onto a screen.)

The surgeon makes a second small incision in the pubic area, inserts special tweezer-like forceps, and grasps the fallopian tubes one at a time. With an electrocauterizing device, the surgeon passes an electric current through each tube in two or maybe three places, which makes them disintegrate. After both tubes have been cauterized, the surgeon removes the instruments and lets the gas out of the abdomen. The small incisions can be sewn up with a couple of dissolving stitches. Laparoscopic surgery is not riskier than regular abdominal surgery, but if injury should occur, the surgeon will have to make a regular abdominal incision to repair the damage.

▶ Can a tubal ligation be performed under local anesthesia?

Usually in this country tubal ligations are done under general anesthesia, because whatever the approach, the surgeon must find the tubes in the pelvis and destroy them. Local anesthesia will deaden feeling in the skin, but it will not help with the nerve endings in the tubes themselves. Still, in countries such as India where tubal ligations are done in large numbers, local anesthesia is frequently used.

▶ How long does it take to recover?

After a laparoscopic procedure you can usually leave the hospital or the surgicenter on the same day and resume your regular activities, including sexual intercourse, in a day or so. The incision site is tender for few days, and you may have some abdominal soreness as well. Many women experience pain from the gas that was pumped into the abdominal cavity. Some even feel shoulder pain, if a small pocket of gas gets under the diaphragm and stimulates a nerve that goes to the shoulder.

A minilaparotomy causes about the same level of postoperative discomfort and, again, you can resume your normal activities within one or two days. Shoulder pain is not an issue, because gas is not used in this procedure.

Joanne, an amateur race-car driver, decided to have a laparoscopic tubal ligation. She was scheduled for a Friday and wanted to know whether she would be in shape to race on Sunday. This was a request I had never encountered before, and while I would not have wanted Joanne out there on the track the very day her surgery was performed, a couple of days later seemed safe.

The surgery went very smoothly and Joanne felt fine almost immediately afterward. On Sunday she drove the best race of her life, came in first, and won a handsome trophy. On Monday she called, wondering whether I could tie her tubes another time, jokingly suggesting the surgery had somehow contributed to her victory!

▶ How reliable is tubal ligation?

Tubal ligation is one of the most reliable forms of contraception, more than 99 percent effective both in theory and in actual use. It has a failure rate between 0.3 and 1 percent. That is, of every three hundred procedures one to three women will become pregnant. Failure does not necessarily mean that the surgery was performed incorrectly; it simply means that the ends of the tubes have somehow managed to find their way back together again. The failure rate is greater in women who are having their tubes tied after a cesarean section or after delivery. During pregnancy the blood vessels are dilated and have more blood flowing through them, so that tissue can rejoin more easily.

▶ What should you do if your tubal ligation fails?

If you have had a tubal ligation and suspect you might be pregnant, call your doctor immediately. You could have an ectopic pregnancy, a fertilized egg that does not make it down the fallopian tube to the uterus but starts developing somewhere outside the uterus. Warning signs include bleeding, especially after a late or light menstrual period, and abdominal pain, which may be sharp and localized on one side of the body. An ectopic pregnancy can be life threatening, so don't delay calling.

▶ How long does it take for a tubal ligation to be effective?

Unlike a vasectomy, a tubal ligation is effective immediately. You may not feel like having intercourse for a day or so after the procedure, but you are protected from pregnancy if you do.

▶ *Should you have a tubal ligation right after having a baby?*

Some physicians recommend performing a tubal ligation shortly after delivery, usually a day or two later, after you have recovered from the delivery. I strongly urge against it. For one thing, the first days and weeks are a vulnerable time in a baby's life. I have seen two heartrending instances of babies who died shortly after their mother had a postpartum tubal ligation.

In a minilaparotomy the incision, though not large, is a real incision and the procedure involves a certain amount of work inside the pelvic cavity. If you wait six or eight weeks, everything inside the pelvis will have gone back to its normal size. The uterus will have shrunk, the blood vessels will have returned to their prepregnant state, and the surrounding tissues (which get softer during pregnancy) will have returned to normal. The operation will be much easier to perform as a laparoscopy.

Finally, tubal ligations have the highest rate of failure if they are done right after delivery, whether the delivery was vaginal or via cesarean section.

So I urge new mothers to wait until their regular postpartum checkup to think about having a tubal ligation, and then perhaps to choose a laparoscopic procedure.

▶ *What are the possible complications?*

Tubal ligation is not a high-risk procedure; only about one in a thousand women who have it encounter significant complications. On the other hand, no surgery is trivial. You can minimize risk by choosing a surgeon who has done the procedure many times before. Don't feel shy or awkward about asking.

Besides the usual hazards of any surgery—unexpected bleeding, infection, and difficulties with the anesthesia—there is a small risk of damage to the bowel, bladder, or blood vessels, because the fallopian tubes are crowded close to these structures in the pelvis.

Heidi, a nurse who worked in the labor room at the hospital where I practice, decided to have a tubal ligation when she was in her mid-30s. An active woman who enjoyed horseback riding and other sports, she was in good physical condition. Heidi almost died during her tubal ligation because she had a rare reaction to the anesthesia, and her heart stopped. Fortunately, we were able to save her.

Carole had a routine abdominal tubal ligation when she was 35. I was a first-year resident at the time and assisted the surgeon performing the tubal, which went very smoothly. Later I went around to check on Carole and found her sitting on the edge of her bed, blue in the face and wheezing. She couldn't catch her breath.

She had a blood clot in her lung, a pulmonary embolus which had formed in her legs or her pelvis and traveled to the lung. I ran to the nursing station, grabbed a syringe of heparin, an anticoagulant, injected it as quickly as I could, and gave her oxygen. When Carole could breathe again, we took her for diagnostic x-rays. Her blood clot was almost the size of a fifty-cent piece, so large that you could see it on the x-ray from across the room. On heparin, her clot dissolved and she recuperated well.

Although complications are rare, and serious complications even more so, these incidents did impress on me the potential hazards of a tubal ligation.

▶ *Can a tubal ligation pose long-term complications?*

Some women, years after tubal ligation, notice heavier menstrual periods, more cramps, and menstrual irregularities. It is difficult to tell whether these difficulties came about simply because of increasing age or because of the tubal ligation. Furthermore, many women who have tubal ligations formerly used birth control pills, which kept their periods light and comfortable. Sometimes I ask women who are using the pill to try a few months without it before having a tubal ligation, in order to see how their periods respond.

▶ *How much does a tubal ligation cost?*

The cost of the surgeon, anesthesiologist, and operating room facility can come to about two thousand dollars, but your insurance will probably cover the procedure. In the past, insurance companies did not usually pay for tubal ligations, but eventually the insurers realized that sterilization is less expensive for them than a pregnancy.

▶ *Are tubal ligations ever reversible?*

Although no one should have a tubal ligation who does not consider it permanent, some women do want their tubes connected again—usually because of major life changes. The surgery to repair the severed tubes is delicate and expensive, and succeeds only about 50 percent of the time. And often insurance will not pay for the procedure.

VASECTOMY

Vasectomy is simpler than tubal ligation and can be performed in an office setting with local anesthesia. Most vasectomies in this country are performed by urologists.

Xylocain, a local anesthetic, is injected into the skin. The physician makes a tiny incision in the skin over the vas deferens, cuts the tube, ties the ends, and puts a stitch or two in the skin to close it. The whole procedure takes twenty or thirty minutes. Most men find it less traumatic than they had imagined.

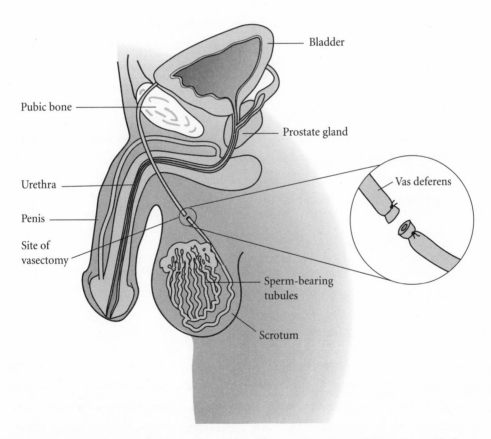

FIGURE 20. A vasectomy carries no risk to internal organs, since the vas deferens is outside the body cavity.

▶ *What are the risks or possible complications of a vasectomy?*

A vasectomy is a low-risk procedure, and most men do not have any problems. Rarely, difficulties with bleeding arise, for example a hematoma (a swollen area filled with blood) or a blood clot in the scrotum. To help avoid these complications, some doctors recommend that men not take aspirin or aspirin-like products for a week before the procedure. Another risk is infection. If an infection develops, antibiotics may be needed, but they are not used routinely. A few men have an allergic reaction to the material used in the stitches, which usually goes away on its own. A few men report a nagging kind of discomfort in the scrotum on one side or the other for several weeks after the procedure, but this reaction also is uncommon.

▶ *How much does a vasectomy cost?*

If a vasectomy is performed in an office setting, as perhaps 99 percent are, it costs in the range of five hundred to six hundred dollars. If it is done in a surgicenter, there is an additional surgical fee for the use of the operating room and possibly for an anesthetic.

▶ *How long is the recovery period?*

After the procedure, the patient can simply get up and go home. The recuperation period is really very short: if someone has a vasectomy on Friday, he should take it easy over the weekend and go back to work on Monday. He should not resume vigorous physical activity—jogging or running, for example—for a week or two.

▶ *Are pain medications necessary after a vasectomy?*

Some men need no pain medication at all; some need only ibuprofen. However, some physicians prescribe stronger pain medication (for example, Percocet).

▶ *How effective is vasectomy?*

Although we really do not know the failure rate because of long-term follow-up issues, the best estimates are in the range of one failure in every one hundred to three hundred operations. These failures result from what is called recanalization of the vas deferens, which means that somehow a passageway opens in the tube that was tied off during the operation. In that case, the ejaculate will contain sperm.

The most common cause of "failure" is that people rely on the vasectomy too soon. Vasectomies are not effective immediately, because sperm in the duct downstream from where the vas was cut have to be ejaculated. Usually the urologist will suggest that the patient come back for a sperm count six or eight weeks after the procedure. A laboratory technician will examine a sample of the ejaculate under a microscope to make sure that all the sperm are gone.

To be absolutely certain that no sperm are still present, some doctors prefer two consecutive negative sperm analyses. The first one is done six weeks after the procedure and the second one two weeks later, a total of eight weeks after the operation. Until two sperm counts have shown that there are no viable sperm in the ejaculate, it is advisable to use backup birth control.

> Abby, who has a family history of high blood pressure, had two children before she was 23. During her first pregnancy, she gained more than forty pounds and did not lose much of the weight afterward. During her second pregnancy, she gained even more weight and her blood pressure got significantly worse.
>
> Therefore she and her husband decide not to risk a third pregnancy. He has a vasectomy, which seems reasonable considering Abby's medical history. Unfortunately, despite our best educational efforts, Abby and her husband do not understand the need to use other birth control methods until his sperm count drops. They decide to celebrate his vasectomy and have sex the next day. She becomes pregnant once again. Her blood pressure is even higher this time.

▶ Can men have erections after vasectomy?

Yes, all the male hormones that account for sex drive and performance and for other masculine physical and behavioral traits remain fully in force after a vasectomy. The only difference is that because the duct to the outside world is blocked, the sperm do not get out of the body. The scar is small and not easily visible, so it is really not evident that the procedure has been done.

The ejaculate itself remains the same to the naked eye. Although a lab technician can see through a microscope that no sperm are present, neither the man nor his partner can notice a difference.

▶ *Are vasectomies harmful to men's health later on?*

There are two myths, both unfounded, that men who have had vasectomies have greater risk of heart attack and of rheumatoid arthritis. No data support these notions. Some studies on macaque monkeys have shown that those with vasectomies had higher rates of atherosclerotic heart disease (in which fat and cholesterol build up inside the arteries) than a similar group without vasectomies, but no studies of humans have yielded similar results.

Other well-designed studies show that there is no documentable relationship between vasectomies and rheumatoid arthritis or prostate cancer. Certainly men who go to their urologists in order to have vasectomies can be diagnosed with other conditions, but only because the physical exam reveals those other problems.

▶ *Are vasectomies reversible?*

A man who has a vasectomy should treat it as permanent. For this reason a few men donate sperm to a sperm bank before the procedure is done. There *is* a surgical procedure for reversing a vasectomy, but it is more expensive and more difficult than the vasectomy itself. It requires a general anesthetic and two or three hours of surgery. The success rate depends to some extent on timing of the reversal. If the vasectomy is reversed within five years, about 80 percent of men do have sperm in the ejaculate, with pregnancy rates approaching 50 percent. However, successful reversals have been reported as late as twenty years after the vasectomy.

NATURAL BIRTH CONTROL

Now used by only about 5 percent of couples in this country, fertility awareness (along with male condoms) was for many years the preferred and sometimes the only method of contraception readily available. Fertility awareness uses the biological rhythms of the menstrual cycle; couples time intercourse for days when conception is unlikely to occur, and abstain from intercourse when conception is likely. The method works on the principle that you are most likely to get pregnant if you have intercourse around the time of ovulation, and it offers three ways of determining when ovulation occurs.

Fertility awareness is not a reliable contraceptive method and you should use it only if you would not be devastated by an unplanned pregnancy or cannot use other methods because of your religious beliefs. *Any* other method, including contraceptive foam, is more effective.

Because your fertility depends not only on when you ovulate but also on the life span of your partner's sperm, which can live inside your body for as long as five and even seven days, an egg is more likely to be fertilized from intercourse that took place before or during ovulation than from intercourse after ovulation (though fertilization can happen a day or two afterward). You need to take this into consideration when planning your "safe" days.

The three techniques for predicting ovulation are the calendar method, the basal body temperature method, and the cervical mucus method. For maximum protection, you should use all three. All demand abstinence from sexual intercourse during a significant part of the month, and all demand accurate record keeping.

THE CALENDAR METHOD

If you have an absolutely regular twenty-eight-day cycle, you will ovulate around day 14 (counting the first day of your menstrual period as day 1). If you have a longer cycle, you will probably ovulate a little later. If you have a shorter cycle, you will probably ovulate earlier.

However, the time between ovulation and the beginning of the next period remains about fourteen days no matter how long or short your cycle; it is the beginning of the cycle whose length varies. So if you have a thirty-five-day cycle, you will probably ovulate on day 21, whereas if you have a twenty-five-day cycle, you are likely to ovulate on day 11. This means that if you know when you ovulate, it is easy to predict when you will get your period. But it does not mean that if you know when your last period began, you know when you are next going to ovulate.

▶ *How does the calendar method work?*

People who use the calendar or rhythm method in its plainest version use a calendar to predict future menstrual cycles, assuming they will be like past ones. These observations can help you guess a couple of days in advance when you probably will ovulate, though no one is absolutely regular every month every year. Use this method in conjunction with the basal body temperature method and/or the cervical mucus method, and if any sign suggests that you might be ovulating, abstain from vaginal intercourse (or use a backup method of contraception).

Kimberley usually has a menstrual cycle that varies between twenty-five and thirty days. If her shortest period is twenty-five days, then she probably ovulates no earlier than day 11; if her longest cycle is thirty days, then she can ovulate as late as day 16. Her fertile period is likely to be between days 11 and 16.

However, because sperm can still fertilize an egg for two or three days after they are ejaculated, to be on the safe side, she should add a couple of days to day 16. And maybe she is ovulating just a littler earlier than she thinks, so she should add a day or so to the beginning of the fertile period, pushing the starting date back to day 9. So between days 9 and 18, Kimberley and her partner should abstain from unprotected intercourse.

▶ How do you find your safe days?

On a regular calendar, circle day 1 of your period, the day bleeding begins. Continue to circle day 1 every month for at least eight months, preferably a year. To determine your safe days, find the shortest cycle on your calendar. Subtract 18 from the total number of days: If your shortest cycle was 26 days, then 18 from 26 leaves 8. Starting with day 1 of your period, count forward 8 days. Mark that date on your calendar with an X or a special color. It is the first day you are likely to be fertile. You should abstain from intercourse beginning on that date (or use backup contraception). The longer the time of abstinence, the more reliable the method. Some people suggest subtracting 21 instead of 18; although you will be safer, you will be able to have intercourse on fewer days.

To find your last fertile day, subtract 11 days from your longest cycle. Say it was 30 days, so that leaves 19. Mark that date on your calendar as well, with another X or another colored mark. It is the last day you must abstain or use backup contraception.

Your safe days are between the Xs (or the colored marks). The other days are unsafe. If any other sign—a change in cervical mucus, or a drop in the basal body temperature, or spotting, or a twinge of ovarian pain—suggests that you may be ovulating, then you must abstain or use backup contraception until you have reached the next safe day.

▶ Why does the rhythm method fail?

If your cycles are absolutely regular and you conscientiously avoid intercourse on your fertile days, the method works reasonably well. It fails when you ovulate much earlier (or later) than you think you will, or when sperm remain potent much longer than you anticipate.

THE BASAL BODY TEMPERATURE METHOD

The basal body temperature (BBT) method works because your basal temperature (temperature at rest) falls during the twelve to twenty-four hours before ovulation; after ovulation it rises. By charting these changes, you can keep better track of when you ovulate. This method is quite accurate in documenting when ovulation occurs, but it is not so good in *predicting* when it will happen.

At a family planning clinic or pharmacy you can buy a special basal body temperature thermometer, for ten to twelve dollars, which comes with charts for recording changes. The scale runs from only 96 to 100 degrees Fahrenheit and shows small fluctuations in temperature. Or you can use a regular thermometer, which costs about a dollar.

Take your basal body temperature every morning before you get up—before you eat, drink, smoke, read the paper, watch television, or have sex. It doesn't matter whether you take your temperature orally or rectally, though rectal temperatures are thought to be more accurate, but be consistent. Record the temperature on your chart and connect the dots, to make a graph showing the temperature changes throughout the month.

When the temperature falls, you are about to ovulate. When it rises (usually a half degree or a full degree Fahrenheit), you are ovulating or have ovulated. The rise may be sudden, making a spike on the chart, or it may be gradual, like steps. The pattern may change from one cycle to the next. Illness, emotional distress, jet lag, or even a poor night's sleep can alter your basal body temperature. So can sleeping under an electric blanket or drinking more than your usual amount of alcohol the night before. Noting these events on your chart will help you interpret the results.

▶ *Which days are safe, according to the basal body temperature method?*

After your temperature has risen and stayed up at least three days, you can assume your safe days have begun. These safe days last until the temperature drop that usually comes before your next menstrual period. You should consider unsafe all the days from the start of your period until the fourth day of the next temperature rise.

Why the long unsafe period? While the egg can only be fertilized for about a day after ovulation, sperm remain capable of fertilizing an egg for two or three days after ejaculation. If you have intercourse a couple of days before ovulation, there is a chance that lingering sperm will be available to fertilize the egg as it is released into the fallopian tube. Sperm can only survive eight hours in the vagina, but in the fallopian tubes they can live five to seven days.

▶ *How long should you chart your temperature before you begin using this method alone?*

Chart your temperature for at least three months before you begin relying on this method. But it is much better to combine temperature charting with another method to help predict ovulation.

CERVICAL MUCUS METHOD

This method, also known as the ovulation method or the Billings method, detects changes in the cervical mucus that occur during the menstrual cycle. The hormones that control the cycle also work on the glands of the cervix that secrete mucus, which helps to lubricate the vagina during intercourse and, depending on the time of the month, helps or hinders sperm in their journey toward the egg. Family planning clinics, including Planned Parenthood and clinics at Catholic hospitals, may be able to help you learn the method.

▶ *How does the cervical mucus change during the monthly cycle?*

During the first four or five days of your menstrual period, the blood flow covers up any changes in the cervical mucus. After the bleeding stops, there are a few "dry days" when little or no mucus is present.

As an egg starts to develop within the ovary, the amount of mucus in the vagina increases and it becomes sticky, cloudy, and yellow or white in color. As ovulation approaches, the quantity continues to increase and the mucus gets clear and slippery like raw egg white. It also becomes elastic and can be stretched between the fingers. These "wet days" are your most fertile.

Four or five days later, the mucus may again become cloudy and sticky, but scantier in volume. There may be a few more dry days before your period begins again. The changes vary from woman to woman and from month to month, although the general pattern holds true.

▶ *How do you chart your cycle?*

As with other methods, you note your observations every day on a calendar. Mark your menstrual period. Note which days are wet, which are dry, and when the color and consistency of the mucus change. It is wise to chart for at least a month before depending on the method, and during that month use backup contraception.

▶ *Which days are safe, using the cervical mucus method?*

With this method the days of your menstrual period are unsafe, especially if you have a shorter cycle, say twenty-one or twenty-two days. It is safe to have unprotected vaginal intercourse during the dry days after your period and before ovulation if you have a long cycle. However, the safe period ends at the first sign of wetness after menstruation. Do not have intercourse during the wet period unless you want to get pregnant.

After ovulation you must refrain from sex for at least three days or until the wet days end, whichever is longer. Naturally, the longer you wait after the wet days end, the safer the method; some doctors recommend waiting three days after wetness ends. It is considered safe to have sex after ovulation when the mucus decreases in volume and becomes cloudy and sticky again. It is even safer to have intercourse on the dry days before the next menstrual cycle.

▶ *What factors can interfere with the accuracy of the cervical mucus method?*

Women who don't produce much mucus may not be able to use this method. Factors that change the natural mucus pattern make the method unreliable: douching; using contraceptive foams, creams, jellies, or suppositories; vaginal infections; sexually transmitted diseases; recent use of hormonal contraceptives (including birth control pills, Norplant, and Depo-Provera); and breast-feeding. Women near menopause may have different and unreliable patterns of cervical mucus, as may women who have had cervical surgery.

▶ *How reliable is the rhythm method?*

Used conscientiously, the rhythm method and its variants (the basal body temperature and cervical mucus methods) are about 80 percent effective, which means that 20 percent of couples using the method will be pregnant within a year. This may seem like a high rate of failure, but it is a lot better than no method at all. Remember that about 85 percent of couples who use no contraception will be pregnant within a year and only about 15 percent will not.

▶ *How much does the rhythm method cost?*

It is one of the least expensive methods of birth control. A thermometer costs between one dollar and twelve. Charts for graphing your cycle cost almost nothing or can be downloaded free from the Planned Parenthood site on the internet (*www.plannedparenthood.*

org). You may have to pay for classes in fertility awareness, though some clinics offer them free; Medicaid may cover the cost of classes in some states when they are taken at a clinic or prescribed by your doctor.

▶ *Is fertility awareness the right contraceptive choice for you?*

If you and your partner are thinking about having a child maybe next year or the year after, but you really would not be distraught if you became pregnant, then the rhythm method is a reasonable choice. The method works best for women who for personal, religious, or health reasons cannot or will not use other forms of contraception, are committed to the method, and understand how it works. They must have the commitment to take their temperature every day, to keep accurate records, and, possibly, to check their cervical mucus. They should have only one sex partner, who is himself committed to the method. Both partners must have the discipline to abstain during the unsafe days (or use backup barrier-type contraception).

This method is not satisfactory if you have more than one sex partner, or if your one sex partner is not committed to the method. Nor is it advisable if you are careless about record keeping, if you don't want to use barrier methods or abstain on unsafe days, or if you take medications that change your cervical mucus, affect body temperature, or cause irregular menstrual periods. If an accidental pregnancy would devastate you, choose another form of contraception.

▶ *What are the advantages and disadvantages of natural birth control?*

It is inexpensive and does not involve last-minute contraceptive effort, but it demands discipline and interferes with spontaneity. Periods of abstention can have negative effects on a couple's sex life, especially since many women most desire intercourse around the time of ovulation—perhaps the body's way of ensuring a next generation.

6 Vaginitis and Urinary Tract Infections

▶ **MYTH** If you have frequent yeast infections, it means that you have HIV.

FACT Most women who get recurrent yeast infections are simply unlucky. However, women with HIV are prone to get frequent yeast infections.

VAGINITIS simply means "inflammation of the vagina," just as appendicitis simply means "inflammation of the appendix." (Vulvovaginitis means that the vulva—the external genitals—are involved, as well as the vagina.) Vaginitis can be very uncomfortable, but it is rarely serious and can usually be treated easily and effectively.

The three major kinds of vaginitis can be categorized by the microorganisms causing them. Yeast infections are caused by overgrowth of a microscopic fungus. Bacterial vaginosis (BV) seems to be caused by bacteria that thrive in the absence of oxygen. Trichomoniasis, discussed in Chapter 7, is caused by a single-celled amoeba-like organism. The symptoms of these infections vary from itching and burning to an unpleasant vaginal discharge to no manifestations at all. Some of the infections are transmitted sexually; others are not. Since treatments vary, it is important to figure out which infection you have.

YEAST INFECTIONS

Yeast infections, among the most widespread of vaginal infections, are fortunately the least harmful. Sometimes they disappear on their own, overcome by the body's natural defenses. If not, they are readily treated with over-the-counter or prescription medications, but they can have a nasty way of recurring.

▶ *What causes yeast infections?*

Under normal conditions, the healthy vagina is populated by millions of bacteria, collectively known as the vaginal flora. These microorganisms, of many different species, usually coexist peacefully; they create an acidic environment that keeps them in balance and fights off hostile invaders. The presence of these microorganisms does not mean that your vagina is "dirty" or "infected," or that your hygiene is poor: after all, your skin and the inside of your mouth both play host to thousands and thousands of microorganisms. Sometimes, however, the ideal balance is disrupted and one species of organism reproduces excessively, or a foreign invader gets a foothold and begins to multiply.

Yeast infections are caused by the overgrowth of fungi that belong to the normal vaginal flora and are usually held in check by "good guy" bacteria, notably members of the *Lactobacillis* family. Because the major culprit is *Candida albicans,* yeast infections are sometimes called candidiasis.

▶ *What are the symptoms of a yeast infection?*

Yeast infections can cause itching, redness, and irritation, both on the external genitals and inside the vagina. The vaginal discharge, usually thick and white, has the curdy consistency of cottage cheese. Inflammation and dryness can make intercourse uncomfortable, although it is all right to have intercourse when you have a yeast infection if it is comfortable for you. Many women find the vaginal symptoms less distressing than the labial itching, which can be intense. Occasionally yeast infections can cause discomfort or pain on urination, or the need to urinate frequently. Sometimes it is difficult to differentiate between a yeast infection and a urinary tract infection.

▶ *How can you be sure your symptoms are caused by a yeast infection?*

Usually your physician can diagnose a yeast infection through a pelvic exam or by examining the vaginal discharge microscopically. If your infection responds in a few days to antifungal medications, then you probably had a yeast infection. If there is any doubt, your doctor can send a sample of the vaginal discharge to a laboratory where it will be cultured for *Candida albicans* or other fungi that sometimes cause yeast infections.

▶ *Who is at risk for yeast infections?*

The most common risk factor is antibiotic use. Maybe your dermatologist has put you on tetracycline for severe acne; while killing off the harmful bacteria that caused your skin problems, the medication also stifled the protective bacteria that check the growth of yeast cells in your vagina. All of a sudden you have a yeast infection. Diabetes can also disrupt the normal vaginal balance, and diabetic women often have recurrent yeast infections that can be difficult to treat. Pregnancy sometimes disrupts the normal balance and predisposes women to yeast infections, though women who have recurrent yeast infections during pregnancy usually have had them previously. Obesity is a risk factor. Overweight women often sweat heavily, providing the warm moist atmosphere that nurtures yeast cells; these women may also be predisposed to diabetes or may have borderline glucose metabolism.

Tight nonbreathable clothing such as lycra encourages yeast growth by providing that warm moist atmosphere. Some people believe that a diet rich in starches and yeast can contribute to an environment conducive to yeast growth.

Emotional stress, which lowers your immune response, can predispose you to a yeast infection, just as it can predispose you to a cold. Women with suppressed immune systems are candidates for all kinds of opportunistic infections, including those from yeast. Although some women with AIDS have frequent yeast infections, the vast majority of women who have yeast infections, even recurrent ones, do not have AIDS.

Since menopause can lead to vaginal dryness and hence vaginal irritation, many postmenopausal women get yeast infections. Women who choose hormonal replacement after menopause are less likely to have recurrent yeast infections because their vaginas are better lubricated and more elastic.

▶ *Do birth control pills make you susceptible to yeast infections?*

No one knows precisely whether oral contraceptive use contributes to yeast infections. Some scientific papers have suggested that birth control pills may increase your susceptibility, and several of my patients swear that ever since they went on the pill, they have had one yeast infection after another. Other women believe that condoms increase susceptibility to yeast infections, possibly because they irritate vaginal tissues.

▶ *Are yeast infections during pregnancy harmful to the fetus?*

Yeast infections, fairly common during pregnancy, are in no way harmful to the fetus. There are treatments that are perfectly safe for mother and child, so it is possible to treat a yeast infection during pregnancy even though it is not harmful to the fetus if you do not.

▶ *Can you get a yeast infection if you are not sexually active?*

Many women who are not sexually active do get yeast infections. I treat several nuns, who get these infections from time to time. A couple of them are overweight, which increases their risk.

▶ *Can you get yeast infections from your sexual partner?*

Yeast infections are not considered STDs, but women can be infected by their male partners. Some of my patients are sure this happens: they take their medication, get cured of their symptoms, but when they resume intercourse with their partner after an infection-free period of abstinence, they immediately get another yeast infection. In these situations it seems useful to treat the man as well. Yeast infections can also be transmitted through oral sex.

Although yeast cells dry out and die when exposed to the air, men can get yeast infections from contact with an infected female partner. The primary symptom is the presence of itchy red patches on the penis. Men are treated with the same oral or topical antifungal medications that are used for women.

▶ *How can you lower your risk for yeast infections?*

There is no surefire preventive, but there are some commonsense steps you can take. Let your vagina "breathe." Don't wear skintight jeans or binding undergarments. Wear cotton panties or panties with a cotton crotch. Don't sit around in a wet bathing suit or sweaty exercise clothes. Don't wear nylon panty hose every day. When you use the toilet, wipe from front to back to avoid spreading yeast and bacteria from the rectum to the vagina. Try to keep your weight in the normal range.

If you are taking an antibiotic orally or vaginally, for a yeast infection or some other problem, try to replenish the natural vaginal flora to help prevent a recurrence. Any yogurt with live cultures contains *Lactobacilli;* you can eat yogurt to get these desirable bacteria into your digestive tract and thence into the rest of your system. Or you can use plain unflavored yogurt as a topical medication: use an applicator (they come with contraceptive foams or other vaginal medications) or even a tampon to get the yogurt up into the vagina. Or use it in a douche solution.

Another source of helpful bacteria is *Acidophilus,* available at health food stores as a powdered supplement to use in juice or water, or as tablets that you take daily. Certain *Acidophilus* products contain a combination of "friendly flora." Some physicians do not believe that these preventive measures do much good, but many of my patients find them helpful.

▶ *Are there any self-help approaches once you already have a yeast infection?*

You can use *Acidophilus* or yogurt to treat yeast infections, just as you would use these friendly bacteria to prevent them.

Another remedy especially helpful for hard-core yeast infections is boric acid, used in homemade vaginal suppositories. This mild acid is sold over the counter in drugstores, usually in the eye-care department, as packets of powder. Do not take it orally. Pharmacists who are skilled in filling capsules may make some up for you. (Your gynecologist may know a local "compounding" pharmacist.) If you are unable to find someone to fill the capsules for you, you can make your own.

To make the suppositories, you will need, in addition to the powdered boric acid, some size o empty gelatin capsules, also available at drug stores or health food stores. Fill the capsules loosely with the boric acid powder and use them as vaginal suppositories, inserting one at night before you go to bed and one in the morning. The gelatin will melt and release the boric acid into the vagina. These capsules are less messy than creams or purchased suppositories, but they do leave a small amount of watery, gritty residue. After a week of this twice-daily treatment, decrease the dosage to one capsule daily for another week.

▶ *Do frequent yeast infections mean you have some serious underlying medical condition?*

Most women who get repeated infections do not have serious underlying diseases; they are simply unlucky. In many cases there is no discernible reason for the recurrences. Nevertheless, when someone tells me she has had a yeast infection every month for the past year, I do consider such predisposing diseases as diabetes or AIDS, but the vast majority of women who have yeast infections have neither AIDS nor diabetes. If you seem to get "yeast" infections frequently, see your health care provider for a culture. What you think is a yeast infection could be something different, perhaps another type of infection or irritation from an allergen.

Cancer of the vulva, which is rare especially in younger women, often shows up with persistent itching, which of course is the main symptom of yeast infections. If you have an area of itchiness that does not go away with a week or two of treatment, or a tender area that does not heal in about a month, be sure to contact your health care provider.

MEDICATIONS

Treating a yeast infection often involves a two-step plan: killing the overgrowth of yeast cells with an antifungal drug, and reducing the itching and burning with an anti-inflammatory. Merely killing the yeast does not always end the itching and burning.

Antifungal drugs, available over the counter and by prescription, come as pills, creams, or suppositories that are inserted into the vagina and allowed to melt. Their primary pharmaceutical agents are miconazole, clotrimazole, and butoconazole. They usually provide relief within a day or so, but since yeast infections are notorious for recurring, be sure to follow the prescribed course for the medication even if your symptoms have disappeared. Creams and vaginal suppositories can leak out of your vagina, but a panty liner will protect your clothing.

Nonprescription medications that kill yeast cells include Monistat (miconazole); Gyne-Lotrimin, Lotrimin, and Mycelex (clotrimazole); and Femstat (butoconazole) and Vagistat. The most commonly used prescription antifungal drug is Terazol (terconazole), which comes in cream or suppository form. If you choose suppository form, be aware that the base in which the medication is used can interact with rubber latex products, such as diaphragms and condoms. So use some other form of birth control while you are taking this medication.

The most widely used prescription oral medication is Diflucan, the trade name for fluconazole. Members of this family of pharmaceuticals are also used to treat serious systemic yeast infections, including infections of the urinary tract, pneumonia, and certain kinds of meningitis. While therapy for these conditions may last days or weeks, a single small dose of fluconazole will usually cure common everyday yeast infections. One 150-mg pill might be the equivalent of three days of over-the-counter therapy. Diflucan does not increase the risk of recurrence, and since most people would rather swallow one pill than use creams or suppositories for a week, it is a useful option. Your symptoms should go away in a few days.

Medications to subdue inflammation include some worthwhile over-the-counter choices. One is a simple antihistamine, such as Benadryl. Some women notice that they feel worse in the morning, even after using an antifungal drug at bedtime, and it is possible that they scratched while they slept. Taking Benadryl at bedtime can help with this problem.

Over-the-counter steroid creams like Cortaid can also relieve inflammation. If you go this route, be extremely careful to avoid the vicious circle of steroid dependency. That is, if you use a steroid cream repeatedly, you run the risk of thinning out the tissue on the vulva and making it dependent on the steroid. If that happens, you experience burning and itching when you do not apply the steroid. If the steroid fails to relieve the itching in two to three days, contact your physician.

If your inflammatory symptoms continue even after antifungal medications kill off all the yeast, your doctor may prescribe a double-acting medication like Mycolog, which contains an antifungal (nystatin) plus an anti-inflammatory. Lotrisone lotion is another combination drug aimed at both killing yeast and taming inflammation; you should only use it for a few days.

BACTERIAL VAGINOSIS

Bacterial vaginosis (also known as bacterial vaginitis), abbreviated BV, is another common form of vaginal inflammation. Its causes are less well understood than those of yeast infections. As researchers have tried to zero in on the microorganism responsible, BV has been renamed several times: *Haemophilus* vaginitis, *Gardnerella* vaginitis, nonspecific vaginitis, *Corynebacterium* vaginitis, and anaerobic vaginosis.

▶ *What are the symptoms of BV?*

The most common symptom in women is a foul-smelling milky or grayish-yellow vaginal discharge. Its distinct "fishy" smell is strongest when in contact with something alkaline, for example semen or soap, so the odor is most pronounced after sexual intercourse and, ironically, when you are trying to wash it away. Sometimes, but not usually, bacterial vaginosis causes vaginal itching or burning.

Men infected with the disease may have a discharge from the penis or they may experience irritation when urinating. Most have no symptoms at all, so pass on the disease unknowingly.

▶ *What causes bacterial vaginosis?*

Although several different bacteria have been associated with this condition, a bacterium called *Gardnerella vaginalis* usually can be cultured from the vaginal discharge of someone with the symptoms of BV. There is some question whether *Gardnerella* actually causes the disease or is simply a marker for it. Is *Gardnerella* merely present in the vaginal discharge that gets cultured to diagnose the disease, or is *Gardnerella* responsible for the symptoms? Many researchers believe that bacteria that thrive in the absence of oxygen are actually the culprits and that *Gardnerella,* which needs oxygen to live, is simply a fellow traveler.

Bacterial vaginosis is often associated with sexual activity and is sometimes considered an STD. Unless the disease recurs, it is generally not necessary to test your partner.

▶ *How is bacterial vaginosis diagnosed?*

Your physician can diagnose bacterial vaginosis through your physical symptoms, including the color and odor of the discharge. Examination under the microscope may show the presence of "clue" cells, that is, cells of the vaginal lining that are dotted with bacteria. If doubt remains, or if you are pregnant, a sample of the discharge will be sent to a laboratory for a culture. Results are usually available in three days.

▶ *Is BV dangerous?*

For most women, BV is an annoyance, something that can easily be treated and will quickly go away (though it may come back). It is not as benign as a yeast infection, however, since bacterial vaginosis has been associated with increased risk of pelvic inflammatory disease. By altering the protective acidity of the vagina, BV may allow the harmful organisms that cause gonorrhea and chlamydia to ascend through the cervix and multiply in the uterus or fallopian tubes.

For pregnant women, BV carries the additional risk of premature rupture of the membranes and thus premature labor and delivery. For this reason, many doctors in the past five or ten years test women for BV both before and during pregnancy.

TREATING BV

The usual medication prescribed for BV is metronidazole (trade name Flagyl). Metronidazole is effective against both anaerobic bacteria and protozoa (organisms like amoebas), so it is used to treat not only BV but also trichomonas and amoebic dysentery. The course of treatment usually runs about a week, with a dosage of 250 mg three times a day or 500 mg twice a day.

Though you can take Flagyl with or without food, you should not drink any alcoholic beverages at all while you are taking it, or for twenty-four hours after your last dose. The interaction may cause severe vomiting, nausea, abdominal cramps, headaches, and other unpleasant symptoms. Flagyl acts like Antabuse, a drug given to alcohol abusers to try to wean them from their habit. Our bodies normally produce an enzyme called acetaldehyde dehydrogenase, which is needed to metabolize alcohol. Flagyl blocks this enzyme. So if you drink alcohol, your blood levels of acetaldehyde rise and rise, which eventually produces nausea and vomiting. Some people get stomach upsets from Flagyl even if they do not drink alcohol. Flagyl may also make your mouth dry or metallic tasting.

Metronidazole is also available as a cream, marketed as MetroGel. It is inserted into the vagina with a special applicator that comes with it. Originally the prescribed course of therapy was one applicator twice a day for five days; now the manufacturer recommends just one application before bedtime. This is considerably more pleasant, since vaginal creams can leak out and be messy. Metronidazole is also used to treat rosacea ("adult acne").

A newcomer to the field of BV therapy, clindamycin, is prescribed for acne as well as for vaginal infections (the anaerobic bacteria that cause both conditions are similar). As a treatment for BV, clindamycin is marketed as Cleocin Vaginal Cream or as vaginal suppositories; as a treatment for acne, it is called Cleocin T Gel. Cleocin is probably more effective than Flagyl against bacteria that belong to the *Mobiluncus* family.

As with metronidazole, the therapy time with clindamycin has been shortened. The old recommendation was to apply Cleocin Vaginal Cream once daily before bedtime for a week. The manufacturer has reduced the course of therapy to three nights, for both cream and suppositories.

▶ *Is Flagyl safe during pregnancy?*

The FDA has given Flagyl a B rating for use during pregnancy, which means that studies done on animals or humans have presented no evidence of risk to the fetus. Some physicians, however, will not prescribe it during pregnancy, especially during the first trimester. If your physician chooses not to prescribe Flagyl, a possible substitute is MetroGel. Like Flagyl, it has received a B rating from the FDA.

▶ *Can you have more than one kind of vaginitis at the same time?*

Unfortunately, it is possible to have mixed infections. For this reason a culture of the vaginal discharge can be helpful, because it can be difficult for your doctor to decide from your symptoms alone exactly what kind of infection you have and what medication would best eradicate it.

URINARY TRACT INFECTIONS

Urinary tract infections (UTIs) are an all-too-common problem for women, afflicting an estimated 26 million American women every year. UTIs are caused by bacteria growing unchecked in the urinary tract, often by *Escherichia coli* (abbreviated *E. coli*), an organism usually found in the intestinal tract.

The seriousness of a UTI depends on whether it affects only the lower urinary tract or the upper tract as well. The lower urinary tract consists of the bladder, where urine is collected, and the urethra, the tube that carries urine from the bladder to the outside of the body. If the infection affects only the urethra, it is called urethritis; usually any infection that involves the urethra also involves the bladder, in which case it is called cystitis.

The upper urinary tract consists of the ureters (two tubes that carry urine from the kidneys to the bladder) and the kidneys, the organs where urine is made. Infections that travel upward and affect these organs and become systemic are known as pyelonephritis. An untreated infection that spreads to the kidneys can lead to kidney damage, which is serious and even life threatening.

The female urinary tract is not an ideally designed piece of plumbing. First, the opening of the urethra to the outside world is near the opening of the intestinal tract where bacteria thrive abundantly. Second, the female urethra is short, which means that bacteria that get into it can easily travel upstream to the bladder. Men have an extra few inches of urethra, which helps protect them from UTIs.

▶ *What puts you at increased risk for a urinary tract infection?*

Sexual intercourse, especially increased activity, is one risk factor. Urinary tract infections used to be called honeymoon bladder or bride's kidney, because women who were having frequent sexual intercourse, perhaps for the first time in their lives, often got these infections. Inadequate lubrication may be another factor.

Hygiene can be a factor. So can some forms of birth control, including spermicidal foams and jellies or condoms, which may irritate the urethra. Using a diaphragm may predispose a woman to infection; it can press against the urethra, making it more difficult to empty the bladder.

Pregnant women frequently have UTIs, in part because the fetus presses on the bladder and prevents it from emptying completely. The hormonal changes of pregnancy may relax the muscles of the urinary tract, which also allows urine to remain in the bladder or ureters. Women near menopause and postmenopausal women are more likely to get UTIs than

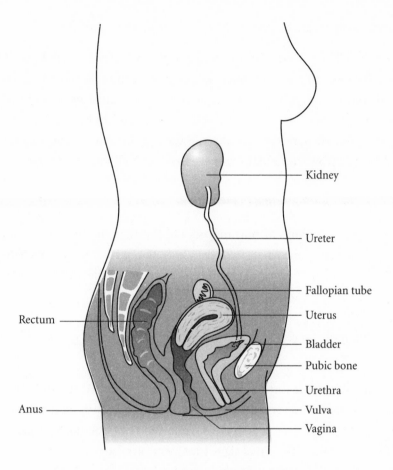

FIGURE 21. In the female urinary tract, infection can spread upward through the ureters and reach the kidneys, causing serious disease.

younger women, because the loss of estrogen at this time of life thins out tissues in both the reproductive and urinary tracts, making them vulnerable to irritation and infection.

Women who have already had one urinary tract infection are likely to have another. Sometimes the repeat infection comes within six months of the first one, sometimes later. Certain STDs, for example, chlamydia and gonorrhea, that cause inflammation of the urethra can lead to UTIs. Finally, some women just seem to get them—perhaps because they are genetically at risk.

▶ *Can physical or anatomical conditions cause urinary tract infections?*

Although most UTIs are caused by bacteria getting into the urethra, a few physical conditions can contribute to infection or cause symptoms similar to those of UTIs. Kidney stones, which are deposits of calcium, can block the flow of urine and cause infection. Another cause of blockage can be a cystocele (a protrusion of the bladder into the vagina), caused by a weakening in the vaginal wall. A diverticulum in the urethra (a pouching out of the wall) can trap bacteria and become a reservoir of infection.

▶ *What are the symptoms of a UTI?*

Painful urination—stinging or burning—is the classic symptom. Often women with UTIs feel an intense urge to urinate frequently, even though there is not much urine in the bladder. The pain may be greatest when the bladder contracts after urinating: it hurts most just as the flow ceases.

▶ *What symptoms suggest that a urinary tract infection has spread to the ureters and kidneys?*

Sometimes it is difficult to distinguish between upper urinary tract infections and those that involve only the bladder and urethra; the symptoms may be the same. However, if you have fever, or flank pain (pain in the side of your midback), you might suspect an upper tract infection. Another suspicious sign is frequent or recurrent infection. Nausea and vomiting can also be associated with a kidney infection.

▶ *What causes repeat infections?*

If the bacteria that caused the original problem were not all killed by antibiotic therapy, they can flourish again once the antibiotics are stopped, causing what seems to be a repeat infection. But sometimes repeat infections are caused by bacteria different from those that caused the first episode.

▶ *How long should you wait before calling the doctor if you think you have a UTI?*

Sometimes UTIs will go away on their own or respond to self-help measures, but if your symptoms continue for more than two days, call your doctor. If you have fever, chills, back pain, or nausea—symptoms of a possible upper tract infection—call your doctor right away. If you have recurrent infections, two or three within a year, even though they are not accompanied by fever or back pain, you should be checked out.

If you suspect you have a urinary tract infection, it is reasonable to give your regular physician a call. If the problem is easily cleared up, so much the better. If you have frequent or recurrent UTIs, then you should probably be referred to a urologist, who specializes in urinary tract problems.

▶ *How can you prevent UTIs?*

First of all, follow your mother's advice about not "holding" urine; go to the toilet often, whenever you feel the urge (if it is convenient). Wipe yourself from front to back after urinating and especially after a bowel movement so that you do not spread bacteria from the rectum to the urethra. Change sanitary napkins frequently during your period. Every time you have intercourse, be sure to get up and urinate afterward, even though falling asleep may be more comfortable. You want to rinse out the bacteria that are trying to climb up your urethra.

If you are prone to UTIs, you probably should not wear panty liners all the time. You might not want to use a diaphragm, spermicide, or condoms (provided you and your partner are monogamous and you do not need protection from STDs). Some women find that avoiding bubble baths and chlorinated hot tubs or swimming pools cuts down on the frequency of UTIs.

Try to drink plenty of water, as much as eight to ten glasses daily. Don't wear tight-fitting jeans or all-nylon underwear (which may create an environment that also contributes to vaginitis and yeast infections). Some women find that it helps to cut their intake of coffee, other caffeinated beverages, alcohol, and spicy or highly acidic foods; these may cause bladder irritation. Avoid using perfumed toilet paper, perfumed bath products and powders, or scented soaps, which can be irritating.

SELF-HELP METHODS

The classic home remedy is cranberry juice, which makes the urine more acid and also seems to make it difficult for bacteria to stick to the bladder wall. Some women drink it as a preventive measure; others use it when they feel the first symptoms of an infection coming on. Blueberry juice also works well, but is not as readily available. Cranberry tablets, with a high concentration of the active ingredient, are available in health food stores. Some women take vitamin C, which also makes the urine more acidic. Drinking a lot of water can help. Try warm tub baths to relieve the discomfort of an infection or a heating pad to relieve abdominal pain.

Other herbal preparations have been proposed, though cranberry juice or supplements are probably most effective. Among the others are buchu (any of three species from the genus *Barosma*) and bearberry (*uva ursi*), which are used in herbal teas. Both are safe in moderate doses and may be effective, though no scientific studies have proved that they are.

▶ *How are UTIs diagnosed?*

In cases where the infection seems related to sexual activity, your caregiver may recommend urinalysis, which can be done in a doctor's office or a medical laboratory. If you have a UTI, the test will probably show white blood cells and bacteria in the urine, both signs of infection.

Sometimes the next step in the diagnosis is a urine culture to reveal exactly which bacteria are causing the symptoms or to rule out other causes (for example sexually transmitted diseases, yeast infections, or vaginitis). Once the culprit has been identified, your caregiver will prescribe an appropriate antibiotic. If you have had UTIs in the past and your caregiver is familiar with your history, he or she may prescribe antibiotics without a urine culture. If you have a new sexual partner, your doctor may recommend a chlamydia test.

If your UTIs keep recurring, a urologist might do a "postvoid residual" test, which uses a catheter to make sure that the bladder empties completely. The physician may examine you to check that your urethra feels normal—for example, has no pouchings (diverticula). If these tests prove normal, an ultrasound might reveal anatomical irregularities in the kidneys, ureters, bladder, or urethra.

TESTING FOR RECURRENT INFECTIONS

As a means of diagnosing upper tract disease, a CT (computerized tomography) scan may show anatomical abnormalities in the kidney itself, or perhaps obstruction or dilation of the ureters, kidney stones, or evidence of scarring from previous disease. If the technology for a CT scan is not available to you, another test called an IVP (intravenous pyelogram) may give the same information.

An IVP is an x-ray test in which dye is injected through a needle inserted into a vein of one arm. The dye, which shows up in strong contrast on an x-ray, circulates through the bloodstream to the kidneys and then is excreted through the urinary tract. X-rays are taken at regular intervals for about an hour after the dye is introduced, to show what is happening in the urinary tract. The test can be performed in the outpatient department of a hospital or at a radiology center.

Another test, a backflow test, in which dye is introduced into the bladder with a catheter, will show whether urine is flowing backward up the ureters.

▶ *What is the next step if these diagnostic tests turn up a kidney stone or some abnormality?*

Many anatomical defects can be corrected surgically. Kidney stones can be removed surgically or dissolved by bombarding them with sound waves, a procedure called lithotripsy, which my patients have told me is somewhat uncomfortable and performed with the use of pain medications.

▶ *Which medications work for UTIs?*

Most urinary tract infections respond to antibiotics. The course of treatment depends on the severity of the infection. One antibiotic favored nowadays is Macrodantin (generic name nitrofurantoin), because it remains concentrated in the bladder. Since it does not appear in high levels throughout the body, Macrodantin is unlikely to destroy the helpful vaginal organisms that fight yeast infections. Other antibiotics include sulfa drugs, trimethoprim, or quinolones. Some physicians use amoxicillin or ampicillin.

Pyridium, a urinary analgesic, is available without a prescription as Uristat. While it does not kill the bacteria that cause the infection, it does relieve the discomfort. (Don't be surprised when it turns your urine orange!) Pyridium does not alter a urine culture, so you can still be tested to determine the exact cause of your UTI even when you are taking pyridium.

Common everyday infections, the kind caused by increased sexual activity, can be treated by short courses of antibiotics, between one and seven days. Repeat infections involve longer courses, sometimes three months or more, to make sure that all the offending bacteria have been killed. After a course of antibiotics, your caregiver may ask for another urine culture to be certain that the infection is gone. Sometimes antibiotics make the symptoms disappear, but the infection can still be detected in the urine sample.

7 Sexually Transmitted Diseases

▶ **MYTH** If you have gonorrhea, you'll have symptoms, so you'll know you
need to get treated.

FACT Eighty percent of women and a large percentage of men with
gonorrhea have no symptoms, so both you and your partner can spread the
disease without knowing it.

SEXUALLY transmitted diseases (STDs) are almost as common as the common
cold. Every year an estimated 15 million Americans contract a disease that is transmitted
by intercourse or other sexual activity. Worldwide, 340 million people annually contract
curable sexually transmitted infections; in addition, an estimated 5 million new cases of
HIV arise each year.

Although we like to think of STDs as happening to other people, they can appear in
anyone who is sexually active, since the viruses and bacteria that cause them are blind to
social and cultural distinctions. They do not discriminate according to education or economic status; they are indifferent to race and to religious, cultural, and political persua-
sions. While teenagers account for about 25 percent of new cases, teenagers and people
younger than 25 for perhaps as many as 67 percent, young people are not especially vulnerable to STDs except in their behavior, in that they are more likely than their elders to
have unprotected sex with several partners.

Some STDs do discriminate along gender lines. These diseases in general are more easily transmitted from men to women than from women to men, and several have more serious consequences for women, causing permanent reproductive damage in women who are undiagnosed or untreated.

It would be comforting to think that sexually transmitted diseases are succumbing to the advances of modern medicine, but unfortunately that is not entirely true. Of the three major diseases tracked in the United States by the Centers for Disease Control and Prevention (CDC), two are generally under control. From 1975 to 1997, gonorrhea declined by almost 74 percent, reflecting a national program for detection and treatment. The rate has risen slightly since then but is holding steady. Syphilis, after increasing dramatically in the late 1980s and early 1990s during the height of the AIDS epidemic, decreased until 2000, when 5,979 cases were reported, the fewest since 1941, the year the government began keeping statistics. In 2001, however, there were 6,103 new cases mainly among gay and bisexual men, raising concern that these groups are becoming less careful about practicing safe sex.

Chlamydia, a disease that was barely known a generation ago, is now the most prevalent STD in the country. The 702,093 cases reported in 2000 are almost double the number of cases of gonorrhea (358,995). Furthermore, chlamydia is on the rise, reported cases increasing from 48 per 100,000 people in 1987 to 257.5 per 100,000 in 2000, with women having a rate of infection four times greater than that of men. Although better screening and better reporting account for part of the increase (and the number of reported cases is probably lower than the number of actual cases), the burden of disease is extremely high.

It is important to remember that STDs travel in groups. If you have one of these diseases, you are at increased risk for others. In part this is because the behavior that exposed you to one disease puts you at risk for others.

The most widespread sexually transmitted diseases are chlamydia, gonorrhea, syphilis, herpes, HPV (human papilloma virus), HIV (human immunodeficiency virus), and hepatitis B. Some of these diseases, notably gonorrhea, chlamydia, and syphilis, are caused by bacteria and often can be completely cured with medication. Other diseases, caused by viruses, remain with you permanently, though they may lie dormant and not show symptoms. Among these are HIV, HPV (which causes genital warts), and HSV (herpes simplex virus), which causes painful blisters on the genitals and elsewhere.

The bacteria responsible for several common STDs can also cause pelvic inflammatory disease, which can affect your uterus, fallopian tubes, or ovaries. PID can cause scarring, and the scar tissue may block the entrance to your fallopian tubes or distort their shape, impeding the journey of the egg from ovary to uterus. PID can also cause chronic

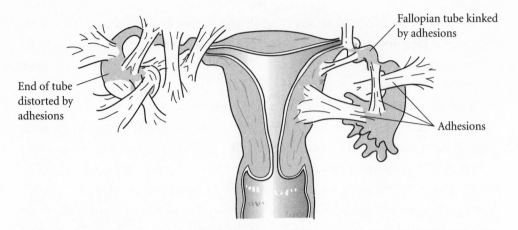

FIGURE 22. Pelvic inflammatory disease can cause scar tissue to develop between organs and cause persistent pain. It can also distort the shape of the tubes or block the entrance to them, causing infertility.

infection, pelvic pain, or tenderness in the abdomen, and a foul-smelling vaginal discharge. Sometimes, however, the symptoms are so mild that they are not noticed.

▶ How can you protect yourself from STDs?

The only 100-percent protection against sexually transmitted diseases is sexual abstinence. Short of that, the best protection is to use a condom plus a spermicide, unless you are absolutely certain you are in a mutually monogamous relationship with an uninfected partner.

TRICHOMONIASIS

Trichomoniasis, infection with the *Trichomonas* organism, is a widespread STD. It does not by law have to be reported to health authorities, so some guesswork is involved in tabulating the number of new cases in the United States each year. Estimates range from 3 million to 5 million new cases yearly, and some data suggest that the incidence is decreasing.

▶ What causes trichomoniasis?

Trichomoniasis, also known as trich (pronounced "trick"), is an STD caused by a microscopic single-celled organism called *Trichomonas vaginalis* that propels itself through its wet microenvironment by means of three whiplike tails called flagella. Like most of the other organisms responsible for STDs, this one is relatively fragile, cannot survive drying out, and can be cured by drug therapy.

▶ *What are the symptoms?*

The usual symptoms in women include a foul-smelling vaginal discharge, usually yellow or yellow-green, which can be thick, thin, or frothy. Sometimes, but not always, the infection causes burning, itching, or redness of the vagina or vulva. It may cause discomfort during intercourse and frequent or painful urination. About 40 percent of women diagnosed with trich have no symptoms and thus can spread the disease without knowing it.

Men can also be infected with trich, but they do not usually have symptoms. If they do, the symptoms include irritation, a discharge from the penis, or a burning sensation during urination.

▶ *How do you get trichomoniasis?*

In the vast majority of cases, trich is transmitted sexually. It is possible, though unlikely, to get it from swimming in a contaminated lake or an inadequately treated pool or hot tub (though the chemicals used to disinfect pools and hot tubs, if used properly, will make quick work of *Trichomonas*). A few cases have been traced to shared washcloths or wet towels, but you cannot get trich from toilet seats or dry linens.

▶ *How is trich diagnosed?*

Your physician can diagnose *Trichomonas* by looking through a microscope at a drop of your vaginal discharge. Its whip-like tails make it easy to recognize.

▶ *Is trichomoniasis dangerous?*

Unlike syphilis, gonorrhea, and chlamydia, trichomoniasis is not dangerous in itself; it does not cause pelvic inflammatory disease, nor does it seem to have consequences during pregnancy. However, trich is often a marker for other STDs, so if you have trich you are at increased risk for diseases such as gonorrhea, for example, which does cause PID. If you have been diagnosed with trich, your physician may want to test you for other STDs by doing a culture of your cervix.

▶ *What is the treatment?*

The best drug for treating trich is metronidazole (trade name Flagyl), which is also used to treat BV. Flagyl has been used for many years and can be administered in several ways. Some physicians like to give 2 gm orally, as a one-time treatment (known as a stat dose). Other physicians choose a longer course, one 250-mg tablet, three times a day for a week, or 375 mg twice a day for a week. Many people prefer the stat dose because it is quickest and easiest.

Metronidazole also comes in gel form (trade name MetroGel) for vaginal use. It is usually effective, though probably not so potent as the oral medication. Recurrence rates are higher with the gel; if you can tolerate the oral form, you are more likely to be cured. On the other hand, the gel has fewer side effects than the oral form. (For the side effects of Flagyl, see Chapter 6.)

▶ *If you are diagnosed with trich, should your partner be treated?*

Trich often seems to be passed back and forth between sexual partners, so most physicians will treat both to prevent reinfection. It is difficult to discover who infected whom, but if one partner is infected, the other probably is as well. If you have more than one sexual partner, all of them should be treated.

> When my colleague Tom diagnosed Camille with trichomoniasis and recom-
> mended that her partner be treated as well. Camille hesitated and then said,
> "Well, I guess I'll need prescriptions for eight gentlemen." Tom wrote out eight
> prescriptions. Later that day the office got a call from Camille. "Better make that
> nine prescriptions," she said. "After I got home, I remembered someone else."
> Sad as this story is, in terms of the diseases being spread around, we appreciated
> Camille's honesty. She and Tom talked about the importance of safe sex, for her
> *and* her partners.

If you continue to have symptoms after you have finished your course of medication, whether it is a stat dose or a longer treatment, your physician may ask for a follow-up visit.

GENITAL HERPES

Genital herpes, like trich, need not by law be reported to the local health department, so estimates of its frequency rest on informed guesswork. More than 40 million Americans may be infected with this disease, and probably five hundred thousand new cases occur annually.

▶ What causes herpes?

Genital herpes is caused by a DNA virus from the family that causes chicken pox and shingles. The particular strain responsible for most genital herpes is called HSV-2 (herpes simplex virus type 2). It is similar but not identical to the virus (HSV-1) that usually causes cold sores, canker sores, or fever blisters in your mouth. Practically everyone has had contact with the oral herpes virus, HSV-1, though not everyone develops symptoms. Once you have herpes, you have it forever, since the virus lives in the nerve roots near the spine. It may exist there in a state of dormancy for long periods and then be exacerbated by cold or sunlight or heat or other causes. Thus people who have had chicken pox may get shingles in later life; and people who have oral or genital herpes may have recurrent outbreaks from time to time.

▶ What are the symptoms of genital herpes?

One of the classic symptoms of genital herpes is a cluster of small blisters or vesicles in the genital area. The blisters may be preceded by pain or itching and first appear as little red bumps that later develop into blisters that rupture and ooze. The initial infection can be very painful. Besides the blisters, you are apt to have aches, fevers, chills, headache, swollen lymph nodes, and maybe even a diffuse rash. If you have had chicken pox, you may remember the general viral feeling. Occasionally I get a phone call at two in the morning from an anxious patient who was taking a shower, felt a "bump down there," and called immediately. If it is her only symptom, she does not have genital herpes.

The other classic symptom is painful urination, which is different from the kind of urinary pain that accompanies a bladder infection. The stinging pain from herpes occurs when the urine touches the infected area; the pain from a bladder infection comes from within the bladder itself as it empties.

Fortunately, herpes is self-limiting. It goes away after a few days. The perineum heals even if you do nothing to treat it. The rash goes away, as do the aches and pains, though sometimes people have nerve-root pain such as sciatica.

Remember, though, that the herpes virus remains dormant in your body and you may suffer recurrences. Repeat episodes are rarely as painful as the initial one, and some people never have recurrences. Usually the frequency of recurrence will decrease with time, and the recurrent episodes will be less painful.

▶ How long does it take the symptoms to appear after infection?

Symptoms tend to appear between two days and a week after the infection, though many women who are infected with herpes are unaware of it.

▶ How do you get herpes?

HSV is fairly transmissible, although you cannot be infected by shaking hands. It is spread by contact between mucous membranes, contact that includes vaginal, anal, or oral intercourse. Accordingly, you can get oral herpes as well as genital herpes in your vagina, or you can get genital herpes in your mouth. It is possible to spread oral herpes to the genital area via your hands, or to spread genital herpes to your mouth or eyes in the same way.

To avoid spreading the virus, try not to touch the sores. If you do, wash your hands well with soap and water. Wash your hands before rubbing your eyes, especially when you wake up. Do not wet your contact lenses with saliva, especially if you have oral herpes; wash your hands before you touch your lenses.

Often patients with genital herpes are anxious to know whether they have HSV-1 or HSV-2, because they think that HSV-1 is acceptable but HSV-2 is "dirty." That is the myth surrounding these subtypes of the virus. In fact, the only real difference between the two is that a child born through a birth canal infected with HSV-1 as opposed to HSV-2 might get less sick.

▶ If you have herpes, can you have sex?

If you have a genital sore, do *not* have sexual intercourse—even with a condom. The virus can spread from sores not covered by the condom, and it can spread in sweat and vaginal fluids to places the condom does not cover. Even with a condom, the activity of intercourse may rub against the sores and they will take longer to heal. Genital herpes can also be transmitted, even though there are no open sores.

▶ How can you protect yourself from getting herpes?

As with any sexually transmitted disease, practicing safe sex is the best answer. If your partner already has the infection, avoid sexual contact when the herpes sores are present, since the disease can most easily be transmitted through contact with the sores themselves. It is possible that using a spermicide may limit transmission of the virus, but a spermicide foam or gel containing nonoxynol-9 plus a condom is a much better choice for protection.

▶ Can herpes spread if there is no active lesion?

Yes; even though you have no symptoms, you may be "shedding" viruses. Medical studies of women who have had past outbreaks of herpes demonstrate this possibility. The women wear tampons specially coated with a culture medium; then the tampons are sent to a lab and cultured for herpes. While the tampons used by women without active lesions grow only a few colonies, they often are still positive. The cultures on women who have active lesions show many colonies of herpes, not just a few. In other words, these women are much more likely to infect their partners.

This does not mean that everyone sheds viruses all the time, or that if you have herpes you can give it to your partner all the time. Many women with herpes infections do not shed. Furthermore, medication can decrease the shedding time.

I do encourage couples to use condoms if one of them has a history of herpes, particularly if he or she has strong feelings about spreading the disease. Sometimes a women will say something like, "I'll kill myself if my new partner gets herpes." If she feels that strongly, then she and her partner should use a condom every time they have intercourse.

If the partners plan to have children, they should know that if the woman develops herpes before delivering her child, it can lead to a cesarean section. If the couple has finished having children, the situation may be different. If one infects the other, it will be annoying and unpleasant—but usually not more than that, unless either feels that transmitting or getting herpes would be intolerable.

DIAGNOSING HERPES

If one of my patients has a painful genital area, blisters, and possibly pain with urination, I do a regular examination in stirrups. Often the skin of her genital area looks very sore and red. I check the blisters to see whether they are clustered, and I feel her lymph nodes, which may be swollen. To make the definitive diagnosis, I have to do a culture, so I gently touch one of the blisters with a Q-tip. If the touch is very painful, then I am quite sure of the diagnosis, but I send the Q-tip off to be cultured. The culture may take one or two days, perhaps a little longer.

Unless the patient's genital area is just too sore, I also check for gonorrhea and chlamydia; we have seen that STDs travel in company, and someone with one is at risk for others. If too painful, I invite her back for a follow-up visit in two weeks to culture for other STDs and discuss long-term management of the disease. I also check her genital area for bacterial infection, which is sometimes present.

If I am reasonably sure the problem is herpes, she and I talk about the problem even before the culture comes back from the laboratory. I also prescribe some painkiller, usually Percocet or codeine. I counsel her not to have sex until a week after her lesions are healed. If she is not already returning in two weeks for cultures, I invite her back so that we can discuss long-term management of her herpes.

▶ Is there a satisfactory treatment?

There are no medications that will cure herpes and make it go away forever. However, there are drugs that will minimize the pain of the symptoms and help prevent recurrences, reducing both their number and their severity.

The parent drug of the family is called acyclovir (trade name Zovirax). Its offspring include valacyclovir (Valtrex), famciclovir (Famvir), and ganciclovir (Cytovene), which is the most potent of the group and used for extremely severe infections. Zovirax and Denivir (which is more expensive) are available as creams as well. Although the tablets tend to act more quickly, some people prefer topical therapy.

In general, these drugs are well tolerated. They do not have severe side effects, like the drugs used for AIDs. They are quite expensive, though your insurance may help defray the cost.

▶ What are the chances that the disease will recur?

Probably 30–40 percent of those who get herpes will never have more than one episode, which gives anyone a fairly good chance of being in the lucky group. For the others, recurrences are likely to be much milder than the first episode. In general, recurrent episodes have only blisters and local pain, without the fever, malaise, rash, or headache of the first episode.

Often recurrences announce themselves by warning symptoms. Some women say they have a stinging feeling or a heightened awareness of the area where the recurrence will be. These warning symptoms are usually local and do not include generalized aches or pains.

▶ *What triggers recurrent episodes of herpes?*

Stress seems to be one factor. If you have herpes, try to decrease the anxiety levels in your life—though this is more easily said than done. The stresses can be physical, for example, surgery, illness, or fatigue. Sunburn or other skin irritation can also lead to a new outbreak of herpes. For some women, menstrual periods seem to stimulate recurrences of herpes. While you cannot stop your periods and the hormonal changes that accompany them, you can prepare for them and minimize the chance of herpes recurrence or reduce its severity.

▶ *Can you take antiviral drugs to prevent recurrences?*

Antiviral drugs will cut down on the severity and the frequency of recurrences. Some women do best by taking these drugs when they have the warning symptoms that a recurrence is coming. Early intervention can help head off a full-fledged, painful outbreak. In fact, some people take antivirals for long periods.

> Last spring Jessica, who had had several herpes attacks, was in graduate school studying for her comprehensive exams. She was working late into the night and in addition to being tired, she was anxious about passing. She knew that she always had flare-ups when under stress, so she asked me whether it would be a good idea for her to take acyclovir prophylactically during the exam period. I agreed emphatically that it was a perfect time for preventive medication. (I gave the same answer to another patient, who was getting married and had invited three hundred people to her wedding.)

▶ *Is it possible to take antiviral drugs indefinitely and prevent further herpes outbreaks?*

My nagging worry, unsupported by scientific research, is that it might be unwise to give on a long-term basis a drug that works by killing cells. Unless your immune system is compromised, herpes is not fatal; it seems reckless to prescribe acyclovir indefinitely, to prevent a few outbreaks.

▶ *Should you have more frequent checkups if you have had herpes?*

An annual gynecological checkup should be sufficient for women who have had past problems with herpes.

▶ *Is it safe to use antiviral medications during pregnancy?*

This is a controversial topic. For many years physicians would not use acyclovir or other antivirals at all during pregnancy. Nowadays it is a viable option for women who are close to delivery and have active lesions. We also follow up: if the patient is still shedding viruses after treatment (even though the lesions are gone), we do a cesarean section.

▶ *Is there any connection between herpes and cancer?*

No, there is not, although for a long time physicians did think that herpes could cause cervical cancer. When researchers performed blood tests on women with cervical cancer to measure the herpes antibody titers, and did the same on women who did not have cervical cancer, many more cancer patients had positive antibody titers to herpes. Therefore, the researchers concluded, herpes caused cervical cancer. However, the risk factors for cervical cancer are the same as the risk factors for herpes: early intercourse and multiple partners. There is also a connection between certain forms of human papilloma virus and cervical cancer, and since we know that STDs travel in company, someone who has herpes is at risk for having HPV as well. So if you have one STD, be sure to have a yearly Pap smear (which is advisable in any case).

▶ *Does herpes contribute to infertility?*

No, it does not, despite what many people think. Herpes will not block your tubes or give you pelvic inflammatory disease. The only way it contributes to infertility is by possibly making you unwilling to have intercourse for fear of infecting your partner.

▶ *Is it dangerous to have herpes if you are pregnant?*

Herpes is not dangerous to the mother during pregnancy, but it can be dangerous to the child if the mother has active lesions at the time of delivery. A baby born under those conditions is at high risk for herpes encephalitis and other herpes infections, so physicians encourage a woman with active herpes at the time of delivery to have a cesarean section. If during her next pregnancy, she does not have herpes at the time of delivery, it is likely that she can have a vaginal birth after the previous cesarean.

Sometimes a woman will request a cesarean section because she has had herpes in the past. I discourage that approach, because with 20 million American women infected with the herpes virus, obstetricians would be performing far too many unnecessary cesarean sections.

THE SOCIAL CONSEQUENCES OF HERPES

Many women are devastated to find out that they have herpes. No one wants to have this disease, partly because it is painful and unpleasant and partly because it carries a burden of social stigma. It has a reputation as a "dirty" disease; according to this mindset, the people who have it are low-class, inferior, evil people. Of course this is not true, but women do feel ashamed of themselves for having it, are very angry at the person who gave it to them, and feel guilty about giving it to someone else.

I have had only one patient who dealt with a herpes diagnosis in a matter-of-fact way. She was a professor of nursing at a prestigious university hospital. When I told her what she had, she said (though in rather stronger language), "Oh dammit, I'm really angry."

Herpes will not kill you and it should not ruin your life. But it may seriously stress your feelings for the person who gave it to you. I have noticed over the years that a relationship in which herpes is diagnosed usually falls apart because the woman does not want to stay with the partner who gave her the disease.

When I am counseling women who have come down with herpes, I try to lighten the psychological burden by pointing out that I take care of many fine, respectable people who have the disease: nursing professors, doctors, lawyers, and a woman who is working on a graduate degree in theology. Chicken pox can happen to anyone; herpes can happen to anyone who is sexually active.

▶ *Should you tell your partner that you have a history of herpes?*

I encourage you to be truthful about the situation, since you would want your partner to be the same with you. Unless you are honest with each other, the relationship will become precarious. Knowing this sometimes helps ease the embarrassment and social pain of being truthful about having a herpes infection.

Sondra was in her 50s, an executive assistant at a large company. She had always put her work ahead of her social life. She had never married and apparently had not had many relationships with men. Eventually she found a man whom she really liked and was very happy.

They had not been together very long when she came down with herpes. She was completely unstrung—by having the infection and also by her partner's unwillingness to be honest with her. In fact, she was so distressed that she wanted me to authorize a medical disability from work for six months. I didn't think I could do so in good conscience; once her lesions healed, she was fine physically. But I recognized that she couldn't deal emotionally with the fact that the second or third serious relationship of her life had soured so quickly. I referred her to a psychiatrist, with the understanding that if the psychiatrist found her emotionally incapable of doing her job, then she could get a statement of disability for that reason (as well as support).

Clearly, a diagnosis of herpes can have a more profound effect than the symptoms of the disease itself.

HUMAN PAPILLOMA VIRUS

Since HPV is not a disease like AIDS or syphilis that legally must be reported, epidemiological statistics are based on guesswork, but HPV is known to be widespread. At least 1 million new cases are reported each year and somewhere between 40 milliion and 50 million Americans are thought to have the disease. In 1997 the *American Journal of Medicine* published an article suggesting that nearly 74 percent of Americans have been infected with HPV at some point in their lives. Since perhaps two thirds of those infected do not have symptoms, HPV is surely more widespread than the numbers suggest. A survey of women of college age showed that 69 percent were infected.

Although HPV is not physically as painful or emotionally as stressful as herpes, it is a more dangerous disease, since it predisposes women to cancer of the cervix or vulva.

▶ *What causes genital warts?*

Human papilloma virus is an umbrella term that refers to a family of about seventy viruses that can cause warts (condylomas) anywhere on the body. These include common warts, plantar warts that show up on the soles of the feet, and even warty growths called polyps that appear on the vocal chords. Only a few subtypes of these viruses are sexually transmitted and cause genital or venereal warts.

▶ What are the symptoms?

About two thirds of individuals infected with the virus have no obvious or visible symptoms. If you do have warts, they can appear on the vulva or around the vagina or anus. They can be inside the vagina or on the cervix, on the groin, or on the thighs. They look like ordinary warts but may be larger, particularly if you are pregnant, or smaller—sometimes so small and flat that they can barely be seen with the naked eye. They can be single or grouped in clumps like cauliflower. Usually painless, they occasionally cause itching or bleeding.

▶ How do you get genital warts?

The disease is transmitted by direct contact with tissue infected with the virus, not necessarily with a visible wart. HPV is usually spread by sexual contact, but it is also possible for warts to be spread from the hands to the genital area by touching. On rare occasions an infected mother passes HPV to her infant during childbirth.

▶ Who is at high risk?

Sexually active men and women who have multiple sexual partners and who do not use condoms are most at risk for genital warts. You are also at increased risk if you have another STD or some condition that suppresses your immune system. White people are more at risk than others. Statistically, people between the ages of 15 and 24 are at higher risk than others, but they are more likely to have multiple sexual partners.

▶ How can you protect yourself from HPV and genital warts?

Use the same safe-sex techniques that protect you against other STDs: use condoms until all the warts have been eradicated. But remember that condoms protect only the tissue that is actually covered. If the scrotum is infected, contact with it may lead to transmission of the disease. In 2002, researchers developed a successful experimental vaccine against one strain of human papilloma virus, an encouraging first step toward the eventual prevention of many cases of cervical cancer.

▶ How is HPV diagnosed?

If you have a visible wart, the diagnosis is usually made simply by observing it. However, if an abnormal Pap smear suggests that you may have genital warts and the lesions are very small, your doctor may use a magnifying glass or a colposcope (a special kind of microscope used for examining the genital area).

▶ How is it treated?

HPV can be treated symptomatically, but it cannot be cured. About 25 percent of patients have recurrent outbreaks of warts within three months of treatment and there is no drug comparable to acyclovir to help ward off these recurrences. Medications and surgical procedures can treat the individual warts as they appear, destroying the skin of the infected area and the warts along with it. Trial and error is necessary until we find something that works.

The classic drug for treating the warts themselves is podophyllin, which is derived from the roots of a plant commonly known as May apple. Painted on small areas of the skin around the warts, it is washed off three or four hours later. Podophyllin cannot remain on the skin too long, nor can it be painted over large areas; it stings severely after a while, and if large amounts are absorbed through the skin, it can have serious side effects, including liver damage. Because of these problems podophyllin is usually administered by a physician in an office setting. It should not be used if you are pregnant.

A newer drug, podofilox (trade name Condylox) has been refined so that it does not get absorbed systemically and does not have the danger of liver toxicity. It comes as a gel, which you can use at home if your warts are on the surface of the skin. It cannot be used for warts on the mucous membranes, and it can irritate your skin. Trichloroacetic acid (TCA) is another medication sometimes used to remove external warts; it too can burn the tissue exposed to it.

Finally, a new cream called Aldara uses interferon, an antiviral protein normally produced by the body in response to viral infection, to stimulate the anti-inflammatory response to suppress the virus. Before Aldara came on the market, some physicians injected interferon into the infected area, but the treatment was expensive, produced adverse side effects, and was not more successful than other treatments. Aldara may cause redness around the area being treated.

Genital warts, like other warts, can be removed by heat or cold. They can be cauterized with an electric current or vaporized with a laser.

▶ *Is there any way to predict whether genital warts will recur after treatment?*

Some people have frequent recurrences; others do not have any. There is no way to predict the future of the disease. Recurrences often seem to come from reactivation of the virus, rather than reinfection from outside sources. You can have your warts completely removed, abstain from sex altogether, and still have a recurrence. People with immune systems compromised by HIV or physically stressful diseases like diabetes do seem to have more recurrences or are more easily infected.

> Rachel had recurrent episodes of genital warts, which kept coming back, no matter how vigorous the treatment. Fortunately her Pap smears have been normal. At one point she had a major flare-up, with many flourishing warts. Soon thereafter Rachel was diagnosed with diabetes. It is certainly possible that her elevated blood sugar levels and her diminished blood flow made her an easy target for infection. Since Rachel's diabetes has been treated and her blood sugars are under control, she has done very well.

▶ *Do genital warts cause cancer?*

Of the seventy varieties of the human papilloma virus (some of which cause genital warts) about three are associated with cancer, generally cancer of the cervix but occasionally cancer of the vagina or vulva. Certain tests, called vira-Paps, can reveal what strain of HPV you have. They are expensive and may not be covered by your health insurance.

If you have HPV, you should be conscientious about getting a yearly Pap smear. If the smear shows unusual changes in your cervical cells, you should have follow-up Pap tests and discuss options with your caregiver.

▶ *Are genital warts a problem during pregnancy and delivery?*

HPV does not seem to have any adverse effects on pregnancy, though pregnancy sometimes causes genital warts to grow rapidly. Babies born to HPV-infected women may have warts on or around their larynx, though that is rare. Podophyllin should not be used as a treatment during pregnancy. Cesarean sections are seldom performed because the mother has genital warts at the time of delivery.

GONORRHEA

Gonorrhea is one of the longest-known widespread diseases to afflict the human race. Fortunately, the advances of modern medicine and the control efforts of the Centers for Disease Control (CDC) have made serious inroads into the spread of gonorrhea in this country. After falling steadily from 1975 until 1997, rates gradually increased by 9 percent and thereafter remained about the same. While gonorrhea must by law be reported to the CDC, many cases probably go undetected or unreported. Estimates place the actual number of new cases anywhere from 600,000 to 2 million per year, many times the reported number (358,995 for the year 2000).

The disease remains one of the major causes of pelvic inflammatory disease, tubal infertility, pelvic pain, and ectopic pregnancy.

▶ *What causes gonorrhea?*

Gonorrhea is caused by a true bacterium named *Neisseria gonorrheae*—for Dr. Albert Neisser, who first described it in 1879. Gonorrhea bacteria live within cells, notably in the cervix in women and inside the urethra in men.

▶ *What are its symptoms?*

Perhaps 70–80 percent of women infected with gonorrhea have no symptoms whatsoever, which is frightening because untreated gonorrhea can cause pelvic inflammatory disease and infertility. Symptoms usually appear within ten days of the infection. They can include increased vaginal discharge, or a painful or smelly discharge; pain on urination; or pelvic pain. Since many women with vaginal gonorrheal infections also have rectal infections, there may be pain or itching in the rectal area. When the infection has been transmitted through oral sex, one symptom may be a very sore throat, like a strep throat.

Occasionally someone has what is called disseminated gonorrhea, which is a general inflammatory reaction. It may include a rash or arthritis, usually in a large joint such as the knee or elbow. Often people with this inflammatory reaction complain of pain in the arm or wrist. Another problem that may accompany disseminated gonorrhea is Fitz-Hugh-Curtis syndrome, a gonorrheal infection around the liver. Its symptoms can mimic those of gallbladder disease or hepatitis. The classic sign of this disease, violin-string adhesions, can be seen only if surgery is performed.

Elissa was about 40 years old when a surgeon colleague referred her to me to make sure her problem was really gallbladder disease. The x-rays did not definitively suggest that disease, although Elissa had several of its risk factors, which we call the five Fs: female, fair, fertile, forty, and fat. Elissa was the right age, she was certainly female, fair, and plump, though she did not have children.

The surgeon wondered whether Elissa might have Fitz-Hugh-Curtis syndrome. I examined her, decided my colleague might well be right, and ordered tetracycline for Elissa, who got better.

Two years later she needed a hysterectomy, which was performed by a partner in my practice. She discovered that Elissa had abscesses on both her fallopian tubes and ovaries, a finding that suggested she had had pelvic inflammatory disease following the gonorrhea.

Although the symptoms of gonorrhea are unpleasant and even painful, they do alert you to the fact that you have an illness. Therefore you are likely to seek help and be treated before permanent damage occurs.

Men infected with gonorrhea usually, but not always, have symptoms: a discharge or drip from the penis, painful urination, or the need to urinate frequently. Formerly it was thought that men always had symptoms, but about fifteen years ago a study of army recruits in basic training (researchers took urethral swabs of every man who walked in the door) found that there was a huge reservoir of gonorrhea in men who had no symptoms whatsoever. This was really bad news, since it meant that men can be carriers of gonorrhea without knowing it.

▶ *How do you get gonorrhea?*

Gonorrhea is transmitted by direct contact from mucous membrane to mucous membrane. It can be transmitted to the mouth during oral sex and to the anus or rectum during anal sex. Newborns traveling through an infected birth canal can get gonococcal eye infections, which if left untreated can cause blindness.

▶ *Who is at high risk?*

Anyone with multiple sexual partners is at increased risk for gonorrhea. Risk increases if you have another STD. Women are at higher risk than men. It has been estimated that a man having unprotected sex once with an infected partner has a 20–25 percent chance of catching the disease, while a woman's risk under the same circumstances is 80–90 percent. Statistically, city dwellers, adolescents, people with past gonorrheal infections, and drug users are at increased risk—perhaps because people in these groups indulge in high-risk behavior.

▶ Will condoms prevent the transmission of gonorrhea?

If used properly, latex condoms can protect against exposure to gonorrhea bacteria. Spermicides may also offer some protection.

▶ How is gonorrhea diagnosed?

The infection can be diagnosed in women without symptoms by culturing tissue from the infected area, usually the cervix. Your doctor will probably also test for chlamydia at the same time.

▶ How is gonorrhea treated?

Because gonorrhea is caused by a bacterium, not a virus, it can be treated successfully with antibiotics. For many years the appropriate drug was penicillin taken as injections, or ampicillin taken as tablets. However, ten or fifteen years ago in this country, the bacterium started to become resistant to these drugs. When the resistance rate reached about 6 percent, physicians changed drugs. Two new families of drugs were introduced, cephalosporins and quinolones. The current drug of choice for gonorrhea is ceftriaxone, given as a single intramuscular injection in the buttocks. Other frequently used drugs are ciprofloxacin and ofloxacin, both given orally in a single dose.

If you are allergic to cephalosporins or quinolones, you can take tetracycline or doxycycline, which are given as pills. Therapy with tetracycline or doxycycline lasts a week; one dose will not cure you.

If you are diagnosed with gonorrhea, you will also be treated for chlamydia. Because these two diseases occur together so frequently, the CDC recommends that any woman treated for gonorrhea should also be treated for chlamydia, whether her culture for that disease is positive or negative. If you are taking tetracycline or doxycycline for gonorrhea, it will halt the chlamydia as well.

Gonorrhea is a reportable disease; your physician is required by law to notify the local board of health of all cases. The CDC recommends that any sexual partner you have had in the past thirty days also be treated. If you do have gonorrhea, your physician will ask about your partners and see that they are treated, either by your doctor or their own physicians.

▶ *Should you have a follow-up visit after you've been treated?*

I always recommend a follow-up culture to make sure the medication has eradicated the infection. Occasionally there are "failures," though in many cases these are probably reinfections. Certainly you should contact your physician if your symptoms persist after therapy.

CHLAMYDIA

Chlamydia is probably the least-known of the common STDs, but it is the most common and one of the most dangerous in terms of long-term implications. In women, chlamydia often leads to pelvic inflammatory disease, which can cause infertility, ectopic pregnancy, and chronic pelvic pain. Statistics gathered by the CDC suggest that about 30 percent of women with untreated chlamydia will become infertile. Because many women have no symptoms at all, this "silent" PID can compromise their fertility without their being aware of it. Pregnant women with chlamydia can infect their infants during delivery.

Unlike gonorrhea and syphilis, which have been around for centuries, chlamydia is apparently relatively new, at least in epidemic proportions. It seems to have been seen first in Scandinavia, and Swedish researchers were the first to document and seriously study the organism that causes chlamydia. It was not until the 1970s that health authorities recognized it as a major concern.

Chlamydia, along with gonorrhea and syphilis, is one of three diseases for which there is a federally funded program of surveillance and control. In 2000, 702,093 chlamydial infections were reported to the CDC, approximately twice the number of reported cases of gonorrhea, and the rate of infection with chlamydia is skyrocketing. Especially distressing is the fact that the highest rates are among adolescents, young women who are most at risk for the damage that can be caused by PID. In view of all these alarming data, it is encouraging that in parts of the United States where programs exist to screen for chlamydia and treat it, the prevalence of the disease has steadily declined.

▶ *What causes chlamydia?*

It is caused by a bacterium called *Chlamydia trachomatis,* which in some ways resembles a virus. Like any bacterium, it has a cell wall that can be attacked by antibiotics; like a virus, it must exist parasitically within body cells to live and reproduce. For these reasons chlamydia bacteria are difficult to culture and to diagnose by cell culture, but relatively easy to treat.

▶ What are the symptoms?

Unfortunately, in 50–70 percent of cases chlamydia has no symptoms; it can go quietly about its work without your ever knowing you have it. When symptoms do appear, they are similar to those of gonorrhea: a discharge from the vagina, pain on urination, pus in the urine, and irritation of the labia or vaginal area. Men may have burning or pain during urination or a discharge from the urethra but, like women, they may have no symptoms. If symptoms of the disease are to appear, they will usually do so a week or two after the infection.

If the disease has progressed from a simple infection of the cervix to involvement of the whole pelvis, symptoms may include general pelvic pain, fever, vaginal discharge, and painful intercourse. It is again possible to have a pelvic infection without symptoms or warning signs.

▶ How do you get chlamydia?

Chlamydia is transmitted through vaginal, anal, or (less frequently) oral sex with an infected partner. It can be spread even when the infected person has no symptoms.

▶ Who is at risk?

You are at increased risk for chlamydia if you have more than one sexual partner, or if your partner has multiple partners. You are at heightened risk if you are under the age of 20, although in part this comes about because people under the age of 20 are more likely to have multiple sexual partners than are older people. You are at increased risk if you are a woman: statistics suggest that men stand a 20-percent chance of becoming infected from one act of unprotected intercourse with an infected woman, whereas 40 percent of women having one act of unprotected intercourse with an infected man will come down with the infection.

▶ How can you protect yourself?

Condoms with the additional use of a spermicide are the best protection against chlamydia.

▶ How is chlamydia diagnosed?

Tests for chlamydia are getting more accurate, more user friendly, and less expensive. The most reliable test used to be a cell culture done in a laboratory of a sample of the secretions from your cervix or urethra. If chlamydia grew in the culture, then you were infected. This test was technically difficult for the lab workers and expensive to the patient.

In the late 1980s, scientists developed tests that use sophisticated techniques to detect bacterial proteins and identify the DNA of the chlamydia organism in genital secretions. These tests, which can be used for both men and women, give results even if no symptoms of chlamydia are present; they are quicker and less expensive than the cell culture tests. The secretions can be obtained by applying a Q-tip to the cervix or, in men, by applying a swab to the tip of the urethra.

Recently, the U.S. Food and Drug Administration (FDA) approved the use of these newer tests on a urine sample. This is a major step in diagnosing chlamydial infection, in that it does not require an invasive sample; it can be used in settings where performing a pelvic examination would not be convenient, for example in college health services or at health fairs. Results from the urine test are available within twenty-four hours and are quite accurate.

The presence of chlamydia can also be indicated by a blood test, which looks for antibodies to the bacteria that cause chlamydia. If you have these antibodies, then at some time you have been exposed to chlamydia bacteria. While this test does not inform you about your present status, it can be useful after the fact in treating someone who turns up with infertility because of damaged fallopian tubes.

A laboratory technician takes a blood sample and tests it for the presence of chlamydia. If it is positive, the technician dilutes the sample and tests again with the half-strength sample. If it is positive again, the technician continues with successive dilutions 1:2, 1:4, 1:8, 1:16, until the test no longer is positive. If you have a titer of 1:1,024, then the original sample had to be diluted ten times before the sample tested negative. That means that the infection is very, very significant. Even if your disease is later cured, you will still test positive for chlamydia, though your titer will probably not be as high.

A few years ago I was asked to testify as an expert witness in a case involving Nancy, who was infertile. She had had pelvic inflammatory disease, which she blamed on having used a Dalkon Shield a number of years before.

In 1986, years before she decided to sue the Dalkon Shield company, Nancy had a chlamydia titer done as part of an infertility workup. Her physician was one of the few at that time who was doing that test, and it came out strongly positive; Nancy had a very high titer of 512, indicating a significant infection.

In 1996, when Nancy was preparing her lawsuit, she had another titer done, inasmuch as she did not believe the first one. This turned out to be a mistake on her part, because the test still showed a titer of 512. Nancy's case was thrown out of court. She could not blame her infertility on the Dalkon Shield if she had had a serious chlamydia infection. Chlamydia, we know, comes from sexual intercourse, not from IUDs.

▶ *What is the treatment for chlamydia?*

The drugs used for chlamydia are similar to those for gonorrhea. Of the recommended antibiotics, most doctors prescribe doxycycline, which can be taken in a seven-day course of treatment, or a newer drug azithromycin (Zithromax), which can be given in one dose. Other drugs used to combat this infection are ofloxacin and erythromycin. Women whose infection has progressed to PID may require intravenous antibiotic therapy.

Once the symptoms have been relieved, a follow-up culture will ensure that the antibiotics have eradicated the disease and that you have not been reinfected. You and your partner should refrain from intercourse during treatment.

▶ *Should your partner also be tested if you have chlamydia?*

If the test shows you have been infected with chlamydia, you should notify all of your sexual partners, so that further spread of this disease can be stopped. You and your partner(s) need to be retested after therapy for a so-called test of cure, to be sure you are no longer infectious.

▶ *Is chlamydia dangerous during pregnancy?*

Yes, chlamydia can lead to preterm birth or miscarriage. Infants born to infected mothers are at increased risk for eye infections and pneumonia. Trachoma, carried by *Chlamydia trachomatis,* is a classic eye infection of the Third World.

SYPHILIS

Syphilis has been around since ancient times and was described in Chinese medical writings as early as 2000 B.C. It was rampant in Europe from the fifteenth century on and has afflicted famous historical and artistic figures, including the composer Franz Schubert. Though the organism that causes syphilis is susceptible to several antibiotics, the disease is still with us today. About fifteen years ago it seemed that syphilis would disappear permanently in this country, just as smallpox has been eradicated in the world; but as the AIDs epidemic intensified in the late 1980s, the incidence of syphilis rose before falling to the lowest levels since 1941 and then rising again slightly. Because syphilis is a disease that must by law be reported to the local board of health and to the CDC and often has serious consequences, epidemiologists believe these figures to be reasonably accurate.

▶ *What causes syphilis?*

Syphilis is caused by a spiral-shaped bacterium (spirochete) named *Treponema pallidum,* which is closely related to the organism that causes Lyme disease. The organism takes a long time to reproduce itself, so syphilis develops slowly.

▶ *What are its symptoms?*

While syphilis is easy to treat, it can be difficult to recognize, in part because it develops slowly and systemically (unlike gonorrhea, for example, whose main symptoms are genital). Syphilis has three separate stages—primary, secondary, and tertiary—whose symptoms are very different.

The main symptom of primary syphilis is a small painless sore, usually only one, that appears between ten and ninety days after contact at the site of the infection—usually, in women, in the vagina, labia, cervix, rectum, or elsewhere in the genital area. The sore, called a chancre, is not a blister but a raised area with a cavity in the middle. Although it may look red and irritated, it does not hurt and it goes away in three to nine weeks, whether treated or left alone. If the chancre appears on the cervix or in the vagina, it may be difficult to notice. It is unfortunate, in a way, that the chancre is painless and goes away without treatment, because these characteristics may keep infected people from seeking medical attention. If untreated, syphilis can become a systemic disease, attacking other body systems.

Secondary syphilis, which can develop in about six weeks (it can take as long as six months) after the primary stage, has symptoms that can be genital or more widespread. The genital symptom is something called a condyloma lata, a big, flat genital wart, larger and wider than the genital warts caused by HPV. Not everyone who has secondary syphilis has a condyloma, but most people have systemic symptoms similar to those of a generalized virus: fever, swollen lymph nodes, and the all-over wretched feeling that accompanies viral illnesses. These flu-like symptoms last between three days and a week, and the other symptoms persist longer.

Another symptom is a generalized rash that resembles the kind that accompanies many allergies. The rash may occur in a number of places on the body, including the palms of the hands and the soles of the feet. While it may seem odd to think of dermatologists dealing with STDs, they do treat syphilis; in Europe they even advertise themselves as "venereologists." The father-in-law of one of my friends was a Russian émigré, a famous dermatologist who lived in Milan in the 1930s and treated Mussolini's children for their recurrent episodes of syphilis.

Secondary syphilis can cause your hair to fall out. Of course, most hair loss is not caused by secondary syphilis, but it is a symptom doctors use to differentiate between other viral illnesses and syphilis.

Then, whether you treat it or not, secondary syphilis goes into a period of dormancy or latency, where it shows no symptoms at all even though the spirochete is still present in the body and would show up on a blood test. This latent period can last as long as ten or twenty years, even the entire life of the infected person. Tertiary syphilis is quite rare nowadays because most infections are caught and treated long before the later symptoms appear.

At any time during the latent period, however, the spirochetes can reawaken to assault and kill cells in any organ system in the body. They may also form gummas, hard nodules under the skin or in the internal organs. Tertiary syphilis can attack the liver or bone or even the brain, where it can cause neurological disorders ranging from staggering to general insanity. Before therapy was available, people frequently died because syphilis attacked the aorta, the big blood vessel leading out from the heart. It would weaken the vessel wall and the resulting aneurysm, a blister-like bulge, could rupture and cause death.

▶ How is syphilis spread?

Syphilis is usually transmitted by direct sexual contact with an infected person who has an open sore. It can be spread from penis to vagina or vice versa. Syphilis transmitted by an untreated infected mother through the placenta to her unborn child is called congenital syphilis and is, fortunately, decreasing nowadays. The *Treponema pallidum*, which thrives in a warm moist atmosphere, can invade unbroken mucous membranes but is unlikely to invade dry, unbroken skin. In rare instances syphilis has been transmitted through deep kissing.

The disease is most infectious during its early stages of infection when there is an open sore, but it is believed that a person can transmit the disease for about four years after being infected.

▶ Who is at risk?

You are at increased risk for syphilis if you have casual sex or multiple sex partners and do not use a condom. You are also at increased risk if you have some other condition that lowers your immune response; people with HIV are especially vulnerable.

▶ How is syphilis diagnosed?

Syphilis is one of the diseases for which widespread testing has existed for many years. A German bacteriologist, August von Wassermann, developed the first blood test in 1907. When you apply for a marriage license, you are required by some states to have a blood test to screen for syphilis. You will also have a blood test for syphilis when you are pregnant. Newborn babies are screened for syphilis, using blood taken from the umbilical cord.

The most commonly performed blood test to screen for syphilis is called a VDRL, named for the Venereal Disease Research Laboratory where the test was developed. The VDRL is a nonspecific test that measures antibodies called cardiolipins, which your body makes in response to syphilis and a number of other inflammatory diseases. A positive VDRL indicates that you could have been exposed to several different diseases, of which syphilis is only one. There is a more specific test for syphilis, which is called an FTA-ABS (fluorescent treponemal antibody absorption test). This test checks specifically for the organism *Treponema pallidum* that causes syphilis, but is so expensive and tricky to evaluate that it is not useful as a general screening test. The FTA test is done to evaluate the VDRL more definitively.

You will want to recognize that a positive VDRL test does not necessarily mean that you have syphilis. The VDRL looks for antibodies that are brought into play by a whole range of diseases; infectious diseases such as mononucleosis can give a positive VDRL, as can hepatitis and collagen vascular diseases such as lupus and rheumatoid arthritis. Because the organism that causes Lyme disease, an infectious disease carried by deer ticks, resembles *T. pallidum*, people with Lyme disease may have positive VDRLs.

I saw my first positive marital syphilis test about twenty years ago, when I had been in practice for only a few years. Claire was an executive at a prestigious local

corporation. She came to the reception desk at the office to pick up the paperwork for the two premarital blood tests required by the state of Connecticut—
one for syphilis and the other for rubella (German measles). Her wedding was
only a few days away.

My secretary handed me the slip from the lab, which previously had always
required only a routine signature. Back before the AIDs epidemic changed
everyone's preconceptions about syphilis and other infectious disease, I did not
expect to see a positive test among my well-educated, middle-class patients, but I
always looked over the results. Claire's test showed a 4+ positive VDRL and a 4+
positive FTA. Tests are graded as strongly positive or weakly positive, and Claire's
tests showed active disease requiring treatment. I knew that this young woman
did not have lupus or another disease that might affect her VDRL. I took Claire
into one of our private areas and broke the bad news.

Claire had no idea. She must obviously have had a rash at some point, which
she attributed to a virus or food she had eaten. It went away and she thought no
more of it. She simply did not remember. I pointed out that if she had a 4+ positive syphilis test, it was highly likely that her fiancé had syphilis as well. When he
was tested, it turned out that he too was 4+ positive on the VDRL and FTA.

I have no idea who gave what to whom, but before Claire and her fiancé could
marry they had to start receiving therapy. We began treatment immediately. I
also sent Claire for a lumbar puncture to test for syphilis in her spinal fluid, because we had no idea how far the disease had progressed or whether it was attacking her nervous system, even though she did not have symptoms. We were
all pleased when the spinal test was negative.

Claire and her fiancé did get married, but shortly thereafter they moved away
from this part of the country, so I do not know whether their marriage survived
this psychological trauma.

I have seen one or two positive tests during pregnancy:

Bethany, an educated and well-to-do interior designer, had a fight with her husband and went off to Acapulco in a huff. While there, she found a lover and had a
sexual adventure, unfortunately unprotected. Shortly after she returned, she realized that she was pregnant. When she was given a blood test for syphilis because of the pregnancy, we discovered that she also had syphilis.

Bethany was able to figure out that she had been pregnant before she went to Mexico, but the test early in her pregnancy saved her fetus from possible serious deformities. She felt guilty during the entire pregnancy, but was fortunate that her behavior did not cause more unhappiness than it did.

Some states require only one syphilis test, given at the beginning of the pregnancy. Because syphilis will not be passed along to the fetus if the mother is treated before the fourth month or so of pregnancy, this early test is crucial. Other states require two tests, one early in the pregnancy and a later one to detect infection that may have been contracted during the pregnancy. I have had a few patients who were negative during the first trimester and tested positive at the end of their pregnancy.

▶ What is the treatment for syphilis?

Fortunately syphilis, unlike some strains of gonorrhea, is still sensitive to penicillin and can be cured in any stage, though organ damage caused by tertiary syphilis cannot be reversed. Nor can we "cure" the malformations caused by syphilis in a baby whose mother was infected. It is critically important to have the disease diagnosed—both for yourself and for your unborn children.

Even before penicillin was discovered, there was therapy for syphilis. It involved the use of heavy metals and had severe side effects. In 1909 a German bacteriologist, Paul Ehrlich, discovered a compound heavily laden with arsenic, which became the first effective treatment. He called it Compound 606, because he found it on his 606th try, and later had it marketed as Salversan. A 1940 movie with Edward G. Robinson called *Dr. Ehrlich's Magic Bullet* dramatizes Ehrlich's unflagging search (which I often use to point out to my students the virtues of patience and determination).

Penicillin brought a real breakthrough, and it is still an excellent drug for therapy. The CDC has developed formulas for dosages, based on the amount of organ involvement. If involvement seems minor, then a shot or two of penicillin may be all that is required. If diagnostic tests suggest that the syphilis spirochetes may be attacking the spinal cord or the brain, then the course of penicillin will be long and massive.

HEPATITIS B

Hepatitis is inflammation of the liver. It can be caused by viruses, bacteria, exposure to toxic chemicals (including alcohol, drugs, and poisonous mushrooms). Hepatitis can get better by itself within a few months or, in a minority of cases of certain types of the disease, become chronic or even fatal.

▶ What causes hepatitis B?

The hepatitis virus occurs in four forms: A, B, C, and D. While hepatitis is not usually thought of as an STD, one of its forms, hepatitis B, can be spread through sexual contact.

▶ What are its symptoms?

Many people who have the virus in their blood have no symptoms, but these carriers can unknowingly spread the virus to others. The symptoms, if they appear, may take up to six months from the time of infection to appear. They generally resemble the symptoms of flu or any viral illness: fatigue, fever, loss of appetite, and aching joints or muscles. In addition, you may have jaundice—which yellows your skin and the whites of your eyes, and darkens your urine. Some people have itching. About 10 percent of people who get hepatitis B develop chronic liver infections that can lead to cirrhosis (which destroys liver cells) and increase the risk of liver cancer.

▶ How do you get hepatitis B?

The virus is easily transmitted; if your sexual partner has it, you will get it. Hepatitis B can also be spread by sharing needles for intravenous drug use and by other contact with contaminated blood. Mothers can transmit it to their children at birth. Hepatitis B can have serious consequences and even be fatal.

▶ How can you avoid hepatitis B?

As with other STDs, condoms are the first line of defense. Fortunately, there is a vaccine for this disease. The possibility of transmitting hepatitis B through sexual activity is one of the motivating factors for immunizing children against this disease. Health care workers who are exposed to blood or blood products should also be immunized, as should anyone of any age who has several sexual partners. College health services may offer hepatitis vaccination. The immunization consists of three shots, the first two a month apart, the third six months later.

▶ How is hepatitis B diagnosed?

Hepatitis is diagnosed through its symptoms (jaundice, an enlarged liver) and through a blood test.

▶ How is it treated?

As with other viral illnesses, there is no cure. Treatment consists of relieving the symptoms—controlling fever with antiviral and anti-inflammatory medications.

HIV/AIDS

The global epidemic of AIDS (acquired immunodeficiency syndrome) is one of the sad facts of life in the twenty-first century. According to a report issued by UNAIDS, the worldwide AIDS program of the United Nations, at the end of 2001 about 40 million people worldwide were infected with this incurable viral disease, including 800,000–900,000 in this country. Every day, 14,000 more people worldwide are infected. Since the epidemic began, about 22 million people, including 448,000 in the United States, have died of HIV infections.

Although no cure for HIV/AIDS has been found, physicians today have better weapons for combating it, including combinations of antiviral medications that prolong life and delay onset of the most devastating stage of the disease. Because of these therapies, HIV/AIDS has dropped from first to fifth place (behind accidents) as the leading killer of people between the ages of 25 and 44, though it is still the leading cause of death among black men in that age group. The CDC reports that during the years 1995–1999, the number of deaths declined 67 percent. However, the number of new cases among women is increasing, and in 2000 women accounted for 30 percent of new cases of HIV infection. African American and Hispanic women constituted 80 percent of these cases reported in women.

Despite the fact that AIDS is preventable, the two types of high-risk behavior that account for its transmission—sexual activity and intravenous drug use—are extremely difficult to change. Sexual activity is powerfully motivated, and intravenous drug use leads to addiction and thus loss of control. But education and understanding have, at least in this country, been able to slow the spread of HIV/AIDS.

▶ *What causes AIDS?*

AIDS is the final stage of infection by HIV, the human immunodeficiency virus. This virus, which is transmitted through bodily fluids, attacks T-lymphocytes, the white blood cells whose job is to fight off infection. In particular, the virus kills off a subspecies of these T-cells called CD4 cells, which have a concentration of about 1,000 per cu mm of blood in healthy people; in some individuals with AIDS, the concentration drops well below 200 per cu mm. As the virus gradually impairs the immune system by killing off CD4 cells, the body falls prey to infections that normally it could easily ward off.

As more has been learned, epidemiologists at the CDC have refined the definition of the disease. People who have the less severe infections that usually precede the onset of full-blown AIDS are said to have HIV, HIV disease, or ARC (an older term, less widely used today, that stands for AIDS-related complex). Nowadays the acronym HIV/AIDS is used to describe the whole process of the disease.

▶ *What are the symptoms of HIV/AIDS?*

Before fully developed AIDS appears, the disease exhibits a number of warning symptoms that include chronic fever, extreme fatigue, unintended weight loss, night sweats, fungus infections (including recurrent yeast infections in the vagina or mouth), swollen lymph glands, and diarrhea.

All these common symptoms can be caused by many different diseases and do not usually indicate an HIV infection. Many women have yeast infections at one time or another; we all experience fatigue; night sweats can be a sign of other diseases or even of approaching menopause. The difference is usually one of degree: we are all prone to fatigue, but the kind of fatigue associated with AIDS is truly debilitating and goes on and on, regardless of whether you get adequate rest.

▶ *How long does it take the symptoms to appear?*

The HIV virus may lie dormant for years before any symptoms appear. The average time between infection and appearance of the first definitive symptoms is about ten years, though men seem to show symptoms more quickly than women.

▶ *Are there symptoms specific to women?*

HIV/AIDS can cause gynecological problems or it can make existing problems difficult to treat. Recurrent vaginal yeast infections that resist treatment can be a sign of HIV/AIDS, as can abnormal Pap smears and pelvic inflammatory disease (PID). Women with HIV/AIDS are at increased risk for infection by the human papilloma virus (HPV), which causes genital warts. Some strains of HPV have been associated with cervical abnormalities and cervical cancer.

▶ *How is HIV/AIDS spread?*

Although the HIV virus can be found in most body fluids of infected people (blood, semen, vaginal secretions, tears, breast milk, saliva), it is relatively difficult to spread: the fluid of an infected person must enter the body of someone who is not infected, usually through a cut or break in the skin or mucous membranes.

HIV/AIDS can be spread by sexual contact, including vaginal and anal intercourse. If your vagina or external genitals have abrasions, sores, or other breaks in the mucous membranes, your risk is greatly increased. If you have another STD, such as gonorrhea, syphilis, herpes, or chlamydia, you are at greater risk for HIV. It is estimated that about two thirds of the people who have HIV/AIDS in this country got it during sexual intercourse with an infected partner. It can be spread from male to male, from male to female, from female to male, and (in theory at least) from female to female.

It can be transmitted through infected needles. Drug users who share needles are at extremely high risk. There have been cases of medical workers being infected through needle pricks from infected patients.

HIV/AIDS can be spread through blood transfusions. In the early years of the epidemic, before the nature of transmission was understood, a number of hemophiliacs, who receive routine blood transfusions, were infected, as were hundreds of people who received transfusions during surgical procedures. Since 1985 all donated blood in the United States has been screened for HIV. The disease can also be spread through artificial insemination, if the donor sperm is infected. All reliable sperm banks, like blood banks, currently screen for HIV, so this is a remote possibility.

The disease can be spread from a pregnant mother to her child, either during pregnancy or during labor and delivery. It can even be spread from mother to child during breast-feeding, though this is rare.

HIV/AIDS cannot be spread by casual contact, for example, by shaking hands, hugging, sharing eating utensils, or telephones. It cannot be spread through exposure to the sweat or tears of an infected person. It cannot be spread through swimming pools in which infected people have swum or through water fountains. It cannot be transmitted through the bites of mosquitoes, ticks, or other insects.

As with many other viruses, people are contagious when recently infected, even before they have symptoms.

▶ Who is at risk for HIV/AIDS?

Most people who have HIV or AIDS got it either by having unprotected sex with an infected partner or by sharing a hypodermic needle with an infected person. Anyone who engages in these activities is at high risk.

▶ Are women as much at risk as men?

When HIV/AIDS first appeared in this country around 1981, it was thought to be a disease that targeted gay males, so during the early 1980s it was sometimes called GRIDS (gay-related immunodeficiency syndrome). This name suggested that women might not be at risk, an assumption that has turned out to be utterly false. As the gay community developed strategies for dealing with HIV/AIDS, the epidemic shifted its focus to intravenous drug users and their sex partners, so today transmission increasingly takes place through heterosexual sex.

HIV/AIDS, like other STDs, is blind to gender and sexual orientation. In 1981 there were 6 reported cases in women. Five years later, 2,000 women had the disease. By 1993, there were 40,000 infected women. The most recent figures (2001 report) from the CDC suggest that between 800,000 and 900,000 people in the United States now live with HIV. Thirty percent of the 40,000 people who are newly infected with HIV each year are women. In Africa, where the epidemic has spread more widely than in the United States, heterosexual contact is the principal means of transmission; men and women are equally affected. Although the impact of the epidemic in the United States is greatest among men who have sex with men, and among racial and ethnic minorities, the number of cases among women and those transmitted by heterosexual activity has increased.

In several ways women are more at risk than men. First of all, more men are infected than women, at least right now in the United States. Therefore women have a greater chance statistically of selecting an infected partner. Second, the female anatomy puts women at increased risk. Seminal fluid, which contains more virus than vaginal fluids do, stays within the female genital tract for hours, giving the virus more time to infect its target cells. Furthermore, the vagina provides more surface area for infected fluids than does the male urethra. Women who have an STD, such as gonorrhea or chlamydia, are even more vulnerable to HIV infection, since inflamed cells become prime targets for the virus.

▶ How can you decrease your risk?

Knowing how HIV/AIDS is spread is the start of an effective defense. Abstinence from sexual intercourse is, of course, the perfect preventive. Unless you are absolutely and totally certain that you and your sexual partner are 100 percent monogamous, practicing safe sex each and every time you have intercourse can reduce risk. Remember that in terms of HIV susceptibility, when you have intercourse you are exposed to everyone your partner has been exposed to. You may be monogamous; but if your partner has casual sex, it is the same in terms of HIV risk as having casual sex yourself.

The CDC recommends that when women are receiving oral sex they use a "dam" (also called a dental dam, or a mouth dam). This device is a thin plastic sheet similar to plastic wrap placed over the woman's genital area. A dental dam can also be made from a latex condom, by snipping off the reservoir tip and making a lengthwise cut to open the tubular part of the condom into a flat sheet.

As far as HIV is concerned, safe sex means using a latex condom and preferably a spermicide as well. People who use intravenous drugs should not share needles with anyone.

▶ Are condoms totally safe in protecting against HIV/AIDS?

Nothing, short of total sexual abstinence, is 100 percent safe. But condoms are the most effective means we have in preventing the spread of HIV/AIDS and other sexually transmitted diseases.

Choose condoms made of latex, which has been shown to prevent the passage of the HIV virus, the herpes virus, and the microorganisms that cause other sexually transmitted diseases. "Natural" lambskin condoms do not offer this degree of protection. The package in which the condoms are sold should state that they prevent STDs; condoms bearing this message have passed tests required by the FDA. The condom should unroll to cover the entire penis.

▶ *Are condoms safe for use during anal intercourse?*

The Surgeon General, who conveys official U.S. public health policy, has said that "condoms do provide some protection, but anal intercourse is simply too dangerous a practice." Condoms may be more likely to break during this type of intercourse because of the greater friction, though using a lubricant may help.

▶ *Will you be better protected using a spermicide along with a condom?*

In laboratory experiments the spermicide nonoxynol-9 has been shown to kill the organisms that cause other STDs; researchers believe it may kill the HIV virus as well. So it is wise to use a spermicide as an added precaution along with a condom, but do not rely on the spermicide alone. Spermicides come packaged with an expiration date; do not use products whose expiration date has passed. Spermicidal creams are not as effective as we once thought, but they still are better than nothing.

▶ *Is one type of unprotected sex riskier than another?*

No accurate statistics are available on the relative risk, but probably anal sex is the riskiest, in that the tissues of the rectum are thinner and more delicate than those of the vagina. Oral sex is probably not riskier than vaginal sex, but the problem is that many people do not use condoms with oral sex and find dental dams unpleasant.

▶ *How is HIV/AIDS diagnosed?*

HIV is diagnosed by a two-step blood test, which is reliable and relatively inexpensive. The first step, called the Elisa (enzyme-linked immunosorbent asssay), looks for the presence of HIV antibodies in the blood. When a virus enters the body, the immune system responds by making antibodies to that particular virus. Some antibodies protect from disease, but the antibodies produced by HIV do not. Nor do they prevent the infected person from spreading the disease. If the test shows that these antibodies are present, the laboratory technicians proceed to step two, the Western blot test, which confirms the diagnosis. Because of the social, psychological, and medical impact of a positive diagnosis, all HIV/AIDS testing programs should include counseling.

▶ *If you have unprotected sex with someone whose history you don't know, can you take any preventive measures before you become HIV positive?*

You can certainly request that your partner have an emergency HIV test. If his test is positive, you can try prophylactic medications. This HIV testing can be done within one or two days, and you can get the results a day or two later.

AZT, which is used to treat HIV, can also be used to help prevent it. As a preventive treatment, it works best immediately after exposure, so if you have had intercourse with a high-risk person, consult your physician or the CDC national AIDS hotline: (800) 342-AIDS. The preventive drugs are reasonably effective but have significant side effects, just like the drugs used to treat HIV/AIDS. Of course, if your partner was recently infected with HIV, the test will not show it; unless your partner is retested a few months later, you will not accurately know his or her status.

▶ *If you think you have been exposed to HIV, should you get tested?*

Yes, and for very good reasons. If you find that you are infected with HIV, prompt medical care can delay the onset of serious symptoms. You can avoid infecting others. If you are thinking about becoming pregnant, you will want to consider the possibility of infecting a child (see Chapter 11).

Some people cope better with knowing than with not knowing. For others, the stress of knowing that they are infected is far worse. They fear that their test results will become public without their permission, and that if the results are known, they will be discriminated against. Even if you decide against testing, you should act to prevent spreading possible HIV to your sex partners.

▶ *If you think you have been exposed to HIV, how long should you wait before being tested?*

Most people who have been infected with HIV produce antibodies within three months. If you were tested shortly after you were exposed and your test is negative, you should have a second test about three months later. Researchers believe that more than 99 percent of infected people will test positive after six months.

▶ *Is the test always accurate?*

Only rarely does the test give a false positive, saying that you have been exposed to HIV when you have not. But if you are tested too soon, the test may register a false negative, saying that you are not infected when in fact you are. This is why is it wise to wait three months before being tested. Sometimes a woman calls me in a panic; she had unprotected sex the night before and is concerned about HIV. I counsel waiting: even though those three months will be difficult and anxious, the test results will be accurate.

▶ *How much does HIV/AIDS testing cost?*

HIV/AIDS testing costs forty to fifty dollars in a commercial lab. Most insurance companies will cover the cost, but will then know your results. Although your insurance company cannot legally drop you as a client because you are HIV positive, it may be worth the fifty dollars to maintain your privacy.

▶ *Can you control who knows the results of your test?*

If there is a reasonable chance your test will be positive, you can have it performed anonymously. Ask your doctor to give you a blood slip giving you a fictitious name or just a number. When you get to the lab, pay with cash, not a credit card or check. Most doctors will cooperate in this respect; if yours will not, find one who will.

If you cannot afford to have the testing done through a commercial lab, try your city or state health department. Most states have HIV/AIDS testing and counseling programs, and most of these programs are either confidential or anonymous. The costs are low, usually five to ten dollars.

▶ *What is the difference between confidential and anonymous testing?*

At the testing center, someone will record your name with the result of your test. The center will keep this record from anyone except medical personnel and the state health department (which does not keep your name, but merely records the number of cases).

Before you are tested, ask who will know the result of your test and how the test result will be stored. If you are comfortable with the confidentiality of what you are told, go ahead with your test; if you are not, go elsewhere.

With anonymous testing, no one knows your name and you are the only person who can tell anyone else the result of your test. Not all states or cities offer anonymous testing.

▶ Where can you go for testing and counseling?

Your options, which depend on where you live and your financial resources, may include your doctor's office, publicly funded state or local HIV testing and counseling centers, hospital clinics, family planning clinics, and some drug treatment facilities. When you are tested, you should also receive counseling, and many testing centers offer it. If you cannot find a facility near you, call the CDC national AIDS hotline: 1-800-342-AIDS.

▶ What kind of counseling do testing centers offer?

Each testing center may have its own procedure for counseling people who come in for HIV tests, but in general the counseling has two main purposes. The first is to make people aware of the need for safe sex. If you are fortunate and your test shows you have not been infected with HIV, you should take advantage of this "second chance." If your test is positive, you need to practice safe sex to protect your partner or partners. If you are considering becoming pregnant at some time in the near or distant future, you should know the implications for your pregnancy and your baby of being HIV positive. If you seek treatment early in your pregnancy, you can drastically reduce the chances that your baby will be HIV positive.

The second purpose of counseling is to let you know that having a positive HIV test is not synonymous with having AIDS. Today's medications can allow people with HIV to live many healthy years after they have been infected.

▶ How is HIV/AIDS treated?

Medical researchers have not only developed new, potent drugs for fighting HIV/AIDS, but they have found more effective ways to use the drugs already available. The first drugs used against HIV were antivirals, the best known of which is zidovudine (trade names AZT and Retrovir), approved by the FDA in 1987. Others include didanosine (trade names ddI and Videx), stavudine (d4T and Zerit), and zalcitabine (ddC and Hivid). All these drugs prevent the HIV virus from multiplying rapidly by inhibiting the production of an HIV enzyme called reverse transcriptase.

In 1995 researchers developed a new class of antiviral drugs called protease inhibitors, which target an HIV enzyme called protease, needed by the HIV virus to manufacture certain proteins. Protease inhibitors include drugs like saquinavir, indinavir, and ritonavir. Their use together with other antiviral drugs resulted in so-called combination therapies that lowered the mortality rate for AIDS about 75 percent between 1995 and 1997. All these powerful antivirals have significant side effects, which can include anemia, damage to nerves (especially numbness of the feet), headaches, fever, inflammation of the pancreas, and liver damage.

Other drugs used to treat HIV include medications that attempt to strengthen the ability of the immune system to fight off the virus, and drugs that treat the opportunistic infections that attack the body when the immune system is weakened.

▶ Are women with HIV/AIDS less responsive to treatment than men?

When HIV/AIDS was first recognized in women, studies showed that in general women did not live as long after diagnosis as men did. The reason for their shorter survival seemed to be that women were diagnosed later in the course of the disease, partly because those who had HIV/AIDS were often poor and unlikely to seek timely medical treatment. Second, women were less likely to get an accurate early diagnosis, because in the early 1980s women were not thought to be especially at risk and often were not tested for HIV.

Now it appears that treatments for women and for men are equally effective; women who receive prompt treatment have the same life span as men who receive similar treatment.

▶ What about pregnancy and HIV/AIDS?

Many questions about pregnancy and HIV remain unanswered. No one knows for certain whether becoming pregnant adds to the health risk of women who are infected with HIV.

The consequences of having a baby infected with HIV are so serious that any woman with HIV who becomes pregnant should consult her physician. Without treatment, about 30 percent of infants born to infected mothers will be infected at birth. However, the risk of having an infected child can be reduced to about 8 percent if the mother takes the antiviral drug AZT during pregnancy. Studies have suggested that AZT does not cause premature labor and delivery, fetal distress, or fetal malformations.

LESBIANS AND STDS

Lesbians are less at risk for certain STDs (HIV/AIDs, gonorrhea, and syphilis) than heterosexual women. Perhaps the microorganisms responsible for these diseases are less easily spread through oral sex and other sexual activities practiced by lesbians than by heterosexual vaginal, oral, or anal sex. Nevertheless, there are risks.

Not much research has specifically focused on woman-to-woman transmission of HIV. A few studies have shown that women who have had sex only with other women (and have not used intravenous drugs) are at low risk for HIV. Still, it is well known that women can spread HIV to men through contact with vaginal secretions and menstrual blood, so it is certainly possible that women can infect one another. Bisexual women (like heterosexual women) should use a condom each and every time they have sexual contact with men or use sex toys. The FDA has not approved as effective any barrier methods for use during oral sex, but women can use dental dams, cut-open condoms, or plastic wrap to help protect themselves from contact with body fluids. Lesbian women, like heterosexual women, should know their own HIV status and that of their partners.

Lesbians frequently have herpes and HPV (genital warts) infections. Herpes and HPV can be spread by skin-to-skin, genital-to-genital, or mouth-to-genital contact, and thus can be spread from woman to woman. Further, many lesbian women have had sexual contact with men at some time in their lives. The viruses causing herpes and HPV remain in the body forever, so it is possible for a woman to get herpes or HPV from a male partner and at a later time pass it on to a female partner. Since HPV can lead to cervical cancer, lesbians and bisexual women, like heterosexual women, should have regular Pap tests.

Chlamydia, gonorrhea, and syphilis are only rarely transmitted between women, though occasional cases have been reported.

BV, which is associated with sexual activity but is not strictly an STD, occurs frequently among lesbians, even those who have not had sexual activity with a man for at least a year. It seems to spread easily between monogamous partners. Trichomoniasis can also be spread from woman to woman.

8 Fibroids and Endometriosis

▶ **MYTH** Both fibroids and endometriosis can lead to cancer.

FACT Both conditions can cause women considerable grief during their reproductive years, and either can contribute to menstrual pain, heavy bleeding, and infertility. But neither will develop into cancer.

BOTH fibroids and endometriosis are fairly common conditions. It is estimated that between 20 and 30 percent of women of childbearing age have fibroids and between 10 and 20 percent have endometriosis. Some women with fibroids have no symptoms; others are made miserable. Likewise, some women with endometriosis do not know they have it, while others suffer severe pelvic pain. Although both conditions can be treated with some degree of success, neither can be prevented.

FIBROIDS

Fibroids, lumps of fiber-like tissue that grow from the wall of the uterus, are seldom dangerous; they will not harm you. Yet they can be distressing. They may cause heavy periods, episodes of bleeding between periods, back pain, and abdominal discomfort. Because of these problems, fibroids are the leading cause of hysterectomies in this country.

Fibroids can occasionally cause difficulties for women who are trying to have children. They can interfere with a pregnancy once it has been established or, rarely, hinder conception by blocking a fallopian tube. Unfortunately, the late 20s into the 40s, the years when many women are trying to start their families, coincide with the years when they are most likely to have fibroids.

▶ What are fibroids?

Fibroids, also called myomas, leiomyomas, fibromyomas, and fibromas, are technically defined as exuberant growths of the smooth muscle wall of the uterus, which is called the myometrium. In medical terms, "exuberant" means excessive growth of basically normal tissue. The tissue may grow too much, but there is nothing pathologically wrong with it. Sometimes fibroids are referred to as "tumors," a word that also implies excessive growth. But the term does not imply that fibroids are a form of cancer.

To the naked eye, fibroids look rather like tan or whitish rubber balls, different in color from the uterus, which is also muscular but pink. The interior often has a whorled appearance. Under a microscope you can see compacted muscle cells, fibrous tissue (hence the name "fibroid"), and collagen, the substance that glues cells together.

FIBROID SIZES AND GROWTH

Fibroids can be small or large, ranging from the size of a pea to that of a small watermelon; they can even be microscopic, though they are not usually diagnosed at that size. Occasionally fibroids reach a weight of twenty-five pounds. Most physicians are only seriously concerned about fibroids when they are the size of a grapefruit or larger—unless they are causing heavy bleeding, pain, or other problems.

Fibroids usually grow very slowly, but they seem to develop according to their own unpredictable pattern. Sometimes a fibroid will appear suddenly, grow slowly to a certain size, and remain unchanged for a long time. Another fibroid may jump to the size of a lemon, stay that way for five years, and then change again. If a fibroid grows very rapidly, say from the size of a lime to that of a cantaloupe in six months, your physician might want to investigate the situation. Fibroids do not usually enlarge this quickly, so the rapidly growing mass in the abdomen might be something other than a fibroid.

Although it is possible for a fibroid to go on growing indefinitely as long as it is being nourished by estrogen, most fibroids stop after reaching a certain size. Scientists do not understand the reason for this growth pattern. Nor can we predict what the eventual size will be. Therefore most gynecologists have a threshold, perhaps a grapefruit-size fibroid, at which they will intervene.

▶ *Do fibroids ever shrink or go away spontaneously?*

After menopause, when the body is no longer producing much estrogen, many women find that their fibroids shrink or disappear altogether. This happy situation does not usually occur in women who are still menstruating. Sometimes fibroids "degenerate," collapse on themselves because they have outgrown their blood supply.

Like ordinary muscle tissue, fibroid tissue needs oxygen. When it fails to get enough, the fibroid can collapse or infarct, causing severe ischemic pain—the kind you get when you have uterine cramps, but much more severe. Once the fibroid degenerates, its tissue gradually disappears and the pain ceases. The process usually goes on for several days, though not for several weeks.

Wendy, who had come to me for her gynecological checkups for a number of years, started having severe abdominal pain rather suddenly when she was in her 40s. She saw her internist, a very good doctor, who decided that her problem was appendicitis, though he was uncertain because her symptoms were not the classic ones. She went to one of the best surgeons in town, who also thought she had appendicitis, and also agreed that her symptoms were not quite the usual ones. Wendy's pain finally got so bad that she went to the emergency room of the local hospital. Since I was her regular gynecologist, she asked if I could examine her, and I came in to the emergency room before the surgery was performed.

There was a lump on the right side of her uterus, without question, and her uterus was tender. The lump was not far from where her appendix was located. I knew she had a fibroid in that area because I had examined her previously. At this point we did an ultrasound and could visualize the fibroid, right where she was feeling the pain. We concluded that her problem was a degenerating fibroid, so we elected to treat her conservatively with bed rest and pain medication. She improved after several days, and when I reexamined her in my office sometime later, the entire fibroid had disappeared. She has been fine ever since.

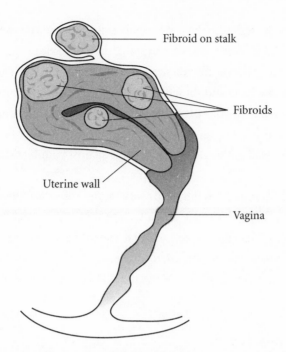

Fibroid on stalk

Fibroids

Uterine wall

Vagina

FIGURE 23. Fibroids may occur anywhere in the uterus or may be attached to its surface by a stalk.

KINDS OF FIBROIDS

Fibroids are classified by their location, which (along with their size) determines the symptoms you may have and the optimum treatment. They can grow on the inner surface of the uterus, in the middle of the uterine wall, or on the outer surface. Some combine all these locations. No one knows what triggers the growth of fibroids, though we do know that they are estrogen dependent. For this reason some researchers have suggested that fluctuating levels of estrogen may have something to do with their onset.

Intramural fibroids grow within the muscular uterine wall (Latin, *mur*) and are extremely common. *Submucosal fibroids* grow beneath the inner lining of the uterus (called the mucosa), displacing it as they grow. They can cause menstrual pain and irregular bleeding. Sometimes a submucosal fibroid develops a stalk, called a pedicle, which remains attached to the wall of the uterus while the fibroid itself may push into the uterine cavity. The uterus may then contract, trying to rid itself of a foreign growth and causing cramping. Women with submucosal fibroids often have erratic bleeding. Submucosal fibroids, even when small, can cause real problems.

Subserosal fibroids grow on the outer wall of the uterus (called the serosa) and can push outward from the wall into the abdominal cavity. Subserosal fibroids are external to the uterine cavity and usually the least symptomatic. They seldom cause bleeding problems because they are outside the main action site of the uterus. However, subserosal fibroids can grow quite large and sometimes press against other organs. If your fibroid is growing off the back wall of your uterus and pressing against your spine, you will probably have a backache. If it is pressing on your rectum, you may suffer from constipation. If it grows on the front wall of the uterus, it can press against your bladder and cause you to urinate frequently.

Other kinds of fibroids exist, but occur very rarely. *Parasitic fibroids* are fibroids with stalks that rest against another organ and attach to that organ, establishing a new blood supply. The stalk that originally was connected to the uterus shrivels away until the fibroid is no longer connected to the uterus. *Interligamentous fibroids* grow between the layers of the ligaments (the strong bands of connective tissue) that support the uterus inside the abdominal cavity.

▶ What is a prolapsed fibroid?

Once in a great while, a fibroid on a stalk may prolapse, or fall down, into the uterus. If this happens, the uterus may try to expel what it perceives as a foreign object. But since the stalk still remains attached to the uterine wall, the whole uterus tends to come along with the fibroid. The woman feels contractions like labor; her cervix actually thins out and dilates. Prolapsed fibroids can be treated either by removing them surgically from their stalks or by hysterectomy.

▶ Why do fibroids cause heavy periods or unpredictable bleeding?

No one knows for sure. Most researchers believe that heavy periods and erratic bleeding occur because the fibroid breaks through the uterine lining, destroying its integrity.

▶ Who is at risk for getting fibroids?

Fibroids are so common that it is difficult to tell whether there is a familial tendency toward them. We do know that young black women are at higher risk than young white women. Almost half of African American women develop fibroids by the age of 50, while only about 20 percent of white women do so. Furthermore, fibroids tend to start earlier and grow faster in black women.

Advancing age is also a risk factor. The older you are (until you hit your early 50s, when menopause usually occurs), the more likely you are to get them. Theoretically fibroids can develop at any age between the onset of menstruation and the menopause, but they rarely appear until the late 20s. (I have only operated for fibroids on one woman who was as young as 23; she was a rare exception.) The incidence of fibroids increases through the 30s and 40s and then declines as estrogen production drops off. Usually no new fibroids appear after menopause.

► *If you have one fibroid, are you at higher risk for additional ones?*

Although no one knows exactly what initiates fibroid growth, experience has shown that certain women are more prone to fibroids than others. If you have one, you may well have more, either at the same time or later.

One of my patients had fibroid surgery three times. When she needed a fourth operation, we decided on a hysterectomy. I asked a colleague, a cancer specialist skilled in complex abdominal surgery, to stand by—not because there was a danger of cancer, but to help with the scar tissue that had built up after the previous surgeries.

► *Do oral contraceptives cause fibroids or make them grow?*

Again, we do not know the exact relationship between birth control pills and fibroids. Some physicians believe that the pills increase fibroid growth; others say their use makes no difference whatsoever.

Women with fibroids seem to have individual responses to the pill. Some women who have heavy bleeding from fibroids find that they do better when they are on birth control pills, although taking them does not shrink the fibroids. Because birth control pills contain synthetic progesterone as well as estrogen, the progesterone may help control the stimulation caused by the estrogen. Women with fibroids who take the pill, for whatever reason, must be monitored by their caregivers.

► *What are the symptoms of fibroids?*

Often fibroids do not produce any symptoms at all, even if they are fairly large; consequently it is possible to have them without knowing it. Certain symptoms, however, are usual. Remember that these symptoms are common and can be caused by other problems. Having backaches or constipation, for example, does not necessarily mean that you have fibroids.

BOX 3.   Classic Symptoms of Fibroids

Heavy bleeding during menstrual periods
Pelvic pressure
Frequent urination
Backaches
Constipation

▶ *How are fibroids diagnosed?*

If a fibroid is large enough, your physician can diagnose it during a pelvic examination. He or she places the fingers of one hand in the vagina and the other hand on top of the abdomen and then palpates the fibroid. What your caregiver is actually feeling is not the lump inside the uterus but the changed contour of the uterus because of the presence of the fibroid. Your caregiver can estimate the size of the fibroid by mentally comparing the way your uterus feels with the feel of a pregnant uterus: the fibroid is about the size of a six-

---

BOX 4.   Fibroid Sizes

Physicians commonly estimate the size of fibroids in terms of the size of a pregnant uterus after a certain number of months. For people who are not familiar with the size of the uterus during the various stages of pregnancy, common fruits are an easier standard of comparison.

Two-month pregnancy: Tennis ball
Three-month pregnancy: Grapefruit
Four-month pregnancy: Cantaloupe
Five-month pregnancy: Honeydew
Six-month pregnancy: Small watermelon

---

month pregnancy, for example. Another common yardstick is to compare fibroids in size to common fruit.

Fibroids can also be diagnosed by means of ultrasound technology. Sonography, as this procedure is called, can confirm that what your doctor is feeling is indeed the uterus with its fibroid (or fibroids), not a growth on an ovary. Sophisticated tests such as MRIs and CT scans will also diagnose fibroids, but they are expensive and expose you to more radiation than ultrasound, which is the preferred diagnostic tool.

▶ *Can fibroids cause cancer or become cancerous?*

In the overwhelming majority of cases, fibroids are not cancerous and do not degenerate into cancer. Certain kinds of cancerous tumors called sarcomas can arise from muscle tissue and occur in many different sites within the body; it is possible, though very rare, to have a sarcoma within the muscular tissue of a fibroid.

TREATING FIBROIDS

The treatments for fibroids range from watchful waiting to surgery. In the past, the standard treatment for fibroids, especially for women who had completed their families, was hysterectomy. Today there are more choices.

▶ *When is watchful waiting a reasonable way to treat fibroids?*

If your fibroid is relatively small and stable, if it does not cause symptoms that you cannot or do not want to tolerate, if it is not interfering with other organs or causing problems with fertility, you have the option of waiting to see what will happen.

Since fibroids are fed by estrogen, women approaching menopause whose estrogen levels are dropping may want to wait until menopause before taking any drastic action to get rid of their fibroids.

▶ *Can fibroids be treated with medications?*

No medication will make your fibroids go away and never come back. The best thing we have so far is Lupron, which I call "menopause in a jar." For as long as you take it, you are in a condition like menopause.

Lupron belongs to a class of drugs called GnRH agonists (chemicals that act like gonadotropin-releasing hormone), and these chemicals act to wipe out estrogen production by the ovaries. Since fibroids are dependent on estrogen, they will shrink away without it. Lupron, although quite effective, is only a temporary cure. The moment you stop taking it, the fibroids will return or grow back to their former size.

> Lisa has fibroids that make her bleed so heavily that her hematocrit (red blood count) is very low. She has become anemic and is tired all the time. Lisa would like to have a hysterectomy; she has two children and doesn't want any more. However, her blood count is so low that the anesthesiologist advises against surgery.
>
> Lupron can be a good temporary solution for Lisa. She can take it to shut down her estrogen production for two or three months, stopping those heavy periods and giving her a chance to build up her blood count by taking a lot of iron. When she has her hysterectomy, chances are she will not need a blood transfusion. Indeed, the Lupron may shrink her fibroid so that the surgery is much simpler and safer.

▶ *Can you take Lupron for a while to keep your fibroids small and under control?*

Since Lupron acts like menopause, it has all the consequences of menopause. It shuts down your menstrual periods; it can cause hot flashes and mood swings. Doctors are concerned about Lupron and osteoporosis: it has been shown that women who stay on this drug for more than six months begin losing bone, so usually Lupron therapy lasts no longer than that. (For more about Lupron, see the section on endometriosis later in this chapter.)

▶ *When do fibroids need to be removed surgically?*

In general, women are alarmed to learn that they have something larger than a grape growing in their abdomen. This is understandable, but gynecologists usually do not feel the need for intervention until much later. Some will tell you to have treatment because you have an eight-week size fibroid. Others will wait until your fibroid is twelve-week size. When I was just starting in practice, I used to intervene when a fibroid reached the size of a twelve-week pregnancy. Now my threshold is a fifteen- to sixteen-week pregnancy unless you are uncomfortable or have warning symptoms.

Factors other than mere size enter this decision, however. The location of your fibroid, your symptoms and willingness to tolerate discomfort, your feelings about surgery, and your age may all enter into your choice. If you are having back pain, urinary frequency, or feel really anxious about something growing in your abdomen, then you and your caregiver may want to do something about the fibroid even though it is still quite small. If, on the other hand, you are not uncomfortable or have a higher tolerance for discomfort than for surgery, and your fibroids do not seem to be pressing against other organs, you can wait longer.

> Lynn, in her early 30s, has a fibroid about the size of an eight- or nine-week pregnancy, which is roughly the size of a tennis ball. She is small and slim; her uterus is anteverted (tilted forward). Consequently there is not much space between the front of her uterus and her bladder. Her fibroid sticks straight out from the front wall of her uterus, pressing against her bladder. Lynn is quite uncomfortable; she feels pressure, abdominal discomfort, and the need to urinate frequently. Even though her fibroid is relatively small, we decide to remove it surgically. Since the surgery, she has felt better and has had no additional problems.

▶ *What kinds of surgery are used to treat fibroids?*

There are two main procedures: hysterectomy, where the entire uterus is removed, and myomectomy, where only the fibroid is removed (the uterus remains intact). Each of these operations has several variations. A third surgical treatment, called transcervical hysteroscopic resection, is used only for very specific types of fibroids.

For women who do need surgery and have finished their childbearing, hysterectomy is the usual choice. It is probably right for you if your fibroids cause symptoms you cannot or will not tolerate, you bleed so heavily that you become debilitated, you have unusually large or extensive fibroids, or your fibroids are causing complications with bladder, bowel, or other organs.

For women who have not completed their families, the choice is more complex.

▶ *What factors weigh in the choice between a myomectomy and a hysterectomy?*

The most serious issue is the question of fertility and future childbearing.

> Debby is 32 years old and has three children. When her third child was born, she decided to have her tubes tied, which worked out well for her. However, she has a sixteen-week size fibroid that causes heavy menstrual periods; she is miserable

every month. The idea of having a hysterectomy is not psychologically problematic for her.

Jessie is also 32 years old. She was married and divorced without having children.
Now she is dating someone new and they are beginning to get serious. She sees
herself settling down and having children at some time in the future. Jessie's sixteen-week fibroid gives her heavy bleeding and uncomfortable pelvic pressure.

Right now a myomectomy would be right for Jessie, though later in her life she might need
a hysterectomy. The important issue here is preserving her fertility.

▶ *How is a myomectomy performed?*

The traditional way is to make an abdominal incision, isolate the uterus from the surrounding organs, and find out where within the uterus the fibroid is located. Then the surgeon makes an incision into the wall of the uterus and removes the fibroid(s) from the
uterine wall or cavity and closes up the incisions with stitches.

Some surgeons now perform myomectomies through a laparoscope or a hysteroscope, fiber-optic devices that can be used to visualize the inside of the abdominal cavity.
The hysteroscope is inserted through the vagina into the uterine cavity. The laparoscope is
inserted into the abdomen through a small incision. If the fibroids are small, this procedure is relatively simple and straightforward. If the fibroids are large, it can be difficult to
remove them through the laparoscope. Surgeons will probably then make an incision in
the vagina and remove large fibroids via that route.

If the fibroids can be removed with the hysteroscope or laparoscope, the recovery period is shorter because there is no major abdominal incision. A relatively new surgical instrument called a morcellator cuts the fibroid into pieces small enough to be removed
through the laparoscopic incision.

Colette, a petite 44-year-old, had all kinds of anxieties and phobias about
surgery. She also had a fibroid that grew to about eighteen-week size, like a small
honeydew melon. She had been living with this fibroid for a long time, but eventually started feeling real discomfort and having very heavy bleeding.

She was willing to have a hysterectomy, but was absolutely certain, for cosmetic reasons, that she did not want to have a standard abdominal procedure;

she did not want a scar. On the other hand, the size of her fibroid made a laparo-scopic removal impossible.

One day she saw a surgeon on television, a doctor on the staff of a hospital near her home. Dr. Jones, a devotee of high-tech surgery, spoke very positively about morcellation. On the strength of his presentation, Colette went to see him. At first she was enthusiastic about his description of the operation, but when she learned that she would be under anesthesia for more than three and a half hours, longer than an ordinary hysterectomy would take, she decided against the new procedure.

She reasoned that it would make little difference in the long run whether she had a laparoscopy with morcellation or an abdominal incision. She was retired, a person who enjoyed a leisurely life at home and had few responsibilities that she couldn't shift around during her recovery period. Without a uterus, she would never have to worry about the fibroids growing back, and she would never have to concern herself about endometrial cancer.

All the same, morcellation can be useful when the fibroid is small but needs surgical intervention.

▶ Are there disadvantages to a myomectomy?

At first glance, it would seem that a myomectomy is always the operation of choice. Why not just remove the fibroid or fibroids and leave the uterus intact?

One major reason for removing the entire uterus is that fibroids can and often do re-cur. Women who have had one fibroid are at increased risk for having more. An estimated 25–50 percent of women who have their fibroids removed by myomectomy have recur-rences.

Myomectomy sounds simple as a surgical procedure, but in fact it can often be more difficult than a hysterectomy and cause more blood loss. Usually more than one fibroid must be removed, and each fibroid has its own blood supply. In a hysterectomy, the sur-geon begins by clamping off the large blood vessels that supply the uterus; once these ves-sels have been clamped, the uterus is removed. In a myomectomy, there is no way to shut down the blood flow to the uterus because the uterus needs its blood supply to survive. The surgeon must dig into the wall of the uterus to remove the fibroid while the blood vessels are intact and still functioning. Because each fibroid is removed individually, the procedure can take longer than a hysterectomy.

Another problem with myomectomy is that adhesions (formations of scar tissue that cause one organ to stick to another) often develop after the operation—for example, adhesion of the uterus to the bowel. Modern surgical techniques can help minimize the problem, but myomectomy still has a reputation as an operation that frequently leads to adhesions.

Although myomectomy is the only surgical choice for a woman who wants to have her fibroids removed and still have children sometime in the future, the adhesions that may result from the operation may diminish fertility.

▶ Can fibroids be removed with laser surgery?

Yes, though laser surgery is not really different from traditional surgery. For surgical purposes, a laser is simply a knife made of a beam of light instead of sharpened metal. While laser surgery is superior to the traditional variety for some procedures, it has no particular advantages for removing fibroids. Often people ask for laser surgery just because they want the newer procedure, but newer is not necessarily better.

▶ Are there other new techniques for dealing surgically with fibroids?

The most recent developments involve cryosurgery, destroying the cells of the fibroids by freezing them. This technique is useful only if the fibroid is small. In general, the procedure is to insert a frozen needle into the fibroid and freeze the adjacent tissue, killing the cells and shrinking the size of the fibroid. If the fibroid is large, the frozen needle may have to be inserted again and again.

FIBROIDS AND FERTILITY

Although many women with fibroids do become pregnant and bear healthy children, fibroids can interfere with fertility, making it difficult to become pregnant or to maintain a pregnancy through nine months. Only a thorough and methodical infertility workup can determine whether fibroids are at the root of the problem.

▶ How do fibroids lower fertility?

Fibroids can interfere with conception by blocking the path of the sperm to the egg, by distorting the shape of the uterus, or by altering the alignment of the cervix, through which the sperm travels on its way to the uterus. Fibroids outside the uterus can press against the fallopian tubes, narrowing them and making it difficult for the egg to travel from the ovaries to the uterus.

Submucosal fibroids, located beneath the inner lining of the uterus, can stretch the lining as they grow, thinning it out and making it less hospitable to the fertilized egg. If the egg does succeed in implanting itself in the lining, it may detach as it grows larger, resulting in a miscarriage.

If the fibroids within the uterus are large, they can take up space intended for the fetus. Fibroids outside the uterus can prevent it from expanding to contain the growing fetus.

▶ Does a myomectomy reduce the chance of getting pregnant?

Myomectomy itself does not have a negative impact on fertility. Still, two issues do generate concern. The first is that myomectomies often result in adhesions. When the surgeon removes a fibroid, there is bleeding from the site where the fibroid was located. Bleeding stimulates an inflammatory response, which in turn stimulates the formation of scar tissue. If the adhesions are located around the fallopian tubes, an area of the pelvis where organs are crowded together, your fertility can be impaired.

The second issue is that women who have had a myomectomy have a significant chance of needing a cesarean section when they give birth. Scar tissue and a general weakening of the wall of the uterus also may put a woman at risk of rupturing the scar during labor. Only the surgeon who performed the myomectomy can tell ahead of time whether the woman will need a future cesarean section. At your postoperative visit, therefore, ask the physician who did your myomectomy whether you should plan on a cesarean section if you do become pregnant.

Jane had a fibroid which grew to about the size of a baseball, during her first pregnancy. She did well during the pregnancy and had a vaginal delivery. Unfortunately, Jane was one of those rare patients in whom the fibroid did not shrink after childbirth. To relieve Jane's symptoms, we did a myomectomy, since she wanted a second child. After a while Jane became pregnant again, but this time I did a cesarean section because I knew that in digging out the fibroid during the myomectomy, I had weakened the uterine wall.

▶ *Is it dangerous to be pregnant when you have fibroids?*

Usually it is not hazardous to go through pregnancy when you have fibroids. However, since fibroids are estrogen sensitive, they are likely to grow during pregnancy, when your body is producing extra estrogen. The fibroids will probably not hurt the baby. Depending on where they are located, the fibroids can make the mother-to-be quite uncomfortable. Back pain, for instance, can get worse if you have fibroids.

Scientific studies have suggested that fibroids may cause miscarriage by interfering with implantation of the fertilized egg in the uterine lining.

Sometimes a fibroid can degenerate during pregnancy, as at any other time. Although the degenerating fibroid is not dangerous to the pregnancy, it can be very painful and frustrating. Pain medications such as Demerol are safe during pregnancy. After delivery, the fibroid tends to shrink.

ENDOMETRIOSIS

Endometriosis, sometimes called endo, is a chronic disease in which the kind of tissue that normally makes up the lining of the uterus (the endometrium) is found other places within the body. Endometriosis is one of the primary causes of infertility and of menstrual pain.

The wandering endometrial tissue can be attached to other organs or implanted within other tissues. Usually endometriosis is confined to the pelvic cavity, with clumps of unwanted endometrial tissue on the ovaries and around the outside of the uterus. Less frequently it is found in the vagina, near the small intestine, bladder, or appendix. But endometrial tissue has been found as far away as the lungs and the nasal passages. It has also been found in skin and in scar tissue remaining after surgery. These occurrences far from the pelvic area are rare.

No matter where it is located, whether in its rightful place inside the uterus or elsewhere, endometrial tissue responds to estrogen stimulation. Every month all the misplaced endometrial tissue acts just like the lining of your uterus: it swells and thickens, gets ready to receive a fertilized egg, and then, responding to hormonal changes, breaks down and sloughs off.

It is this monthly cycling that leads to the symptoms associated with this disease: men-

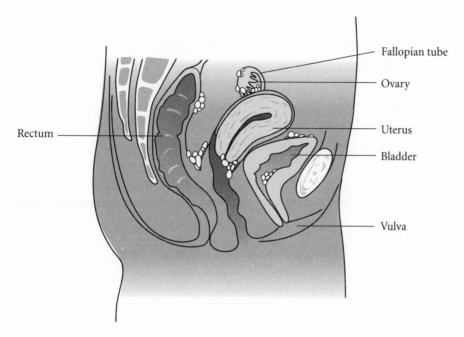

FIGURE 24. Common sites of endometriosis in the pelvis.

strual pain, pain during intercourse, and infertility. Endometriosis can cause inflammation, internal bleeding, and the formation of scar tissue or blood-filled cysts.

▶ What causes endometriosis?

No one really knows the answer to this crucial question. There are several contending theories, but no single one accounts for all the places in the body that endometrial tissue may appear. It is suggested that endometriosis is a disease of the immune system, that it is a genetic disease, or that it is an inflammatory disease. Some researchers hypothesize that the endometrial tissue may migrate through the lymphatic system to other sites in the body. Others suggest that a hereditary tendency plus an immune reaction to one's own tissues may bring on the disease. Still others believe that environmental factors, for example exposure to the pesticide dioxin, may contribute to endometriosis.

One of the oldest explanations is the menstrual backflow theory, according to which some of the flow from your menstrual period, including bits of endometrial tissue, backs up through the fallopian tubes and enters the pelvic cavity. The bits of tissue then implant themselves on nearby organs and begin to grow. However, this hypothesis cannot account for endometrial implants in sites far from the pelvis, such as the lungs or nose; nor can it account for the fact that the cervix and other locations regularly exposed to the menstrual flow rarely get endometrial implants.

I am inclined to favor the "potential tissue" theory, which is based on embryonic development. The tissue that lines many of the body cavities is called "totipotential" tissue because it can develop into anything—it has the potential to become any other kind of tissue. According to this theory, this totipotential tissue that covers the lining of the lungs, for example, lies dormant until a girl begins producing estrogen; then, in the presence of estrogen, it gradually changes into endometrial tissue. The answer may lie in a combination of these theories, and several disease-causing mechanisms may be at work to account for endometrial implants in the distant places they have been found.

▶ Who is at risk for endometriosis?

Endometriosis appears to be more common now than when first described in 1920, perhaps because we have better tools for diagnosing it, but also because current social patterns favor later childbearing. The "typical" woman diagnosed with endometriosis is in her late 20s or early 30s and does not have children. Endometriosis used to be thought a disease primarily of white women, but as more black women have begun pursuing careers and putting off childbearing, the incidence has risen in them as well. For unknown reasons Japanese women are more at risk than Caucasians. In parts of the world where the culture emphasizes early childbearing, endometriosis is rare. Endometriosis is more common in women whose sisters or mothers have the disease, but it is certainly not a genetic disease like hemophilia, whose inheritance can be predicted with some statistical certainty.

▶ Does endometriosis always get worse with time?

Because endometriosis is primarily a disease of women of childbearing age that responds to estrogen, it goes on as long as a woman produces estrogen. Generally the longer it goes on, the worse it gets; but this is not always the case. Some researchers estimate that only between 25 and 40 percent of women with mild endometriosis go on to have more severe stages of the disease.

Two natural occurrences interfere with the progress of endometriosis. Menopause, after which the ovaries no longer produce estrogen, usually brings relief, although some women do have endometriosis later in life. Pregnancy, during which the usual balance of hormones is altered, also can stop the advance of the disease.

▶ *Why does it get worse over time?*

When the endometrium itself breaks down every month, it has somewhere to go: it flows out the vagina. But the blood and debris formed by misplaced endometrial tissue may have no natural exit. If the endometrial implants are inside the pelvic cavity (but outside the uterus), the tissue simply bleeds into whatever tissues surround it. This process, which goes on every month unless treated, can cause inflammation and pain, and eventually will produce scar tissue.

Early on, endometriosis may appear as little speckles or flecks of tissue, scattered here and there in the abdominal cavity. Over time, as scar tissue develops, the patches of endometrial tissue may cause one organ to adhere to another. These adhesions may, for example, glue the ovaries to the back wall of the pelvic cavity. Sometimes more advanced endometriosis forms a cyst, called an endometrioma or a "chocolate cyst," filled with dark blood that looks like chocolate syrup. Chocolate cysts can be very large, as big as basketballs. They are fragile and, unlike other kinds of cysts or tumors, are difficult to remove surgically in one piece. These masses may change the position of the uterus or push against the fallopian tubes, distorting the normal pelvic architecture. If the tumors and scarring build up, they may "freeze" or "fix" the reproductive organs in place and interfere with their functioning.

In 1985 the American Society for Reproductive Medicine established a system for categorizing, or staging, endometriosis, so that physicians would have a standard way of describing its severity. Although the guidelines are somewhat controversial, the simplified version in Box 5 gives a general picture of the stages of the disease.

▶ *What are the symptoms of endometriosis?*

Although up to 30 percent of women have no symptoms, the three classic symptoms of endometriosis are menstrual pain, pain on intercourse, and infertility. Your personal symptoms depend on where the wandering endometrial tissue has landed. If it is in your pelvic cavity near the uterus, you may feel abdominal tenderness or have painful menstrual periods with or without heavy, irregular flow. You may have pain between periods, just after your period ends or before it begins. You may have pain with intercourse. By contrast, if you have a large endometrial cyst on your ovary, you may have no symptoms at all.

If endometrial tissue has lodged in your nasal passages, which happens rarely, you may have nosebleeds around the time of your period. If it has landed in your lungs (also

BOX 5. Stages of Endometriosis

STAGE I: MILD

Small scattered implants on lining of pelvis or surface of ovary

No scarring

No adhesions

No endometriomas (endometrial cysts)

No involvement of bowel

STAGE II: MODERATE

One or both ovaries involved, small endometriomas (endometrial cysts)

Mild adhesions

Endometrial implants may show scarring

Ligaments supporting uterus may be involved

No involvement of bowel

STAGE III: SEVERE

Large endometrial cysts

Involvement of both ovaries, ovaries fixed in place by adhesions

Fallopian tubes blocked or fixed in place

Uterus pushed out of its normal position or fixed in place

Bowel, bladder, or ureters involved

very rare), you may have bleeding into your lungs, a condition known in medical terms as catamenial hemothorax, and cough up blood during your periods.

Strangely, there is no correlation between the severity of your symptoms and the severity of the endometriosis. Sometimes people with tiny endometrial implants have a great deal of pain. Or women with huge masses of endometriosis may have no symptoms.

▶ Can endometriosis turn into cancer?

Endometriosis is not the same thing as endometrial cancer, which is a malignant disease of the actual lining of the uterus. Nor is endometriosis a disease that is likely to turn into cancer. Although it is possible for an endometrial implant located in the ovary to become malignant, it is very rare.

▶ If you have endometriosis, are you more at risk for PMS or other menstrual problems?

There does seem to be some correlation between PMS and endometriosis. The link may be physiological, since endometrial tissue is hormonally active and PMS seems to be hormone dependent. There may also be a psychological link. If you know that your period is going to start next week and you are going to feel awful or even be in acute pain, then it is reasonable that you may be depressed and anxious at the prospect. If your endometriosis is causing infertility, the anxieties surrounding that issue may stress and depress you.

▶ How does endometriosis interfere with fertility?

Infertility is one of the hallmarks of endometriosis, but no one is sure exactly why or how endometriosis prevents conception. Sometimes the causes seem to be mechanical. Maybe the endometriosis blocks the fallopian tubes or causes adhesions that interfere with the process of fertilization; or perhaps endometriosis invades the ovaries so that they are unable to function properly.

Sometimes a woman having difficulty getting pregnant may appear to have no blockages caused by endometrial tumors. Her fallopian tubes are open. Her pelvis does not contain large endometrial implants. Yet she does not become pregnant.

It is possible that endometriosis causes something to go wrong with ovulation. Many researchers believe that endometrial implants are not chemically inert; rather, they are producing hormones or other substances that may interfere with ovulation. This theory also helps explain why women who have endometriosis experience increased pain with their periods: the endometrial implants may be producing extra prostaglandins, the hormonelike substances that cause menstrual cramping.

▶ How is endometriosis diagnosed?

Your medical history is an important tool in diagnosing endometriosis, but the best way to confirm any suspicion is through laparoscopy, a minor surgical procedure, that is performed under anesthesia and involves only a small incision (see Chapter 12). If the endometrial implants are small, your doctor may use laparoscopic tools to remove the endometriosis at the time of the diagnosis.

If the endometrial implants are large enough to distort or enlarge your uterus or change the size of your ovaries, your physician may feel thickening around the ovaries or around the back of the uterus during a pelvic exam. While a pelvic exam can suggest that endometriosis is your problem, other conditions might cause the same physical signs; the only certain diagnosis is through laparoscopy. Ultrasound will pick up cysts or large implants, but if your endometriosis is in the form of scattered bits here and there, ultrasound probably will not be helpful.

Magnetic resonance imaging is probably better than ultrasound for diagnosing endometriosis, but it costs more than a thousand dollars a test.

▶ What are the treatments?

Just as there is no definitive theory that explains why endometriosis happens, there is no "cure" that will make it will disappear forever. There are, however, different treatments, some of which deal with the pain that accompanies the disease and some of which focus on reducing or getting rid of the endometrial implants.

▶ Are there self-help measures that will help with the painful periods caused by endometriosis?

Self-help tactics, similar to those for ordinary menstrual pain or PMS, include dietary and lifestyle measures. They are more likely to be helpful during the early stages of the disease. Remember to exercise, for exercise stimulates the brain to produce endorphins, the body's natural painkillers and mood lifters. Ibuprofen and other over-the-counter medications can also be useful. (See the discussions of cramps and pain in Chapters 3 and 4.) If these drugs do not do the job, your doctor can prescribe more powerful nonsteroidal anti-inflammatory medications. Some women need narcotic painkillers such as codeine, or narcotic painkillers combined with other drugs.

▶ What treatments will get rid of endometrial implants?

There are two routes for reducing or getting rid of endometrial tissue outside your uterus: you can use hormonal treatment to shrink the implants, or you can have surgery to remove them. The two approaches can be tried separately or they can be combined. The choice of treatment depends on the severity of your symptoms and your interest in having children in the future.

▶ *How do you treat endometriosis when fertility is an issue?*

There is no easy answer to this question. One choice is to remove surgically as much of the endometriosis as possible and to repair, if possible, the damage the disease may have inflicted on the uterus, fallopian tubes, and other structures. If your endometriosis has resulted in adhesions that have attached an ovary to the side of your pelvis, or in a large cyst of endometriosis sitting on top of an ovary, surgery can repair these problems and enhance your fertility.

The second choice, obviously, is hormonal therapy. The problem here is that the therapy that shrinks the endometriosis also prevents pregnancy.

HORMONAL TREATMENT

As we have noticed, two natural events—menopause and pregnancy—have a beneficial effect on endometriosis. Hormonal therapies generally mimic one of these conditions.

In recent years researchers have developed a class of drugs called GnRH agonists, which can be used to induce pseudomenopause. The prototype of this drug is leuprolide, which is marketed as Lupron. It behaves like menopause by shutting down the ovaries, but the action is fully reversible: once you stop taking Lupron, your ovaries return to normal and go about their business.

Lupron works by temporarily depriving the ovaries of two hormones that regulate the production of estrogen and progesterone. These hormones that push the ovaries to do their work are called luteinizing hormone (LH) and follicle-stimulating hormone (FSH); they are secreted by the pituitary gland, near the base of the brain. As long as your ovaries are being stimulated by LH and FSH, they will release eggs and produce the estrogen and progesterone needed to build up the endometrium in preparation for fertilization. Lupron works at the pituitary level to bring this cycle to a standstill.

Pseudopregnancy is a second hormonal approach for shrinking endometriosis implants, one that has been used for years. Formerly, women were given high doses of estrogen and progesterone to simulate the hormonal state of pregnancy; today, we use ordinary birth control pills, which contain much lower doses of estrogen and progesterone than earlier treatments. Women who try this therapy take the birth control pills continuously; they have no menstrual periods, they just continue on the pills week after week with no break. A marketing study done by the makers of Lupron has shown it to be more effective than birth control pills. However, Lupron costs about ten times as much and is probably not ten times more effective.

▶ *How do you take Lupron?*

Lupron is given as an injection, once a month, usually for six months. If you dislike getting shots, and some people do, you can take a similar drug as a nasal spray. It is called Synarel (generic name, nafarelin) and is not quite as potent as Lupron. There is also an implant called Zoladex (generic name, goserelin), placed under the skin of the abdomen, which is effective for a month.

▶ *What are the disadvantages of Lupron?*

Lupron brings with it the symptoms of estrogen deprivation, which means that you will have all the annoyances of menopause. You will not have to bother with menstrual periods, but you may get hot flashes, sleeplessness, and headaches. You may have mood swings and vaginal dryness. If you take the drug for an extended period, you may begin to experience significant bone loss, as do menopausal women who are not on hormone replacement therapy. This is why the treatment is usually limited to half a year. Once you stop taking Lupron, all these symptoms disappear.

Lupron is expensive, costing between three hundred and four hundred dollars monthly. Most insurance companies will cover it if you are being treated for the pain of endometriosis, because it is a recognized treatment for a recognized disease. Some insurance plans, however, will not cover Lupron if your endometriosis is being treated because you are infertile.

▶ *Does Synarel have the same side effects as Lupron?*

Because Synarel works in more or less the same way as Lupron, it brings similar side effects. For two months after you start using it, you may have irregular vaginal bleeding. After that, periods usually stop altogether. If yours do not, or if you have bleeding between your periods, call your doctor.

▶ *Do Lupron and Synarel provide contraceptive protection?*

Remember that neither Synarel nor Lupron is a reliable contraceptive. Use barrier methods, not birth control pills or other hormonal contraceptives. If you do become pregnant while taking Synarel or Lupron, you should notify your doctor and stop treatment immediately.

▶ *What can be done about the hot flashes and other symptoms produced by Lupron or Synarel?*

Every so often someone is absolutely miserable with hot flashes because she is taking Lupron. Giving her a small amount of estrogen in what we call add-back therapy can control the hot flashes, but it may also undo some of the benefits of the Lupron treatment.

▶ *Does endometriosis come back after hormonal treatment?*

Yes, when the hormonal treatment is stopped, endometriosis can come back. However, many women remain free of it for several years. There is no reason you cannot have another course of therapy with either Lupron or Synarel if your endometriosis returns. Several of my patients have been "frequent flyers" in this respect, but I notice that often at this point women will opt for surgery.

▶ *If your endometriosis comes back after treatment, will it return in the same places?*

Not necessarily; it can appear in new places or return to the old sites. For this reason, if you have a laparoscopic diagnosis or choose major abdominal surgery, which allows your doctor to visualize your endometriosis, he or she may diagram on your medical chart where the endometriosis is located. Then if you have another procedure at some time in the future, it will be possible to make a comparison with your past condition.

Kristine was in her late 20s when I saw her during my first year of medical practice. She was a beautiful woman with a very pleasant personality. She came to me in December and had a totally normal pelvic exam.

Six months later she came for another pelvic exam. This time she had a very large mass in her abdomen, which had us all worried. I was afraid she had cancer, so I asked the head of oncology at the hospital to stand by—just in case. We took her to the operating room and opened her up. It saddened me to do so, because she was young and attractive and I didn't want to leave her with a large surgical scar. It turned out that she had an endometrioma the size of a basketball on one of her ovaries. That ovary was not salvageable—there just wasn't any ovarian tissue left—but her other side was fine.

After the operation I went upstairs to where her longtime boyfriend and her family were anxiously waiting. "I have good news," I told them. "Kristine does not have cancer; it was endometriosis."

"However," I said to her boyfriend, "since I know you two want a family at some point, you should get married this week and start a family as soon as possible. You have been together for ten years; that's long enough!"

I was really concerned that she would develop an endometrioma on the other ovary and lose her fertility altogether. So that time I was a matchmaker. Kristine and Eddie got married and they have two lovely children. She does have a scar on her abdomen, but compared to a loving husband and two children, it's a minor consideration.

The severity of Kristine's disease made the choice easy. She had to have surgery to remove the mass. When the amount of disease is smaller, treatment options are trickier, because treating the endometriosis means giving therapy that precludes pregnancy. All the drugs we use to treat endometriosis prevent pregnancy, mainly by shutting down ovulation.

So we face a choice: Is it better to suppress ovulation for six or nine months, hoping to decrease the amount of endometriosis, and then try for a pregnancy afterward? Or is it better to keep on trying for pregnancy, even knowing that you may be less fertile than the average woman? I have had patients who were suppressed and got pregnant right afterward. And I have had patients who were not suppressed and became pregnant anyhow within a couple of months of their diagnosis.

Joy came in for a fertility workup. After trying the other less invasive tests, we did a laparoscopy and found that Joy had endometriosis. I had previously operated on her sister for the same problem. Joy chose to be suppressed hormonally, and after six months of treatment began again to try to get pregnant. Six months after she went off the hormonal therapy, she succeeded. But she might have succeeded anyway, without the hormones.

▶ *If endometriosis makes intercourse painful, how can you become pregnant?*

You probably just have to bite the bullet. You can use painkillers to dull the discomfort of intercourse in order to get pregnant. Talk the situation over with your partner and with your physician, who may be able to prescribe something—perhaps codeine—that will help you. Because your uterus may be scarred or glued in place by adhesions, trying different positions during intercourse may help the discomfort.

▶ *If birth control pills are used to treat endometriosis, might they have a protective effect against getting the disease in the first place?*

My own intuition is that they might, though there are no scientific studies to support my belief. If pregnancy deters endometriosis, then birth control pills, which create a hormonal state that resembles pregnancy, could be helpful.

SURGICAL TREATMENT

There are several surgical options to remove endometrial implants if hormonal therapy does not do the job for you. If your endometriosis is diagnosed through laparoscopy, and there is not very much of it, your physician may simply remove it at the time of diagnosis, using either electrocautery, which burns away the tissue, or a laser, which cuts it away. These procedures can be done through the laparoscope and do not involve a major abdominal incision.

A newer technique involves a tool called an argon beam coagulator, nicknamed ABC. This device, which can be manipulated through the laparoscope, is similar to a laser but a bit safer to use. It can be utilized both to zap the endometriosis and to control bleeding within the pelvis.

If your endometriosis forms a large cyst or mass, or is widely scattered throughout your pelvis, or lies near some sensitive organ, then working through the laparoscope may not be practical or safe, and traditional abdominal surgery—called a laparotomy—is necessary.

▶ *Is laparoscopy a hospital procedure?*

In the past, laparoscopy was done in a hospital setting with operating room personnel, including an anesthesiologist and a gynecological surgeon. Usually hospital laparoscopy involved general anesthesia.

In these days of cost-conscious medicine, laparoscopies are sometimes performed with minimal anesthesia in surgical centers or doctors' offices. Instead of a general anesthetic that puts you to sleep, your doctor will give Novocain to anesthetize your skin plus some light sedation to make you drowsy and unaware of what is happening. Instead of a regular laparoscope, which is perhaps 1 cm in diameter, your doctor will use a smaller instrument that is only about 3 mm in diameter. This tiny laparoscope is helpful for visualizing the abdomen, but it is not as useful as the larger version for actually removing endometriosis. Nevertheless, it can give an idea of what stage your endometriosis has reached and whether your therapy is helping.

▶ *When is traditional abdominal surgery necessary for endometriosis?*

When your endometriosis is very widespread, when there are large masses of endometrial tissue (for example, cysts on the ovaries), or when your endometriosis is in a place where it is not safe to use a laser (near the bowel or the ureters), your surgeon may want to get at the endometriosis through an incision in the abdomen. Traditional surgery is also used when adhesions have attached several organs to one another. In addition to removing the endometriosis, your doctor may want to get rid of any adhesions and scar tissue that could be contributing to pain and infertility.

If you have already completed your family or do not wish to have any (more) children, the surgical treatment for endometriosis may be hysterectomy.

▶ *Does endometriosis grow back after it has been surgically removed?*

Yes, sometimes it does, just as it sometimes returns after hormonal treatment. Studies have suggested that in about 20 percent of women who have their endometriosis surgically removed, the disease recurs. Also, most women who become pregnant after surgery do so in the first fifteen months. As with hormonal treatment, the endometriosis does not necessarily grow back in exactly the same places.

▶ *Is it useful to combine surgery and hormonal therapy?*

Surgery can be used alone or in combination with hormonal therapy. Surgical treatments can be conservative, merely trying to get rid of the offending endometriosis, or they can be radical, removing the uterus, ovaries, and fallopian tubes. Surgery gets at the root of the problem, quickly and effectively removing wandering endometrial tissue that causes pain and infertility. Often physicians use hormonal therapy along with surgery to prevent recurrence.

▶ *What are the advantages of laparoscopy?*

If the implants are small and easy to get at, laparoscopic surgery has many advantages. The incisions will be minimal: there will be one incision for looking around with the laparoscope and, if the endometriosis is to be removed, one or more "ports" for the surgery. After inserting the laparoscope into the abdomen, usually just below the navel, the surgeon can use either laser surgery or electrocauterization to remove small growths of endometriosis and adhesions or other scar tissue.

It is possible to treat the endometriosis at the point of diagnosis, in which case you do not have to go into the clinic or hospital twice. Laparoscopy can be done in a surgicenter instead of in a hospital by your gynecologist or another specialist. The procedure can take less than an hour or several hours, depending on the severity of your endometriosis. It is far less expensive than major surgery. You do not end up with a large scar on your abdomen. There are less likely to be complications or formation of internal scar tissue. The recovery period is shorter and easier than with major surgery.

▶ What are the risks?

Although its risks are minimal, laparoscopy is still surgery. There can be complications with the anesthetic. Nearby organs are at risk of damage from the heat of the laser or cauterizing device.

▶ How much does laparoscopy cost?

The laparoscopy itself costs somewhere between fifteen hundred and four thousand dollars, depending on how much surgery is involved (and where you live); in addition, there will probably be hospital or surgicenter charges. Your insurance usually covers much of the cost.

▶ What are the advantages of laparotomy?

Because the incision is large, the surgeon can see all the endometriosis in your abdomen at one time, instead of looking at one nickel-size area and then moving on to another. He can work carefully around vital organs and remove large cysts or masses of endometriosis in one piece without cutting them into smaller bits, which is necessary if they are to be removed through the laparoscope.

▶ What are the disadvantages?

Laparotomy involves a longer hospital stay, usually a couple of days, and is therefore more expensive than laparoscopy. Recovery is slower and more painful. This kind of surgery is more traumatic to the body and more invasive, so there is greater danger of infection. As with any surgery, anesthesia carries its own risks.

▶ Can a laparotomy improve fertility?

In many cases laparotomy is highly successful in enhancing fertility. The surgeon can remove the endometrial tissue found outside the uterus and repair the adhesions formed by scarring. She can remove ovarian cysts, sparing the ovaries if possible, and free up the fallopian tubes and uterus if they are surrounded by endometrial implants.

▶ How much does a laparotomy cost?

The surgeon's fee will be somewhere in the neighborhood of fifteen hundred to four thousand dollars; there will also be the cost of the hospital stay, which may be as long as three days. Because endometriosis is a recognized disease, your health insurance will probably cover the surgery.

▶ When is hysterectomy the right choice for treating endometriosis?

Occasionally endometriosis is so severe that hysterectomy is appropriate. The women who select this operation generally have completed their families or do not want children. Occasionally the endometriosis becomes a threat to health; sometimes repeated surgery has not succeeded, and the endometriosis has reached a stage where living with it is intolerable. In these cases hysterectomy is again the right choice.

The decision to have a hysterectomy is serious. You should be certain that you are finished with your childbearing. You should also be sure you are emotionally ready for the procedure.

9 Cervical, Ovarian, and Endometrial Cancer

▶ **MYTH** If your Pap smear is abnormal, you will probably get cervical cancer and end up having a hysterectomy.

FACT This seldom happens. An abnormal Pap smear does not necessarily lead to cervical cancer, which develops slowly and when detected early is readily cured.

CANCER, especially breast cancer, is the disease women fear above all others. One reason I became a gynecologist is that I have a reasonable chance to heal many people. Most gynecological cancers can be detected early and have high cure rates. The most common cancers that afflict the female reproductive system, in order of frequency, are breast cancer, endometrial (uterine) cancer, cervical cancer, and ovarian cancer. Cancer of the fallopian tube does exist, but it is very rare.

CERVICAL CANCER

Cervical cancer, which most often afflicts women in their 30s and 40s, is a relatively rare form of cancer that usually grows very slowly. The American Cancer Society estimates that each year about 13,000 new cases are diagnosed and 4,100 women die of the disease. Because widespread Pap smear testing allows the disease to be caught in its early stages, invasive cancer has become much less frequent; both the incidence rate and the death rate have declined over the past three decades.

▶ *What is cervical cancer and what causes it?*

Although the cervix (the neck of the uterus as it opens into the vagina) is really part of the uterus, most cancer of the cervix is quite distinct from uterine cancer because the cells involved are very different.

The lining of the uterus is made up of glandular tissue, whereas the outer part of the cervix (the ectocervix) is covered with squamous tissue. Glandular tissue is composed of large, chunky column-type cells; squamous tissue is made up of flat cells. Squamous cell carcinoma is the most common type of cervical cancer. Adenocarcinoma of the cervix, which resembles cancer of the uterus and affects the columnar, glandular cells covering the inner part of the cervix, is the least common.

Before puberty, the cervix is covered with cube-shaped cells. Right after puberty, the cervical cells transform themselves from these columnar cells to flatter squamous cells, a process technically called squamous metaplasia. If the cells being transformed during squamous metaplasia receive an insult of some kind, abnormal cells can develop later. But the impact of these abnormal changes will not show up for years, even decades. Researchers are still trying to fathom what kind of agents initiate, however slowly, cancerous changes in the cervix. Are these agents chemicals or viruses or bacteria? Scientists only know that the substances that trigger the changes are associated somehow with sexual intercourse.

Right now the leading candidate is the human papilloma virus (HPV), the same virus that causes genital warts. Often women who have cervical cancer have had episodes of genital warts, and researchers have actually been able to grow strains of the wart virus from tissue samples of women who have cervical cancer. Yet having genital warts does not necessarily lead to cervical cancer. More than seventy strains of the condyloma or papilloma virus can produce genital warts; only about three can cause cancer. Many, many women carry HPV, just as many people carry some other virus that does not necessarily make them sick. Some experts believe that 100 percent of women who are sexually active in the United States have been exposed to the human papilloma virus. Most women mount their immunological defenses and have warts at worst, but often no symptoms at all.

There are other theories about the cause of cervical cancer and the final answers are not in, except that we do know cervical cancer has something to do with sex. We just don't know what. The older a woman is when she begins having intercourse (that is, the further she is from puberty when her cervical cells are changing), the less likely she is to get cervical cancer. Because the cells seldom change quickly from totally normal to cancerous, yearly Pap smears allow early diagnosis and treatment.

▶ How is cervical cancer diagnosed? Does it have symptoms?

Most cervical disease in this country is diagnosed through Pap smears before it becomes cancerous. At this stage the disease usually has no symptoms, although under the microscope the cells will show abnormalities.

The classic symptom of established cervical cancer is vaginal bleeding, usually slight. It may occur after intercourse or upon severe exertion. While women with endometrial cancer often have heavy menstrual periods, women with cervical cancer seldom have that problem. Sometimes there is watery discharge, which may smell bad. Sometimes cervical cancer has no symptoms at all until it is fairly advanced.

HOW CERVICAL CANCER DEVELOPS

Cervical cancer develops gradually, starting with changes that result in atypical cells (atypia)—they are not normal but not cancerous either. They can spontaneously revert to normal. At first these changes take place only on the surface of the cervix, but they can penetrate more deeply into the cell layers as time goes on if they do not revert to normal. The atypical cells may progress to a state of precancerous change, referred to as dysplasia. When the changes are confined to cell layers above what is called the basement membrane, the condition is fully curable by local therapy. This stage is not yet cancer. In the next stages, the precancerous abnormal cells visible under a microscope have not become invasive cancerous cells with the ability to spread, but they can develop into a local condition called carcinoma in situ. You and your doctor have plenty of time to deal with these changes; they occur slowly, often over a period of years, and it is highly unusual for somebody to proceed from mild to moderate to severe dysplasia to carcinoma in situ to cancer in a matter of months. All the same, you should continue having Pap smears every year; if you do, your chances of getting invasive cancer will be almost zero. Even at the level of mild dysplasia, the cervix can heal itself spontaneously, so some doctors recommend observation only. Once moderate or severe dysplasia is diagnosed, most doctors recommend intervention.

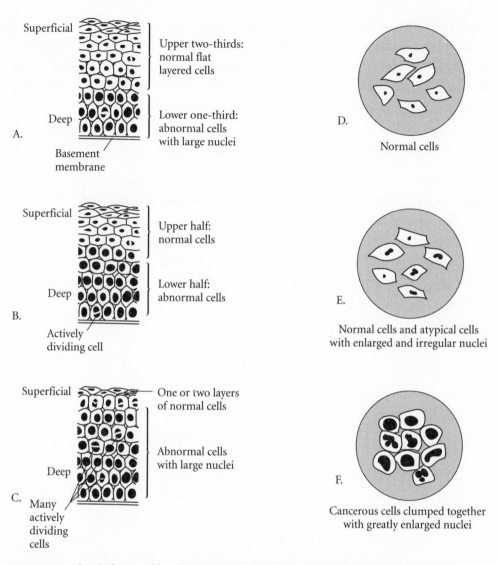

Superficial

Upper two-thirds:
normal flat
layered cells

Deep

Lower one-third:
abnormal cells
with large nuclei

A.

Basement
membrane

D.

Normal cells

Superficial

Upper half:
normal cells

Deep

Lower half:
abnormal cells

B.

Actively
dividing cell

E.

Normal cells and atypical cells
with enlarged and irregular nuclei

Superficial

One or two layers
of normal cells

Abnormal cells
with large nuclei

Deep

C.

Many
actively
dividing
cells

F.

Cancerous cells clumped together
with greatly enlarged nuclei

FIGURE 25. Cervical cancer, like other cancers, develops by a series of gradual cellular changes. A, normal cells; B, normal cells and atypical cells with enlarged and irregular nuclei; C, cancerous cells clumped together with greatly enlarged nuclei.

Microinvasion is a stage of minimal penetration of the basement membrane, which falls between carcinoma in situ and stage I cancer. Though technically invasive, these cancers are still relatively easy to cure. Stage I cervical cancer is confined to the cervix and the uterus. Stage II cancer has spread locally to the top of the vagina. Stage III cervical cancer has spread a little farther, sometimes to the lower part of the vagina, toward the side walls of the pelvis, and sometimes to the ureters, which enter the bladder right next to the cervix. Stage IV cervical cancer has spread still further, perhaps involving the bladder or the rectum.

YOUR PAP TEST

There are several systems for classifying the results of Pap tests, so the terminology can be confusing. Talk to your doctor about the precise meaning of your test results.

One system for grading Pap tests is the Bethesda System (TBS). Its categories refer to the kinds of cell changes and the extent of the cervix affected by these changes. (The ratings in parentheses refer to the former grading system which rated Pap tests in classes I–V.)

Normal: No evidence of malignant cells (class I).

Atypical cells of undetermined significance: The cells look strange (that is, abnormal) but probably are not precancerous. This category is sometimes called reactive cellular changes. The changes can be brought about by infections such as herpes, chlamydia, or yeast infection (class II).

Low-grade squamous intraepithelial lesions (SIL): These abnormal changes in the squamous cells are not invasive but can become so over time, although sometimes the abnormal cells spontaneously change back to normal cells (class III).

High-grade intraepithelial lesions: High-grade SILs are less likely than low-grade SILs to disappear without treatment and are more likely to eventually develop into cancer if they are not treated. However, treatment can cure *all* SILs and prevent true cancer from developing. A Pap smear cannot show for certain whether a woman has a high- or low-grade SIL (class IV).

Invasive cancer (likely to be spreading into the cervix and potentially beyond): I have never had a patient with a Pap smear that showed invasive cancer. The one such patient whom I did see during my residency (twenty-five years ago) was a woman with four children who had not had a single Pap smear since delivering her last child ten years previously (class V).

The most confusing Bethesda System category for cells of the outer cervix is *atypical squamous cells of undetermined significance,* which is often abbreviated as ASCUS and pronounced "ask-us." Pathologists use the category when the Pap test fails to reveal whether the abnormal cells are due to inflammation or to a precancer.

The Bethesda System is not the only classification method for reporting Pap test results. An earlier system referred to dysplasia, which literally means "abnormal growth." Changes in cervical cells were classified by degree, as showing mild dysplasia, moderate dysplasia, or severe dysplasia.

Another term you may hear is cervical intraepithelial neoplasia (CIN). The "intraepithelial" means that the changes are in the epithelium or outer layer of the cervix; these changes are not deep, they are not invasive cancer. The word "neoplasia" connotes unusual cell changes but in this context does not imply invasive cancer. While CIN is definitely not cancer, it is often classified in grades, as is cancer: CIN 1 means mild dysplasia, CIN 2 is moderate dysplasia, and CIN 3 is severe dysplasia.

Some physicians refer to severe dysplasia as carcinoma in situ. I dislike using that terminology, because the word "carcinoma" makes people anxious. Carcinoma in situ and severe dysplasia are essentially the same thing: the "in situ" means that the carcinoma is not invasive. If you take care of it, you should be cured, and unless you have HIV infection, you should never have to worry about the disease again.

▶ *Who is at high risk for cervical cancer?*

Although we are unsure about the agent that causes precancerous changes to cells of the cervix, we do know that women who have been exposed to multiple sexual partners or who started intercourse during their teens are at increased risk of cervical cancer unless they protect themselves with condoms. Because your cervical cells are changing during your teens, you are more at risk if you have intercourse at that time. If you start having intercourse at age 22, most of these changes will have already happened, so you are at lower risk. In this sense, sex can give you cancer; it does matter how many different sex partners you have had and how young you were when you began having intercourse. Early childbearing seems to be a risk factor, but if you have children when you are 20, obviously you have been having sex early. Some factor in childbirth itself seems to increase risk, so that women who have had many children are at higher risk than women who have had only one or two.

Thus, a woman who had intercourse first at age 24 with her husband, who remained her only sexual partner for the rest of her life, is a low-risk candidate—unless her husband has had multiple partners. If that is the case, he increases his wife's risk for cervical cancer.

TABLE 3. Classification of Pap Test Results

PAPANICOLAOU CLASSIFICATION SYSTEM	OLD SYSTEM	BETHESDA SYSTEM
Class I	Normal	Within normal limits
Class II	Atypical	Benign cellular changes (or) Atypical squamous cells of undetermined significance (ASCUS)
Class III	Dysplasia	Squamous epithelial cell abnormality
	Mild	Low-grade squamous intraepithelial lesion (SIL)
	Moderate	High-grade SIL
	Severe	High-grade SIL
Class IV	Carcinoma in situ	High-grade SIL
Class V	Invasive squamous cell carcinoma	Squamous cell carcinoma
	Adenocarcinoma	Adenocarcinoma

Women who have had other sexually transmitted diseases, such as chlamydia and HIV infection are at increased risk. Hispanic, Native American, and African American women have a higher incidence of cervical cancer than do white women, probably because these groups have less access to health care. Diets low in fruits and vegetables have been associated with an increased risk of cervical cancer and several other cancers. Smoking increases risk, because it exposes the body to carcinogenic chemicals that are absorbed by the lungs and carried in the bloodstream throughout the body. Tobacco by-products have been found in the cervical mucus in women who smoke, and researchers believe that these substances damage the DNA of cells in the cervix and may contribute to the development of cervical cancer. Some researchers believe that a diet deficient in vitamins A and C may contribute to the development of cervical cancer, though this has not been proven.

Women whose mothers took DES (diethylstilbestrol) during pregnancy are at slightly increased risk of cervical cancer. This synthetic estrogen was given during pregnancy to prevent miscarriage and other complications, though there was never convincing evidence that it did so. The Food and Drug Administration advised against its use during pregnancy in 1971 and banned its use as a growth hormone for livestock in 1979.

▶ Does genital herpes increase the risk of cervical cancer?

People used to think that genital herpes set you up for cervical cancer, because data showed that women with herpes had a higher incidence of cervical cancer. The current thinking is that the risk factors are similar. Women with herpes are likely to have multiple sex partners, early intercourse, and several children, all of which put these women into a high-risk category for cervical cancer. But the herpes virus itself does not seem to be the culprit.

▶ Are abnormalities of the cervix forerunners of AIDS?

While HIV-positive women are at increased risk for cervical cancer, women with cervical dysplasia are not necessarily at higher risk for AIDS. Cervical dysplasia is much more common than AIDS, and the vast majority of women with cervical dysplasia do not have AIDS. If you do have cervical dysplasia and are worried about AIDS, have an HIV test.

▶ What should you do if your Pap smear is abnormal?

If your Pap smear shows a mild abnormality, your doctor may recommend repeating the test in a few months. Often the immune system will "fix" the questionable cells, making them revert to normal. If the next smear, say three months later, is still abnormal, your gynecologist will probably suggest looking at your cervix with a colposcope, a sort of giant microscope. The procedure can be done in the doctor's office without anesthesia.

Through the colposcope abnormal tissue really looks different from normal tissue, with different blood-vessel patterns and cells that vary in shape, size, and perhaps density. During the procedure your doctor will snip off (biopsy) bits of the most irregular-looking tissue and send them to a pathologist, who will examine them under a regular microscope and tell your gynecologist what is going on. Sometimes the problem will turn out to be an inflammation that is not linked to cancer, or an infection with the condyloma virus, that caused an abnormal Pap smear but no worrisome cellular changes. The biopsy will probably be a little uncomfortable, but not as much so as an endometrial biopsy.

▶ *What is the treatment for precancerous cervical changes?*

If the changes in your cervical cells are only mildly abnormal your doctor may suggest watchful waiting, examination under the colposcope, plus more frequent Pap smears to make sure that the cells revert to normal. Laser surgery, cryosurgery, or the loop electrical excision procedure (LEEP) are other possibilities. Some women, who have severe dysplasia and painful menstrual periods, opt for a hysterectomy if they have finished their families, but few women end up with a hysterectomy because of dysplasia.

CRYOSURGERY AND LASER SURGERY

Cryosurgery is surgery that involves freezing. The physician takes an instrument that looks like a wand and places it against the abnormal area on the cervix. Compressed nitrous oxide gas flows through the tip of the wand, making it very cold and freezing the cells, until the abnormal area becomes a little iceball on the cervix. The frozen area is allowed to thaw and is then refrozen, a process that kills the superficial cells, which are sloughed off. The body generates new, healthy cells with no abnormalities.

Laser surgery too kills the superficial cells so that the body sloughs them off. It utilizes heat rather than cold and actually vaporizes the diseased cells. Both cryosurgery and laser surgery can be done in an outpatient setting or in a physician's office.

CONE BIOPSY

Some physicians recommend cone biopsy, a procedure that surgically removes a chunk of the diseased tissue. It is a little more complicated than cryosurgery or laser surgery, and a bit more aggressive in that more tissue is removed. A cone biopsy can be done either with a cutting tool—a scalpel or a laser—or with an electrical wire. The choice depends on the condition of your cervix and your gynecologist's preference. Either procedure can be done in an office setting, though most are performed in a surgicenter using a little sedation. Usually the sedation is a local anesthetic such as Novocain for your cervix and something like intravenous Valium to calm your nerves. Some women elect to have general anesthesia. Using a scalpel (a "cold-knife conization") or a laser, the surgeon removes a small, cone-shaped wedge of cervical tissue and puts a few stitches around the area where the tissue was removed.

The newest technique, one that physicians are increasingly choosing, is a loop electrical excision procedure, or LEEP. A very hot tungsten wire with electric current passing through it is used to take out a cone-shaped wedge of tissue. The wire cuts through the tis-

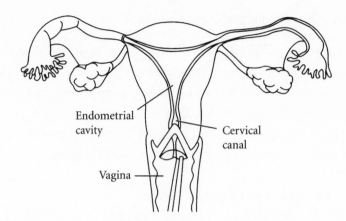

Endometrial cavity

Cervical canal

Vagina

FIGURE 26. A cone biopsy involves removing a cone-shaped wedge of the inner cervix to eliminate and evaluate precancerous cervical changes.

sue easily and cauterizes the blood vessels at the same time, thereby controlling bleeding. Unlike a laser, the hot wire does not char the edges of the incision.

▶ What are the risks of cone biopsy?

These different procedures for cone biopsy are all comparable in terms of cure rates or complications after surgery. As with any surgery, make sure your operation is performed by someone who has done it many times. The risk of infection or bleeding is always present in surgery; but with cone biopsies, that risk is slight.

Many women have a cervical or vaginal discharge for days or even a few weeks after a cone biopsy. The amount of discharge and the time it lasts differ from woman to woman, rather than from one type of procedure to another. The most significant discharge, however, does seem to occur after cryosurgery.

▶ How long does it take to recover from a cone biopsy or LEEP?

Since these procedures are minor enough to be done in a surgicenter or doctor's office, the recovery period is short—aside from the vaginal discharge. You can continue all your usual activities, except that you should abstain from intercourse while your cervix is healing, a period of two to three weeks. Usually your physician will check you after this time to be sure you are healing well. A Pap smear will not give any useful diagnostic information until your cervix is fully healed.

▶ *Will a cone biopsy affect my fertility?*

A cone biopsy will not affect your fertility or harm your cervix so that it is unable to sustain a pregnancy. Women who have had a cone biopsy rarely have problems giving birth.

▶ *When should you have another Pap smear after a cone biopsy?*

Most physicians recommend waiting about three months, but even then your cervix may not be completely healed and the Pap smear will not be readable by the pathologist. The first accurate postoperative Pap smear generally shows that the abnormal cells are gone. After that, most physicians recommend a repeat Pap test more frequently than once a year, perhaps every six months for a year or two; thereafter, if nothing abnormal turns up, it is common to space the Pap smears further apart again.

▶ *Is a hysterectomy ever done because of cervical abnormalities?*

Some old-time physicians do not believe in cone biopsies and prescribe hysterectomy instead. If your doctor recommends a hysterectomy for precancerous cervical disease, get a second opinion. If you have symptoms in addition to your cervical dysplasia, a hysterectomy, which removes the entire uterus including the cervix, may be a better choice than a cone biopsy.

> Daisy has menstrual periods that last ten days, with heavy flow and clotting. She doesn't want more children, and she is really incapacitated with her periods. She is not particularly reliable about following instructions or taking medication. Her last Pap smear showed that Daisy also has cervical dysplasia.

A hysterectomy for Daisy would solve several problems at once. Instead of removing part of her cervix and letting her cope with the heavy periods and birth control, a hysterectomy would give her permanent sterilization and solve her bleeding problems as well.

A hysterectomy may also be necessary if cervical changes have progressed beyond carcinoma in situ. If you prefer conservative therapy—a cone biopsy, for example—you need to follow up and be reliable about coming in for examinations. If you do not want to take that responsibility, then conservative therapy is not right for you.

▶ *Can you get a tubal ligation while you are having a cone biopsy?*

Some women who need a cone biopsy ask for a tubal ligation at the same time. They would prefer not to have a hysterectomy, a personal preference that should be respected, but they would like sterilization. Fifteen years ago I seldom did a cone/tubal, because these two very different procedures achieve the same result as a hysterectomy. Today I do perform them together. The procedures are simple enough that doing both at the same time is not a problem. In general, recuperation from a cone/tubal is rapid. A hysterectomy is major surgery and requires a much longer recovery time.

▶ *What are the therapies for more advanced stages of cervical cancer?*

Most women with cervical cancer are diagnosed early through Pap smears or because they have unexplained vaginal bleeding. There are two options for treatment of stage I cervical cancer. One is radiation therapy, which is quite effective. The other is radical pelvic surgery, which involves removing the uterus and taking out the lymph nodes next to it.

Surgery as a treatment for cervical cancer has the advantage that it does not interfere with the ovaries, because they are not involved with the disease; estrogen, made by the ovaries, does not stimulate cervical cancer. Most women who get the disease are fairly young and have functioning ovaries, which can continue to work normally after the surgery. Radiation therapy, on the other hand, will shut down the ovaries forever and cause artificial menopause, which is not desirable in younger women. The surgical approach can usually maintain normal sexual function by keeping the top of the vagina intact and unscarred.

Many physicians recommend some radiation therapy in addition to surgery, because of the risk of involvement of lymph nodes that have not been taken out. And some new approaches involve chemotherapy.

▶ *What are the survival rates for stage I cervical cancer?*

Ninety percent of women treated for stage I cervical cancer (when the disease is still localized) will be alive five years later. In fact, if you have lived five years beyond your treatment, you are likely to live a great deal longer because cervical cancer, unlike some other cancers, generally recurs quickly if it recurs at all. HIV-positive women have less reassuring survival rates.

▶ *What kind of physician should treat someone with cervical abnormalities?*

Any board-certified gynecologist should be able to treat cervical dysplasia and do a cone biopsy or other appropriate therapy. If the cancer has spread beyond the cervix, it is wise to consult a specialist—a gynecological oncologist or someone who works with one. Obviously, radiation therapy should be directed by a specialist in this field. Surgery for invasive cancer should be performed by a specialist with considerable experience in cancer surgery—not necessarily someone board-certified in gynecological oncology, but someone skilled in radical pelvic surgery. The kind of radical hysterectomy appropriate for invasive cervical cancer is technically more difficult than a simple hysterectomy for fibroids or for early endometrial cancer.

OVARIAN CANCER

Ovarian cancer ranks third among gynecological cancers, after breast cancer and uterine cancer, accounting for only about 4 percent of cancers among women. Each year approximately 23,000 women are diagnosed with ovarian cancer and 14,000 women die of it. Ever since the comedian Gilda Radner died of ovarian cancer in 1989, this disease has received a lot of media attention. It is not its frequency but its mortality rate that makes ovarian cancer so threatening.

Generally, ovarian cancer is discovered late. While most uterine and cervical cancer is discovered while women have stage I disease, about 70 percent of ovarian cancers do not show up until the disease has reached stage III. Women who develop cancer of the cervix or uterus tend to bleed unexpectedly and women with breast cancer often feel a lump or see a change in their breast. Screening tests—Pap smears and mammograms—often pick up these diseases in their very early stages. With ovarian cancer, women seldom have unexpected vaginal bleeding and usually do not feel a mass in their abdomen. But if ovarian cancer is discovered early, while it is still localized in the ovary, the cure rate is about 95 percent.

▶ *What are the warning signs of ovarian cancer?*

The symptoms that send women to seek help are usually the signs of extended disease. Most common is a sense of abdominal fullness or bloating, caused not by the size of the abdominal mass, but from fluid collecting in the abdomen. Most women regularly feel fullness or bloating at some time of the month, which makes it difficult to diagnose ovarian cancer. So if you are more than 30 years old and have vague digestive symptoms (stomach discomfort, gas, distension) that persist and cannot be explained by another cause, talk to your gynecologist about the need for an evaluation for ovarian cancer.

▶ Who is at risk for ovarian cancer?

The main risk factor is being female. Older women are at higher risk, because the incidence of the disease peaks between the ages of 70 and 75. (Compare cervical cancer, which peaks in women's 30s and endometrial cancer, whose highest incidence is in women's 40s.) Therefore, older women should continue to see their gynecologists even after menopause. About 2 in 10,000 women between the ages of 30 and 50 will develop ovarian cancer, while 4 in 10,000 who are older than 50 will get the disease.

Women with a family history of ovarian or breast cancer have increased risk, as Gilda Radner's case indicates. If your mother or sister had ovarian cancer, your risk increases slightly and signals that you should be closely followed; having a strong history, with several afflicted relatives, puts you at substantially increased risk. The families in which ovarian cancer is an ongoing problem tend to have numerous members affected, not just one or two.

> Erin's mother had ovarian cancer and her mother's sister died from it. Her mother's sister's daughter—Erin's cousin—was recently diagnosed. With this kind of strong family history, it is clear how to proceed. Erin had her second child when she was about 30. She waited until the infant was getting along well enough that Erin could go to the hospital and have her ovaries removed. All the physicians treating Erin and Erin herself felt that this was unquestionably the right move.

Women who have had breast cancer are also at increased risk, partly because some of the risk factors for breast cancer are the same as those for ovarian cancer. Furthermore, inheriting the genes that predispose women to breast cancer puts them at risk for ovarian cancer as well. There are some familial syndromes that involve colon and endometrial cancer. If your family has a history of several of these different cancers, point this out to your gynecologist.

Other risk factors include never having children or having children late in life, using fertility drugs but not getting pregnant, and early menarche and/or late menopause. Some researchers believe smoking slightly increases risk, although not so much as with lung or bladder cancer. Industrialized countries have higher rates of ovarian cancer than developing countries, and it is more common in white than in African American women. Some researchers believe that a high-fat diet raises risk, and the American Cancer Society recommends a diet low in fat, particularly animal fat.

Some studies have suggested that using talcum powder on sanitary napkins and in the genital area slightly increases risk, though other studies find no such links. In the past, talcum powder was sometimes contaminated with asbestos, a known cancer-causing mineral, but for more than twenty years body- and face-powder products have been required by law to be asbestos free.

GENES AND CANCER

Scientists believe that the BRCA1 and BRCA2 (or Breast Cancer 1 and 2) genes are responsible for nearly all cases of "inherited" ovarian cancer and approximately half of all cases of "inherited" breast cancer. In addition to determining such things as height and eye color, genes instruct the body in building proteins, the chemical substances that keep it in working order. Sometimes an error in a gene causes it not to do its job properly, and this genetic defect can lead to disease (see Chapter 10).

▶ *Can you lower your risk for ovarian cancer?*

The factors that reduce risk for cervical cancer—postponing your first intercourse, limiting the number of sexual partners, and using condoms for protection—unfortunately will not help prevent ovarian cancer. However, using birth control pills may offer significant protection. Women on the pill are about 50 percent less likely to get the disease than comparable women who are not. This protective effect seems to last for a considerable time after a woman has stopped taking oral contraceptives. If you are anxious about getting ovarian cancer, talk to your doctor about taking birth control pills.

Women who have never been pregnant are more at risk than women who have had at least one child, although of course avoiding ovarian cancer is not in itself a valid reason to have a child. Breast-feeding also reduces risk. Researchers believe that the ovarian changes that eventually lead to cancer come about because of ovulation; by reducing the number of times you ovulate, you reduce the number of times these ovarian changes can take place. Pregnancy, breast-feeding, and oral contraceptives all block ovulation.

FAMILY HISTORY

The Gilda Radner Familial Ovarian Cancer Registry at the Roswell Park Cancer Institute in Buffalo, New York, is a data bank of familial histories. (The hotline and Web site are given in the Resources section at the back of this book.) The head of the registry is Dr. Steven Piver, whose job it is to supply any information you may need. When I called him about Erin, he concurred in our decision, believing strongly that she was at such high risk that she should have her ovaries removed even though she was still a young woman.

▶ *Do women without a strong family history of ovarian cancer get the disease?*

Yes, familial cases make up only a small percentage, somewhere between 5 and 10 percent, of women who get ovarian cancer. Fortunately, if you have just one relative who has had ovarian cancer, perhaps your mother, you are not at greatly increased risk. Your mother— or your cousin or sister—might be one of the many nonfamilial, sporadic cases that turn up, so you are not genetically at risk. If, on the other hand, you have several relatives who have had ovarian cancer, then you probably *are* at increased genetic risk. Sad to say, you are not home free just because you do not have a relative who has had ovarian cancer.

▶ *Do fertility drugs increase the risk for ovarian cancer?*

Considerable controversy has erupted over whether fertility drugs, for example Clomid and Pergonal, increase the risk of ovarian cancer. Large-scale studies suggest that it is not the Clomid or Pergonal that increases the risk, but the fact that women who have never been pregnant are at higher risk.

All the same, some connection may exist between fertility drugs and ovarian cancer, because women who get the disease are women who have ovulated often. Women who have many children have lower risk of ovarian cancer because they did not ovulate during their pregnancies. As we have seen, birth control pills also limit the incidence of ovarian cancer. Therefore it is reasonable to assume that a medication that increases ovulation may increase later ovarian problems.

On the other hand, in order to become pregnant you do have to ovulate. Sometimes women tell me that they don't want to take Clomid or Pergonal because they have heard that these drugs increase the risk of ovarian cancer; but they *do* want to get pregnant. They cannot have it both ways. They can take birth control pills, which reduce the risk of ovarian cancer but also reduce to nearly zero the chances of getting pregnant.

▶ *Are there ways to detect ovarian cancer early?*

Most ovarian cancer that is picked up early is found during routine pelvic exams. The American College of Obstetricians and Gynecologists recommends an annual pelvic exam to screen for ovarian cancer.

Some people believe that ultrasound technology can detect ovarian cancer, but its uses are limited. For one thing, ultrasound is not cost effective as a screening tool. A pelvic exam with ultrasound costs somewhere between two hundred and three hundred dollars. If the ovarian tumor is so small that a gynecologist cannot feel it, the ultrasound scan may not pick it up either. The situation is different with mammography, where breast-cancer tumors too small to be felt often show up on x-rays. However, ultrasound is useful in determining the nature of an ovarian growth. If during an exam your physician notes a mass on your ovary, ultrasound can help determine whether it is benign or malignant. Fluid-filled cysts are much less likely to be cancerous than those with solid matter inside.

Certain blood tests look for cancer markers, but these are not reliable enough for routine screening. One is called a CA-125 test; a newer one is the CA19-9. These tests look for high blood levels of the carbohydrates CA-125 and CA19-9. Women with ovarian cancer have elevated blood levels of these carbohydrates. Yet the correlation is not like the firm association between, for example, spina bifida (a condition in which the neural tube does not completely close during fetal development) and alpha fetal protein. If a fetus has an incompletely closed neural tube (the channel that holds the spinal column), the mother shows an elevated blood level of alpha fetal protein because the protein, made by the fetus, leaks out from the open neural tube and gets into the mother's blood, where it can be measured.

The test gives many false positives (false alarms) and false negatives (false reassurances). Women who have endometriosis often have elevated CA-125. So do some women with fibroids or chronic thyroid disease. On the other hand, many women who do have cancer of the ovary have perfectly normal CA-125 levels.

Thus, CA-125 tests are not reliable enough for screening, but they are useful in special situations. Suppose someone has had cancer of the ovary and her ovaries have been removed. After the surgery, her CA-125 level goes down. Her doctor can use the test as a way to check for recurrence of the disease. Or suppose someone has a familial history of ovarian cancer that is not clear-cut:

Sofia's mother had ovarian cancer as a young woman and maybe great-aunt
Natasha had it also. Since she lived in Russia and the stories describing Natasha's

symptoms are hearsay (no one in American ever met her), Sofia is not sure whether she died of ovarian cancer or something else. Sofia is anxious; she hasn't had her children yet and doesn't want to have her ovaries removed.

How can Sofia's doctor monitor her closely? We can increase her pelvic exams to two per year. Or we can alternate a pelvic exam with an ultrasound every six months. And we can follow her CA-125 level to see whether it changes.

▶ *Are all ovarian tumors cancerous?*

Definitely not. If your doctor says you have a mass on your ovary, chances are that it is *not* malignant. The overwhelming number of ovarian masses are benign, even in women as old as 60.

▶ *Are there different kinds of ovarian cancer?*

Yes, there are almost forty different kinds, but a few predominate. The ovary is made up of three kinds of tissue: the epithelium, which is the capsule surrounding the ovary; the tissue of which the eggs themselves are composed; and the inner stromal tissue that supports the eggs.

About 85–90 percent of ovarian cancers are epithelial tumors, on the outside rim of the ovaries. The most common of these are called serous cyst adenocarcinomas. "Serous" means that the tumors contain fluid or serum. The "adeno" root indicates that the tumor arises in glandular tissue. Some cancerous tumors of the epithelium contain a jelly-like substance; these are called mucinous cyst adenocarcinomas. Both mucinous cyst adenocarcinomas and serous cyst adenocarcinomas can have solid material inside them.

Tumors of the inner structure of the ovary are called stromal tumors. These tumors can make hormones and may cause hormone-related problems. For example, tumors in the granulosa cells (that surround the eggs as they mature) produce estrogen. Women with such tumors may have vaginal bleeding, because they are producing very high levels of estrogen. Women who have a different type of stromal tumor that produces testosterone may notice problems of masculinization: excessive facial hair, acne, and aggressive behavior. These tumors are rare, but are occasionally seen in older women.

Tumors of the egg tissue itself are called germ cell tumors or egg tumors. The most common are cystic teratomas, also called dermoid cysts. They are very rarely cancerous and are most common in younger women. They can have almost any body tissue inside

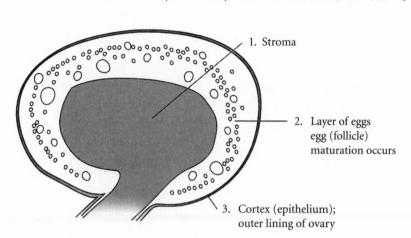

1. Stroma

2. Layer of eggs
   egg (follicle)
   maturation occurs

3. Cortex (epithelium);
   outer lining of ovary

FIGURE 27. The normal ovary contains three types of cells. The central supporting layer is made up of stromal cells; the cortical cells form the covering of the ovary (the epithelium). Between these two layers the egg cells (follicles) perform the actual business of the ovary.

them, including hair, teeth, or cartilage. After all, the egg is a totipotent cell, able to make any kind of cell found in the body; it makes sense, therefore, that disordered egg cells can also make body tissues. Because the diseased egg cells are not fertilized, they are not "turned on" in the normal way. Indeed, scientists do not know what turns them on and makes them start dividing. These tumors used to be diagnosed by taking an x-ray and looking for teeth within the ovarian mass. Once I had a patient who had a whole palate in a cyst.

▶ *Can any tests determine without surgery whether an ovarian mass is cancerous?*

Recently developed tests can differentiate fairly effectively between malignant and benign growths. The Doppler flow study measures the blood supply to the ovarian mass. If the mass has normal flow characteristics and no signs of increased blood flow (which indicates the presence of rapidly dividing cells), it almost always proves to be benign. The test sometimes shows false positives, whereby it indicates that an ovarian mass has increased blood flow, but the mass turns out not to be cancerous at all.

▶ *If a physician recommends ovarian surgery, is cancer the likely diagnosis?*

While some physicians are beginning to rely more heavily on tests such as the Doppler, it is often difficult to tell with certainty whether a tumor is benign or malignant without resorting to surgery. The only absolutely sure diagnostic method is to remove the tumor or cyst and send it to a pathologist who can determine what is going on. If your doctor recommends surgery, there is still a very good chance that your condition is benign.

When one of my patients has to have ovarian surgery for diagnostic reasons, I do prepare her for the possibility of cancer, however. It is psychologically important to realize that the possibility exists, even though chances are that she does not have cancer.

THE STAGES

The stages of ovarian cancer are similar to those of uterine or cervical cancer. Stage I disease is confined to the ovaries. Stage II disease extends through the pelvis to the uterus and fallopian tubes. Stage III disease involves spread through the pelvis to more remote pelvic organs such as the omentum, the apron of fatty tissue that surrounds the intestines. Stage IV disease has spread beyond the pelvis to distant tissues, for example the lungs.

With endometrial or cervical cancer, the physician can often tell how far the cancer has advanced. Because the gynecologist has already done a D&C or taken a Pap smear, the extent of the disease may be fairly evident before any surgery. With ovarian cancer this is not the case. Not until the surgery is performed can the physician know the extent of the disease.

▶ *If your doctor recommends a bowel prep before surgery, does that mean she thinks you have cancer?*

Because ovarian tumors can attach themselves to the intestines or other internal organs, I often recommend a bowel prep to clear out the bowel before diagnostic surgery. If someone's tumor has adhered to her intestine, the surgeon may have to peel it off. For that reason it is advisable to have the bowel completely prepared. Very few people end up with a colostomy or removal of part of the intestine, even if they have ovarian cancer. Today for a bowel prep, most physicians recommend a liquid laxative such as citrate of magnesia or a preparation called Go Lightly. Occasionally a bowel prep will also include oral antibiotics.

▶ *What is the usual surgery for ovarian cancer if a woman has completed her family?*

For women who have completed their childbearing, the usual surgical procedure is to remove both ovaries, the uterus, and the fallopian tubes. Often women wonder why they should have all these organs removed when the mass is only on one ovary. There are several reasons. First, women who have completed their families or who are menopausal have no need to preserve reproductive function. Second, a hysterectomy may avoid repeat surgery. Suppose the surgeon removes the ovary, has a tissue sample known as a frozen section examined during the operation, and the pathology report comes back benign. Later, when the pathologist examines the entire sample, a spot of cancer turns up somewhere else in the ovary that was removed. (In a small percentage of cases this does happen.) A second surgery will be needed.

It is also possible that cancer is developing in the second ovary, even though that ovary looks normal. In a small percentage of cases the disease is bilateral; someone who has had an ovarian cancer in one side has a higher chance of developing it on the other side later, even if she does not have any active disease at the moment. So there is reason to remove both ovaries.

Why take out the uterus also? Occasionally there is microscopic spread of cancer to the uterus. Beyond that, many older women who have their ovaries removed are candidates for estrogen replacement therapy. If their uterus is removed, they will not have to take progesterone to protect them from uterine cancer.

At the beginning of the operation, the surgeon will wash out the interior of the pelvic cavity with water, which is then collected and examined to see whether there is evidence of cancerous cells floating anywhere in the pelvis, cells that could attach themselves to some organ and start cancer elsewhere. These floating cells are called washings; their presence suggests higher risk for the spread of disease.

Most surgeons will also sample some lymph nodes in the pelvis during the operation and send them to the pathologist. Their condition will help decide the course of subsequent therapy—whether to have chemotherapy or radiation. Sometimes the surgeon will remove some of the fat inside the pelvic cavity. Because the omentum is a favorite place for ovarian cancer to spread, the pathologist will check some of the fat cells for evidence of disease.

▶ *What is the surgical routine if a woman has not completed her childbearing?*

Each woman must discuss her situation at length with her gynecologist. If at all possible, the surgeon will take out only the cancerous ovary, removing only what is absolutely necessary to cure the disease. If the patient has completed her childbearing, her options depend on the type of tumor. The gynecologist may recommend removing the remaining ovary and possibly the uterus and fallopian tubes, since her previous ovarian cancer places her in a higher risk category.

Sadly, there are times when the ovaries cannot be saved because the tumor has spread. All doctors who treat cancer would recommend removal of the cancerous tissue at the expense of childbearing.

> Jane had a worrisome 10-cm ovarian mass, roughly the size of a large orange. Because there was no chance of saving the ovary that had been invaded by the tumor, the surgeon removed the ovary as well as the tumor. The tumor turned out to be not cancer but a cyst of endometriosis, which would have had to be removed in any case.
>
> Unfortunately, Jane's other ovary was missing. Although she was cured of her disease, she went on to sue the surgeon for making her infertile, though chances are that the large endometrial cyst kept the ovary from functioning and, considering the size of the cyst, there was no way to save the ovary. Jane testified under oath that she would rather have kept a cancerous ovary than be infertile. Despite the unrealistic nature of her allegation, the jury awarded her $375,000.

▶ *If the physician recommends chemotherapy, does it mean that he could not remove all the cancerous cells?*

Many physicians recommend chemotherapy as a preventive step, even though they are quite certain that they got all the cancer and there is no evidence that the cancer has spread. In some cases the surgeon is unable to remove all the cancer. Chemotherapy may well be recommended in such a situation. It is worth knowing that chemotherapy often dissolves the remaining tumor and that there are recently developed chemotherapies to which ovarian cancer is extremely responsive. One of the reasons for ovarian cancer's bad reputation is that in the past none of the available therapies worked.

Chemotherapy can still be difficult to endure and can have significant side effects. There is no way to prevent hair loss, although lost hair invariably grows back. The agents for chemotherapy are changing all the time, and there have been significant break-throughs in nausea medications. A wonderful (and expensive) drug called ondansetron almost always prevents nausea in chemotherapy patients. Many HMOs will pay for its use.

▶ *What kind of follow-up is done after chemotherapy?*

After several rounds of chemotherapy, perhaps six months to a year after the original op-eration, the physician may want a second look at the interior of the pelvis, to see whether the disease has completely cleared up.

There are two possibilities. Some physicians recommend a laparoscopy, the kind of procedure that is used when someone's tubes are tied with the aid of a laparoscope. The physician makes a small incision, inserts a long tube with a light into the pelvic cavity, and looks around to see what is going on. The older standard procedure was a second-look la-parotomy. The physician reopens the old incision and looks at the organs in the pelvis, tak-ing biopsies to see whether any evidence of cancer remains. Even if the second-look oper-ation does not reveal any cancer, the physician occasionally recommends several more rounds of chemotherapy to make sure that all the cancer is truly gone.

If the cancer is still present at the time of the second-look operation, then the physi-cian will recommend more cycles of chemotherapy and perhaps a third-look operation. This may seem like heavy-duty therapy, but the reason for the second-look operation is that ovarian cancer is obscure and hard to track. The doctor wants to be certain that the disease is no longer present.

The surgery for a second look is apt to be much less intense than the original opera-tion. With a hysterectomy, women should allow at least six weeks for recuperation; after a second-look procedure, women seem to be pursuing their normal activities in three or four weeks.

▶ *What kind of doctor should perform the pelvic surgery for women who have not finished their childbearing?*

Over the past two decades, attitudes toward surgery and ovarian cancer have changed. Twenty years ago the standard recommendation was that if a woman had ovarian cancer, her ovaries, fallopian tubes, and uterus were removed—no exceptions. Physicians have become more open-minded and try to adapt their recommendations to the specific cir-cumstances. If a woman wants to have children, often the surgery can be restricted to the diseased ovary with a very careful follow-up. Many women who have had ovarian cancer do subsequently have children, even women who have had chemotherapy.

For this reason younger women should be particularly careful about who operates on a pelvic mass. The surgery is probably best performed by a gynecologist, not a general surgeon. In some parts of the United States general surgeons routinely do these operations, but they may not be as knowledgeable about the latest thinking on conserving ovarian function as gynecologists, who are specialists in this field.

ENDOMETRIAL CANCER

Endometrial cancer, also called uterine cancer, usually announces itself by irregular bleeding—sporadic spotting that comes for a few days, goes away, and then comes back again. Sometimes uterine cancer causes heavy bleeding during periods. The cancer grows slowly and is likely to be diagnosed early. When the disease has not spread beyond the uterus, the five-year survival rate is 96 percent.

The principal risk factor for this disease, aside from being female, is age. Most women who get this disease get it after menopause. Ninety-five percent of endometrial cancers occur in women aged 40 or older, and the average age at diagnosis is 60. The relatively few young women who do get endometrial cancer often have problems with ovulation (no menstrual periods, widely spaced or sporadic periods) and some have the masculinizing symptoms of excessive androgens (male hormones). Underlying all these factors is long-term exposure to estrogen, especially without the balancing power of progesterone.

Obesity is also a critical risk factor, because fat tissue makes estrogen. A woman who is seriously overweight is a candidate for endometrial cancer in that her uterine lining is being constantly stimulated not only by the estrogen produced by her ovaries, but also by the estrogen manufactured by her fat. Even after menopause, when her ovaries no longer produce estrogen, her fatty tissue is still at work. Women who are twenty-one to fifty pounds overweight triple their risk; women more than fifty pounds above their normal weight increase their risk tenfold.

Other risk factors include diabetes and high blood pressure, which sometimes but not always are linked to body weight. If you are obese, you are at increased risk for high blood pressure and diabetes; but if you have one of these conditions even if you are not obese, you are still at higher risk for uterine cancer. For example, if you are a slender diabetic, your risk of uterine cancer is somewhat increased. If you are an overweight diabetic (weight control is a problem for many diabetics), you are at significantly increased risk.

Not having children increases risk. If you have had four pregnancies, you are at much lower risk for uterine cancer than someone who has had one child. During pregnancy the hormonal balance shifts toward more progesterone, reducing your endometrial cancer risk. Delayed childbearing also seems to increase risk but not greatly. Women who are at high risk for endometrial cancer are also at increased risk for breast cancer, because the risk factors are similar.

Reliable studies suggest that birth control pills protect you against both uterine and ovarian cancer. Protection is greater if you take oral contraceptives for a long time, and this benefit continues for at least ten years after you stop taking the pill.

An endometrial biopsy or an ultrasound scan can diagnose the condition. During an endometrial biopsy your physician uses a sharp tool or tiny suction device to sample the tissue of your endometrium, which is sent to a pathologist for evaluation. The procedure can be done in the doctor's office. An ultrasound done through the vagina will show the thickness of the endometrium, a clue to whether or not it is cancerous.

Emma, the mother of three, started having heavy bleeding when she was 30 years old. Emma weighs about 350 pounds, and so my first guess was that she had uterine cancer, at least in its beginning stages. An endometrial biopsy confirmed my guess; she had endometrial hyperplasia, a precursor stage that was not yet actual cancer. I did not want to perform a hysterectomy because Emma's weight increased her surgical risk, so I started progesterone therapy. After a few months the progesterone made her hyperplasia disappear.

Emma was still spotting between periods, even though biopsies showed that her precancerous condition was gone. Then we discovered that Emma had a small fibroid, only about 1 cm in diameter, under the lining of her endometrium. We removed the fibroid using a hysteroscope. Today she is fine and has no more spotting.

▶ *How does endometrial cancer develop?*

Before a full-blown cancer of the endometrium develops, the tissues go through precursor stages, just as they do with other cancers. Cancer is classified according to its location and how far it has spread.

Adenomatous hyperplasia is overgrowth of the glandular cells that make up the lining of the uterus. There are more than the normal number of glandular cells in a given sample of uterine tissue, but all of the cells look normal.

Adenomatous hyperplasia with atypia means that there are more than the normal number of glandular cells in a given tissue sample, but that some of these cells look atypical—not normal, but not cancerous. It is adenomatous hyperplasia with atypia that may lead to endometrial cancer.

Adenomatous hyperplasia, even with atypical cells, can be treated without surgery, usually with progesterone. Since adenomatous hyperplasia seems to be a condition of excess estrogen, the addition of progesterone will bring the hormones into balance and actually reverse some of the hyperplasia changes. The customary approach is to try progesterone and have a biopsy in another three months or so to see whether the overgrowth is gone. Because this kind of cancer is not ordinarily fast growing, you and your doctor have the luxury of time to try medical approaches before resorting to surgery.

THE STAGES

As with most gynecological tumors, there are four stages of uterine cancer. Stage I disease is basically confined to the body of the uterus and is the easiest to treat. Stage II disease involves the uterus and also the cervix. Although the cervix can be considered part of the uterus, lymph nodes lie close to the cervix and if these are involved, it is possible for the cancer to spread from this location. In stage III disease the cancer has spread beyond the uterus and cervix to other pelvic organs, to the ovaries, to the tissue around the uterus, or to lymph nodes outside the uterus. Stage IV disease has distant metastases. Fortunately we see very little stage IV disease, since the vast majority of women who have endometrial cancer discover it during stage I, while the disease is curable.

TREATMENT

The classic therapy for stage I disease is a hysterectomy. Unless there is a very good reason for not doing so, the ovaries are also taken out, since the estrogen they produce stimulates cancerous cells. If cancerous cells are left anywhere in the body, estrogen will cause them to grow. Sometimes the surgeon will take out a few lymph nodes. The uterus is sent to a pathologist, whose report will determine whether follow-up therapy is needed.

10 Breast Health

with Kristin Zarfos, M.D.

▶ **MYTH** Taking birth control pills can give you breast cancer.

FACT Most experts believe that taking birth control pills does not increase your risk of breast cancer, even if you have a relative who has had the disease and even if you take the pill for many years.

BREAST cancer is probably the disease women in the United States fear most. Although coronary artery disease is the leading killer of American women, affecting about 2.5 million and killing about 500,000 every year, breast cancer has a more fearful image. Excluding skin cancers, it is the most widespread form of cancer among women in this country and the second most lethal (after lung cancer). According to the American Cancer Society, an estimated 192,000 American women are diagnosed with breast cancer every year and 40,200 die of it. Even when it is not lethal, the consequences of this disease—the possible surgical loss of a breast and the physical and psychological aftereffects—are profoundly disturbing to most women.

BREAST CANCER

FACTS AND FIGURES

Breast cancer in this country has been on the rise since about 1940, growing about 4 percent yearly during the 1980s. The increase leveled off in the 1990s and the incidence currently stands at about 101 cases per 100,000 women. Much of the increase took place among older, postmenopausal women; women are living longer, and mortality from other diseases has gone down. In other words, women are living long enough to get breast cancer. Only about 5 percent of breast cancer occurs in women younger than 40, and only 25 percent in women younger than 50.

One statistic that gets a lot of attention is that the lifetime risk of getting breast cancer rose from 1 in 9 in the early 1980s to 1 in 8. The change comes about partly because in the early 1990s the National Cancer Institute changed its statistical pool, including cancers diagnosed in women over the age of 85, a group at relatively high risk, and extending the statistical lifetime to 110 years (an age most women will not attain). While the 1-in-8 figure is frightening, it does not mean that of any group of sixteen women sitting together in a room, two will get breast cancer. It does mean that each baby girl born in America has a 1-in-8 chance of getting breast cancer at some point in her lifetime if she lives to be 110. Her chance increases significantly with age.

If you are between the ages of 20 and 24, the chance that you will get breast cancer during the next ten years is only 1 in 2,500; if you are 60, that risk rises to 1 in 29. No matter how you slice the statistical pie, the fact remains that breast cancer is a serious disease that affects many women.

▶ Why has the incidence of breast cancer risen in this country?

As we have seen, one reason is that the accounting rules of the National Cancer Institute have changed slightly. Other reasons may be nutrition and changes in dietary habits: women who are better nourished often begin to menstruate earlier (see Chapter 3) and thus have a longer exposure to estrogen than women who begin to menstruate at age 15 or 16. Delayed childbearing also increases risk, and women are now marrying later, having fewer children, and having them later. It is also possible that environmental pollutants contribute to breast cancer, though the links have not been firmly established.

Another important reason is that people are living longer, which makes them vulnerable to many kinds of cancer. The population as a whole is aging. From 1970 to 1990, the number of American women who were between 20 and 39 years old rose substantially, leading to an increase in the number of breast cancers diagnosed at those ages. If age-specific breast cancer rates are applied to the female population for 1970, 1980, and 1990, the resulting numbers of breast cancer cases are 5,120, 7,800, and 10,050, respectively. These increasing numbers could give the impression of an epidemic in younger women if the increase in population is not taken into account. The same reasoning can be applied to older groups of women, who are statistically more likely to be diagnosed with breast cancer.

One of the most significant factors is increased detection because of widespread mammography. Breast cancer now is often detected earlier when it is more treatable; though more cases are discovered, fewer women die of the disease. Between 1950 and the late 1980s, the rate of mortality from breast cancer was more or less stable. Between 1990 and 1994, breast cancer mortality declined 5.6 percent, the largest short-term drop in more than forty years.

Then too, more treatment choices have become available. Many women who are diagnosed with breast cancer will not have to have a mastectomy. Instead they will probably face a combination of surgery, radiation, and/or chemotherapy.

KINDS AND STAGES OF BREAST CANCER

The working machinery of the breast consists of lobules, the glands where milk is made, and ducts, the passageways through which the milk passes on its way to the nipples. The breast also contains fatty tissue, ligaments that support the ducts and lobules, blood vessels, and lymphatic vessels. Lymphatic vessels are similar to veins, except that they carry lymph instead of blood. Lymph is a clear fluid containing the waste products of tissues and large numbers of white blood cells that fight infection. Cancer cells can enter the lymph vessels. Most of the lymphatic vessels of the breast lead to lymph nodes in the armpits.

Cancer can occur either in the ducts or the lobules, but ductal cancer is the most common and worrisome kind. Fortunately, with better technology and more accurate mammograms, we are finding ductal cancer earlier than we did in the past.

▶ How does breast cancer develop?

Like other cancers, breast cancer develops through a series of gradual changes, which progress from normal breast tissue to full-fledged cancer. The first step is proliferative fibrocystic disease, also called hyperplasia (a word that simply means "overgrowth"). This condition is not cancerous: the cells divide faster than normal cells, but are otherwise normal.

The next stage is called atypical hyperplasia. The cells are growing and dividing abnormally fast (hyperplasia), and some of the fast-growing cells have unusual characteristics (atypia). The presence of hyperplasia with atypia is an early warning that the breast is

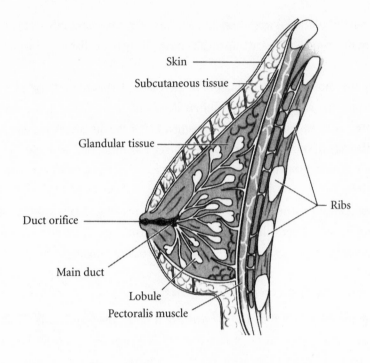

Skin

Subcutaneous tissue

Glandular tissue

Duct orifice

Main duct

Lobule

Pectoralis muscle

Ribs

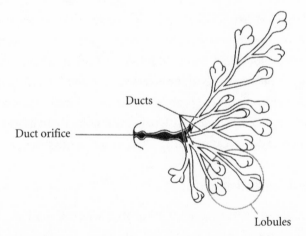

Ducts

Duct orifice

Lobules

FIGURE 28. A, the structure of the breast; B, one lobe, with its ducts and lobules.

at increased risk for developing cancer, but it is not in itself cancer. Women who have this condition are about four times as likely to get breast cancer as women who do not; they should be extremely vigilant about breast exams and have more frequent mammograms than women less at risk. But most of the time, women with atypical hyperplasia can live normal lives without overwhelming anxiety.

The next development is carcinoma in situ. Cancerous changes occur within some of the cells of the breast, but these abnormal cells do not invade their neighbors. In the next stage, invasive carcinoma, the abnormal cells invade nearby tissue and may also infiltrate blood vessels or lymph nodes. The sequence of changes, from normal to cancerous, is the same whether the cancer is in the ducts or in the lobules, though the prognosis is different.

Ductal Carcinoma

A carcinoma is a cancer that begins in the lining layer (epithelial cells) of organs. At least 80 percent of all cancers and almost all breast cancers are carcinomas. Ductal cancer is the development of malignant cells within the ducts that carry milk.

Another name for ductal carcinoma in situ, sometimes abbreviated DCIS (in which the cancerous changes remain confined to the ductal cells), is intraductal carcinoma. It has a very good prognosis: if the cancer is removed, the disease is cured. If the cancer has become invasive, the prognosis is more difficult.

Lobular Carcinoma

Lobular carcinoma, which develops in the lobules where milk is produced, has the same two stages as ductal carcinoma: either it is confined to the lobule itself—in situ lobular carcinoma—or it has spread to adjacent blood vessels or tissue and become invasive.

If an in situ lobular carcinoma is removed, the disease is cured and no further cancer treatment is necessary. However, women who have had in situ lobular carcinoma are at about 33 percent increased risk for developing breast cancer, either in the breast that was previously involved or in the other one. Lobular carcinoma that has invaded nearby cells, blood vessels, or lymph nodes must be treated more aggressively.

Inflammatory Carcinoma

Inflammatory carcinoma, the third kind of breast cancer, originates in the lymphatics within the underlying layer of the skin and is quite rare, accounting for only about 1 percent of breast cancers. Inflammatory carcinoma looks like a hot, red area on the skin of the breast. Often the skin looks textured or pitted, like the skin of an orange; sometimes the breast develops ridges and small bumps that look like hives. These symptoms are caused by cancer cells blocking lymph vessels in the skin over the breast.

RISK FACTORS

A risk factor is something that increases your chances of getting a disease, but having one or more risk factors does not mean that you will necessarily get the disease. Some women with several risk factors do not get breast cancer, while most women who do get the disease have no risk factors beyond being female. Some risk factors are beyond your control; others depend on your lifestyle and are within your power to change.

Those You Cannot Control

The greatest risk for breast cancer is being female. Although men do get breast cancer, they account for only 1 percent of cases. The second greatest risk is age: the older you are, the greater your risk. About 77 percent of women with breast cancer are over 50 when diagnosed. Women in their 20s account for only 0.3 percent of breast cancer cases.

Other risks include having a first-degree relative—a mother, sister, or daughter—who has had breast cancer. Family risk may have to do with genetic inheritance, but it can also be explained by similar lifestyles among family members and an inherited predisposition to the influence of those lifestyle factors (for example, obesity and early menstruation). Another risk factor is a personal history of breast cancer: if you have had cancer in one breast, you have a threefold to fourfold increased risk of developing a new cancer in the other breast, a cancer that is not a recurrence of the first tumor.

North American and European women have a higher rate of breast cancer than do women living elsewhere, though when women from countries with lower risk move to the United States their rates of breast cancer increase. White women are at slightly higher risk than African American women, although the latter are more likely to die of the disease, probably because they have less access to health care and are diagnosed later. Asian American or Hispanic American women have lower risk. Certain ethnic groups, for example Ashkenazi Jews, are at slightly higher risk.

Lifetime exposure to estrogen is a risk factor, and women who began to menstruate early or had late menopause are at increased risk, as are women who have never had children.

▶ *Does having had a breast biopsy in the past increase breast cancer risk?*

Having had a previous breast biopsy does not in itself increase cancer risk. Furthermore, if the biopsy showed only fibrocystic changes without proliferative breast disease, there is no increased risk. If the biopsy was diagnosed as proliferative breast disease without atypia, there is perhaps slightly higher risk; but if the biopsy showed hyperplasia with atypia, the risk is definitely increased.

▶ *Is there a gene for breast cancer?*

In 1994 researchers identified two genes, BRCA1 and BRCA2, whose mutated forms contribute to inherited breast cancer; in the future many more contributing genes will probably be discovered. Every person has two copies of the BRCA1 gene in the cells of his or her body, one inherited from each parent. Usually both genes function normally, but in some people one copy carries a mistake (something like a misspelling). This alteration can occur at hundreds of different sites along the BRCA1 gene, and some of these changes are associated with increased risk of developing breast or ovarian cancer, and cancers of the colon and prostate.

▶ *How do the genes for breast cancer increase risk?*

It is believed that the normal forms of BRCA1 and BRCA2 help prevent cancer by producing proteins that keep cells from dividing and growing abnormally. However, if a person has inherited a mutated gene from either parent, these cancer-inhibiting proteins are less effective or produced in smaller amounts, and the chances of developing cancer increase. Women with these defective genes are at very high risk for breast or ovarian cancer, a risk as high as 85–90 percent over a lifetime.

If one of your parents has a defective BRCA1 or BRCA2 gene, there is a 50-percent chance you may inherit their defective copy. If you do, then each of your children has a 50-percent chance of inheriting it from you.

Remember that the genes do not cause breast cancer. If you have inherited a mutated form of these genes, you have an increased susceptibility to breast cancer, but you will not necessarily get it. At present it is impossible to predict the percentage of women having inherited one of these genes who will actually develop breast cancer, and it is equally impossible to assess any individual woman's risk. The altered gene is not the sole cause of breast cancer, merely a contributing factor. Only 5–10 percent of breast cancer is believed to be inherited and of these hereditary breast cancers, altered forms of BRCA1 and BRCA2 are associated with only 40–50 percent of these cases.

▶ *How common are these genes?*

It is estimated that somewhere between 0.04 and 0.2 percent of women in the general population carry the mutated form of BRCA1; the mutated form of BRCA2 is less common. The prevalence of BRCA1 and BRCA2 mutations among women of Ashkenazi Jewish descent is estimated at 1–2 percent, depending on whose statistics you accept.

▶ *How important is family history as a risk factor?*

You are at increased risk for breast cancer if a first-degree relative—mother, daughter, sister, and maternal aunt (your mother's sister)—had breast cancer. If your maternal grandmother had breast cancer, you should be especially careful about doing your monthly self-exams and getting your annual physical exam and mammogram. Some physicians do not include maternal aunt and maternal grandmother as first-degree relatives, but I believe they are worth considering. Having one of these relatives with breast cancer means that you might possibly carry a gene for the disease, though probably your risk is not so high as that of women whose mothers, daughters, or sisters had breast cancer.

▶ *Does the age at which your relatives had breast cancer make a difference in your risk level?*

Some physicians believe that your risk is lower if your relative had breast cancer when she was postmenopausal or elderly, but you may still carry the gene for breast cancer even if the disease did not show up in your relative until she was older.

▶ *If your mother had breast cancer, should you have genetic testing to see whether you have inherited the gene for the disease?*

Genetic testing uses a blood sample to analyze DNA and determine whether you carry the mutated form of BRCA1 or BRCA2. The test is expensive, and your insurance may well not pay for it.

There are several issues you should consider before you are tested. Genetic testing can show whether you have inherited the mutated form of BRCA1 or BRCA2, but it cannot predict whether you will actually get breast cancer.

It is worth asking yourself what you would do if you discover that you carry one of these genes. Would you, as some women choose to do, have your breasts surgically removed preventively, so that you will not get the disease? Would you have that procedure even if you knew, as is the case, that about 5 percent of women who have both breasts removed because they have a strong family history of breast cancer still get the disease?

Privacy is another crucial issue, as with HIV testing. You cannot be absolutely certain that your test results will remain private. Suppose your insurance company learns that you carry the mutated form of BRCA1. It is certainly possible, though illegal, that you will be discriminated against because of that knowledge and have difficulty getting health insurance or be forced to pay more for your coverage.

▶ *Are women who have had other forms of cancer at increased risk for breast cancer?*

Women who have had breast cancer seem to be at somewhat increased risk for colon cancer. Women with inherited mutations of the BRCA1 or BRCA2 gene have an increased risk for developing cancer of the ovary.

▶ *Are daughters of women who took diethylstilbestrol (DES) at increased risk for breast cancer?*

No, their daughters are not at increased risk, nor are the women who took DES. However, women whose mothers took DES are at slightly increased risk of cervical cancer.

Those You Can Control (or Influence)

▶ *Does smoking increase the risk of breast cancer?*

While no scientific study shows unequivocally that smoking increases your risk for breast cancer, there is overwhelming evidence that smoking negatively affects your immune system. Many researchers strongly believe that a healthy diet helps boost the immune system and thus helps prevent breast cancer. It makes sense to avoid smoking.

▶ *How does pregnancy protect against breast cancer?*

Researchers suspect that during pregnancy breast cells differentiate into new forms, which may be more resistant to the effects of stimulation by estrogen. Researchers also believe that the different forms of estrogen produced during pregnancy, primarily estriol, may be protective.

▶ *Does breast-feeding decrease the risk of breast cancer?*

Although the answer is not definitively known, one study suggests that women who breast-feed for as little as four to six months during their lifetime have as much as a 20-percent decrease in breast cancer risk. The decrease is even greater for women who breast-feed before the age of 20. Other studies find less protection or none at all. Surgeons who do numerous breast cancer operations and see many cases of the disease generally believe that breast-feeding does offer protection against breast cancer, though their evidence is based on experience and is not rigorously scientific.

▶ *Do birth control pills increase the risk of breast cancer?*

No solid evidence links oral contraceptive use to increased breast cancer risk. Even women who took the high-dose birth control pills of the 1960s do not seem to have a higher risk.

▶ *Does estrogen replacement therapy (ERT) increase the risk of breast cancer?*

Long-term ERT use, say ten to fifteen years, may increase breast cancer risk. However, recent studies suggest that the increased risk may disappear when the ERT is stopped. The studies that do indicate an increase in risk do not show higher mortality, so the kinds of cancer associated with ERT seem to be among the less dangerous forms of the disease.

▶ *Does drinking alcohol increase the risk of breast cancer?*

Alcohol does seem to be linked with increased risk of breast cancer, and there is evidence that alcohol increases blood estrogen levels. Women who have one alcoholic drink a day have a very small increase in risk compared to nondrinkers; those who have two to five drinks daily have about one and a half times the risk.

▶ *What is the relationship between obesity and breast cancer?*

It has often been suggested that there is a link between obesity and breast cancer, especially in older, postmenopausal women. The relationship is complex, perhaps influenced by factors such as whether a woman has gained weight in later life or has been overweight since childhood. Remember that fat tissue produces estrogen, so that extra weight you are carrying around makes you a walking estrogen factory.

▶ *Are there any environmental pollutants that increase the risk of breast cancer?*

Current studies do not clearly show a link between breast cancer risk and exposure to environmental pollutants such as the pesticide DDE (chemically related to DDT) or PCBs (polychlorinated biphenyls).

PREVENTION

▶ *What can you do to protect yourself against breast cancer?*

As we have seen, many of the risk factors involve things you cannot change: your age, your sex, your heredity. Others, like the age at which you marry and have children, depend on a number of psychological, social, and economic factors. Your best bet is to cut down on the risk factors you can control and to follow the recommended guidelines for early detection.

▶ *Can you reduce your risk of breast cancer by diet?*

Having a diet high in fat may contribute to breast cancer. In fact, having a high-fat diet is not beneficial to your health in other ways. The standard dietary recommendation for general health is to eat five servings of fresh fruits and vegetables every day. The known vitamins in fruits and vegetables and the known fiber content are thought to protect against all kinds of cancer.

The type of fat you eat is at least as important as the total amount. Monounsaturated fats, including olive oil and canola oil, are linked to lower risk, while polyunsaturated fats, such as corn oil and tub margarine, and saturated fats, the kind found in meat, are associated with increased risk.

Although the data are controversial, some researchers believe a substance called lycopene in tomato sauce lowers breast cancer risk. Recently there has been scientific interest in flax seeds. Researchers have experimented with adding ground flax seeds to the diet, though the benefits have not been proven. Soy products seem to have a protective effect. Studies have shown that women from Asian cultures have a much lower incidence of breast cancer than women of Western cultures, but this advantage recedes when Asian women adopt a European or American diet.

Oily fish such as salmon and tuna that contain omega-3 fatty acids seem to be advantageous. Their use in preventing breast cancer cannot be proven, but they have other benefits and are worth emphasizing in your diet.

▶ *Does exercise have any influence on breast cancer risk?*

This is a relatively new area of research and more work needs to be done. However, some research shows that women who exercise have less breast cancer than women who do not. This is true of both older postmenopausal women and women in the 15–44 age group. Some studies suggest that strenuous exercise in youth has a lifelong protective effect. Certainly obesity increases the risk of breast cancer, and exercise is one way to fight off extra weight.

▶ *What about the drug tamoxifen as a cancer preventive?*

If you are at high risk for breast cancer, perhaps through your genetic background, talk to your doctor about taking tamoxifen as a cancer preventive. Tamoxifen is an antiestrogen drug used for many years to prevent the recurrence of breast cancer in women who had already had it. An American study completed in 1998 showed that women at high risk for breast cancer, whatever their age, substantially decreased their chances of getting the disease by taking tamoxifen. In fact, tamoxifen's effectiveness in preventing breast cancer was so obvious that the study was stopped even before the allotted time had elapsed. Interestingly, the findings of European studies were more ambiguous.

The company that manufactures tamoxifen, AstraZeneca, has promoted a scale for calculating risks called the Gail Model Risk Assessment Test. It factors in a woman's age, her age when she had her first menstrual period, her age when her first child was born, the number of first-degree relatives who have had breast cancer, the number of previous breast biopsies, and the presence (or absence) of atypia in these biopsies.

My own feeling is that every woman considering this preventive therapy should sit down with her physician and have a thorough discussion of all the pros and cons. It is fine to have a risk scale, but you cannot use it arbitrarily to decide who should use tamoxifen and who should not.

▶ *Does tamoxifen have side effects?*

One side effect is that tamoxifen can put women who are close to menopause (perimenopausal) into premature menopause. Tamoxifen blocks the action of estrogen, and estrogen is important at many sites in a premenopausal woman's body.

A second side effect is it slightly increases the risk of uterine cancer. Women with a strong family history of uterine cancer or other risk factors for this disease must take these risks into consideration before starting tamoxifen. Every woman taking tamoxifen should have a gynecological exam at least every year and perhaps every six months.

Another risk is the development of deep-vein thrombophlebitis (inflammation of the veins and the formation of blood clots there). These clots can move through the circulatory system to the lungs, where they can be life threatening. So if a woman has a tendency to this condition or has had it previously, she should carefully consider whether tamoxifen is right for her.

▶ How long can you take tamoxifen?

The standard recommendation for women who have had breast cancer is five years of therapy. Researchers are currently trying to develop a timetable for preventive tamoxifen therapy.

▶ Does it matter when in your life you start tamoxifen?

This is a very important question, and the answer depends heavily on childbearing priorities. If a woman wants children, she should not use tamoxifen until she has finished her family.

▶ Are there drugs other than tamoxifen that might help prevent breast cancer?

Current drug trials are comparing tamoxifen with a close relative, raloxifene, in terms of breast cancer prevention. Raloxifene was designed to prevent osteoporosis and has only been studied in postmenopausal women. The results of these trials are yet to come, so at present tamoxifen is the drug of choice.

SELF-EXAMINATION AND MAMMOGRAMS

The three approaches to early detection of breast cancer are self-examination, examination by a physician, and mammography. No single method alone is sufficient. All women should conscientiously pursue all three.

Monthly self-examination should begin at puberty. You know your breasts and their shape and feel better than anyone else. Although you may not know what a malignant lump feels like, you can detect subtle changes and, if you notice something different, have the change evaluated promptly by a physician.

Once you start to menstruate, you should have a yearly breast exam in conjunction

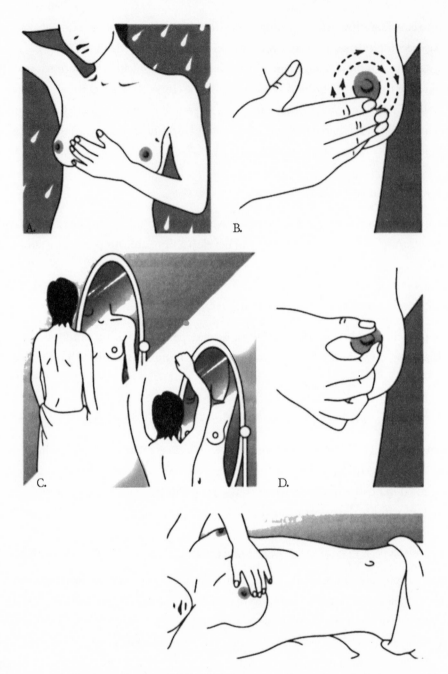

FIGURE 29. A. Check your breasts while bathing; lumps are often easier to feel when your skin is wet.

B. Place your right hand behind your head and use the sensitive finger pads of your left hand to feel

with your regular physical or gynecological exam, preferably by the same person year after year, so that he or she can get to know the character of your breasts and notice if something changes. Such stability can be difficult to achieve in this day and age, when HMOs make it hard to see the same provider year after year.

The third step is mammography, which can find lesions or lumps that may be too small or too subtle to feel. Even though mammograms do not pick up all lumps, including 7–10 percent of the breast cancers that can be felt, mammograms are far from useless. You must couple them with self-examination and examination by your doctor to get maximum protection.

▶ When should you do your monthly breast exam?

If you do your breast exam at the same time each month, it will be easier for you to identify any changes. The best time is right after your menstrual period, when your breasts are least tender and least lumpy. If you have gone through menopause already or are pregnant, simply pick a convenient day of the month—maybe the first day—and examine yourself then.

▶ How do you do a breast self-exam?

There are five steps to a thorough exam. One of your goals is to familiarize yourself with the geography of your breasts, so that you notice any changes that occur.

▶ What are the symptoms of breast cancer?

The classic symptom of breast cancer is a lump in the breast. You should also report to your caregiver any changes in the contour or shape of the breast, changes in the character

---

the right breast as you check for thickening, lumps, or other changes. Then use your right hand to examine your left breast in the same manner.

C. With your hands at your sides, examine your breasts in a mirror, looking for any change in size or contour or for dimpling of the skin. Raise your hands over your head and again look for changes. Place your hands on your hips with your shoulders forward to reveal dimpling.

D. Gently squeeze each nipple and check for discharge. Is the nipple retracted or puckered? Are there sores or scaling of the skin in the area of the areola or the nipple itself?

E. Lie flat and put a pillow under your right shoulder. Place your right hand under your head and use your left hand to feel the right breast and armpit for lumps. Then place your left hand under your head and use your right hand to examine your left breast and armpit. Move around the breast in a circle, up-and-down line, or wedge pattern. Be sure to check the same way every time; examine the entire breast area, and remember how your breast feels from month to month.

of the breast tissue (for example, thickening), a retracted nipple, dimpling of the skin, and bleeding from the nipple or any other drainage, even if it is clear. Report these signs right away, even though the odds are strongly favorable that the changes you notice are not cancerous.

Breast pain is not usually related to cancer, especially in younger women. Only about 6 percent of women with breast cancer have pain.

▶ What percentage of breast lumps are cancerous?

Fibrocystic breast disease is a very common condition in which the breasts are generally bumpy and lumpy, and it is the cause of the vast majority of lumps in younger women. About half of all persistent breast lumps in women older than 50 (the average age of menopause) are cancerous and about three quarters in women over 70. The odds are much better for younger women.

▶ Is there any way to tell by feel whether a breast lump is benign or cancerous?

There is no sure way to tell by physical examination alone whether a lump is cancerous. Cancerous lumps are often very hard and difficult to move under the skin; some have irregular edges. In medical terminology these lumps are called "discrete," because they feel very different from the surrounding tissue.

"Vague" lumps are less distinguishable from their surroundings and usually less hard. If someone has a vague lump in her breast and is a heavy caffeine drinker, her physician may take her off caffeine, give her vitamin E and vitamin B, and see whether the lump goes away. If your doctor makes these suggestions, follow them conscientiously for a cycle or two. If the lumps disappear, so much the better. If they remain, see your doctor for a follow-up exam.

▶ Are breast lumps that develop during pregnancy or during breast-feeding more likely to be cancerous than lumps that develop at other times?

It is certainly possible that lumps that develop at these times are related to the hormonal changes that come with pregnancy or nursing, but see your physician right away to make sure they are not cancerous.

▶ *If you have previously had breast cancer, is there any danger in becoming pregnant?*

This is a controversial area and needs to be addressed individually by each woman who has had breast cancer and is considering becoming pregnant. Age, family history, how advanced the previous cancer was when discovered, and other emotional and personal considerations enter into the decision. Each woman needs careful counseling to review all the factors that have surrounded her breast cancer. Of my own patients, three who had had breast cancer later had children; all did beautifully and are now in good health.

▶ *Does breast cancer discovered during pregnancy have a bad prognosis?*

People used to think that breast cancer diagnosed during pregnancy was extremely dangerous, but current thinking has softened this view somewhat. If the cancer is found early in the pregnancy, the woman must go seven or eight months without treatment if she wants to preserve the pregnancy. Obviously a pregnant woman cannot have chemotherapy or radiation. The prognosis also depends on how early the cancer is found and how advanced it is at the time of discovery.

▶ *How often should you have a mammogram, and when should you start?*

I recommend an annual mammogram for women older than 40. We know that for women in their 50s yearly mammograms can improve the cure rate by 30 percent and for women in their 40s by 15 percent. Even 15 percent is a significant improvement.

If some symptom like a lump or discharge has shown up on an earlier examination, or if you have a strong family history of breast cancer or some other risk factor, then your care should be individualized and your age at the first mammogram customized to your personal circumstances. If, for example, your mother had breast cancer while she was in her 30s, you might start having mammograms at that age.

The scheduling of mammograms for women in their 40s is a controversial issue. The American Cancer Society recommends a baseline mammogram at 40 and annual mammograms thereafter. The American College of Obstetricians and Gynecologists, the professional association for these physicians, suggests a mammogram every other year for women in their 40s. The position of the National Cancer Institute is that you do not really need annual mammograms until you are 50. Since breast cancer risk rises with age, yearly mammograms for women over the age of 50 are universally recommended.

▶ *Are mammograms painful?*

While no one thinks that mammograms are fun or comfortable, the peace of mind a favorable mammogram report can bring is certainly worth the momentary discomfort. Some women with very small breasts find mammograms painful; so do some women with very large breasts. To minimize the discomfort, you can cut down on caffeine for a few days before the exam, which will also make the x-ray easier to read.

▶ *How reliable are mammograms?*

Everyone has heard stories of women whose mammograms gave false negatives (did not find existing breast cancer). Research has shown that mammography has a sensitivity (ability to detect existing cancer) of up to 94 percent, which means that about 6 percent of cancers will not be found. On the other hand, mammograms have a specificity (ability to find an absence of cancer when the woman being screened does not have the disease) of greater than 90 percent. Mammography can detect a cancerous growth as much as two years before it can be felt by a manual exam. However, mammography may not be able to detect a growth in dense breast tissue, the type of tissue often seen in young women's breasts.

▶ *Are mammograms safe?*

Since 1992, when the Food and Drug Administration required hospitals, breast clinics, and other facilities to meet specific standards in order to offer mammography, the quality and the safety of mammography has improved. The guidelines assure that the mammography equipment is safe and uses the lowest possible dose of radiation.

Many people are concerned about exposure to x-rays, but the level of radiation in up-to-date mammograms does not significantly increase the risk for breast cancer. A woman who receives radiation therapy for breast cancer will receive several thousand rads (a measure of the energy absorbed from radiation). A woman getting yearly mammograms from age 40 until age 90 will receive 10 rads total. The amount of radiation to which you are exposed during a single mammogram equals the radiation you get flying from New York to Los Angeles.

BOX 6. When Your Mammogram Gives the Wrong Answer

False negatives (missed diagnoses) occur when mammograms appear normal even though breast cancer is actually present. False negatives are more common in younger women than in older women. The dense breasts of younger women contain many glands and ligaments, which make breast cancers more difficult to detect in mammograms. As women age, breast tissues become more fatty and breast cancers are more easily "seen" on the mammograms. Screening mammograms miss up to 25 percent of breast cancers in women in their 40s, but only 10 percent in older women.

False positives occur when mammograms are read as abnormal but no cancer is actually present. For women of all ages, between 5 and 10 percent of mammograms are abnormal. Most abnormalities are not confirmed as cancer. Like false negatives, false positives are more common in younger women than in older women. About 97 percent of women aged 40–49 who have abnormal mammograms turn out not to have cancer, as compared with about 86 percent for women 50 and older. But all women who have an abnormal mammogram need to undergo follow-up procedures such as repeat mammograms or biopsies.

▶ *Do you need a mammogram even if you have no family history of breast cancer?*

Absolutely. Most women who develop breast cancer do not have a known family member who has had the disease.

▶ *Do breast implants interfere with the accuracy of your mammogram?*

Women with breast implants must be particularly vigilant about breast self-examination, yearly exams, and mammograms. The implants can obscure portions of the breast tissue that need to be examined.

The capsule of the implant holds either a silicone gel (no longer on the market, but still present in implants done before 1992) or a saline (salt water) solution. Over time the capsule can leak, and the leakage can appear as a lump in the breast. Even though you suspect that your implant has sprung a leak, have the lump evaluated by your doctor. Do not assume that the implants have caused any changes you notice in your breasts.

▶ Can you have a mammogram if you are breast-feeding?

Yes, although the breast tissue is very dense at this time and the density might hide a lump or other lesion. There are other ways to evaluate the situation using ultrasound or perhaps even a biopsy. I usually recommend waiting three to six months after your baby is weaned before having a routine mammogram; however, if you notice a lump or some other change, be certain to notify your doctor.

▶ What tests other than mammograms can be used to detect breast cancer?

Mammograms are still the most accurate way to detect breast cancer, though some newer techniques can be used to supplement them. If we want to know whether a breast lump is filled with solid matter or fluid, ultrasound can help. Sound waves can outline the area whose texture differs from the surrounding tissue, but ultrasound does not detect the kind of small calcium deposits that often appear on a mammogram, sometimes triggering a diagnosis of breast cancer.

Magnetic resonance imaging (MRI) is another new technique, touted by the press as marvelous and less painful than mammography technology. MRI is useful for finding out whether a breast implant has developed a leak, which can help determine whether a breast lump is caused by leakage or something more worrisome. In terms of evaluating breast tissues, pointing out areas in the breast that may be suspect, or suggesting whether suspicious tissues are actually cancerous, MRI is still an experimental technique.

Thermograms, which measure heat production by tissues, were popular for a while on the premise that cancer produces heat. However, the sensitivity of these tests did not ultimately prove helpful in screening for breast cancer.

So mammograms remain the principal test for breast diagnosis. No replacements appear on the immediate horizon. However, one radiologist at the University of Arkansas is using MRI for diagnosis. While this technology is still in the research stage, it holds out the promise that women might not need surgical biopsy to diagnose or rule out cancer. At present, MRIs are too costly to be used as a screening tool for the general population: a single study costs more than a thousand dollars. If they can be made more cost effective, MRIs could be a satisfactory tool for diagnosing lumps that are too small to be felt.

BREAST BIOPSIES

Biopsies are tissue samples taken for diagnostic purposes. They can be used either to determine the cause of an abnormality that shows up on a mammogram but is too small to feel, or to ascertain the nature of a lump or lesion that is large enough to be felt. If you have had a previous baseline mammogram, the trouble spots can be compared to the earlier image.

Changes that show up on mammograms include deposits of calcium in the breast tissue. Sometimes these calcifications indicate that cells are rapidly dividing (as cancer cells do). Although 80 percent of the calcifications that show up on mammograms are benign, any new cluster needs to be evaluated.

If a change shows up through physical examination of the breast (for example, a new lump, asymmetry, or an unusual density in the breast), sometimes further mammographic views, perhaps from different angles, will clarify the problem. If these additional views do not explain the nature of the change, or if the change or lesion is still worrisome, then we try a biopsy. Depending on the kinds of changes, different kinds of biopsies can be taken.

One kind of biopsy, called a stereotactic biopsy, is a needle procedure that uses computerized technology to take small samples of tissues for purposes of diagnosis. The mammographic x-ray machine serves as a basis for finding the tissues that need to be sampled but are too small to be felt. Stereotactic biopsies are usually performed by radiologists.

Another kind of biopsy, a minor surgical procedure, is called a needle localization biopsy. It is done either because the woman prefers not to have a mammographically localized biopsy, or because the location or character of the lesion rules out that procedure. This kind of biopsy is usually an outpatient procedure, often done in the x-ray department of a hospital. It involves removing the entire area of concern, not just taking needle-size samples of the tissue from that area.

The breast is anesthetized and a guide needle is inserted into the area to be biopsied. Once the guide needle is in place, the patient is taken to the operating room and given a mild intravenous sedative so that she feels no pain and is not frightened during the procedure. The surgeon then puts some Novocain into the location indicated by the guide needle and surgically removes the area of concern. Usually the incision is only about an inch and a half long. After the surgery there is only a little discomfort and not much deformity.

▶ *What kinds of biopsies are done for lumps or lesions that can be felt?*

If there is a lump in the breast, a mammogram and an ultrasound can help determine its nature and find other lesions that may be too small to feel. A biopsy can be performed, if further investigation seems necessary.

One choice is a needle biopsy. The breast is anesthetized with a local anesthetic and a needle is inserted into the lump to sample a piece of the tissue. This sounds like an easy approach, but the surgeon must be very careful; since only a small sample is taken, there is a possibility that cancerous tissue is present but the needle has not hit it. The surgeon has to advise the patient whether to go a step further and have an excisional biopsy.

This excisional biopsy, also called an open surgical biopsy, is the second kind of biopsy. It is performed pretty much like a needle biopsy. The patient goes to the operating room and receives intravenous sedation. The breast is anesthetized with a local anesthetic and a small incision is made; the entire lump is removed. This procedure usually takes about an hour. There is not much pain afterward, not much deformity, little risk of infection—less than 2 percent—and an equally small risk of bleeding at the biopsy site.

An excisional biopsy is the best way to be absolutely sure of the nature of the lump. Sometimes a large lump may have a small bit of cancer inside. If the whole lump is removed and examined by a pathologist, we can be sure that we have not missed a cancer.

▶ *Which is better, a needle biopsy or a surgical biopsy?*

My own preference is for an excisional biopsy. One of the worst things I can do for a woman is to have her undergo a needle biopsy, reassure her that her lump is benign, then discover six months or a year later that in fact the needle missed some cancer. If the test gave a false negative in this way, an easily cured tumor might have become more difficult to treat.

If a woman has a lump that looks cancerous to her examining physician, and its location and nature make it easy to sample with a needle, then it is wise to counsel the patient before surgery to avoid two procedures and proceed with the one that burdens her less. The needle biopsy can make the diagnosis immediately. Occasionally the surgeon will then recommend radiation therapy before surgical excision if the tumor is large.

▶ *Are biopsies safe during pregnancy?*

Yes, they are safe during the second two trimesters of pregnancy—both to mother and to fetus. If a biopsy is needed during the first trimester, it is safe provided that it is done under local anesthesia.

▶ *What is the procedure if an ultrasound suggests that the lump is a cyst?*

The treatment may be as simple as putting a needle into the cyst and draining the fluid. If the cyst goes away completely, your physician will schedule a follow-up visit in a month to be sure that fluid has not accumulated again. If the cyst does not disappear when it is drained, the area needs to be biopsied again—either with a needle biopsy or with an open surgical biopsy.

▶ *What can a pathologist tell about the tissue sample from a biopsy?*

At a very basic level, a pathologist can tell whether tissue is benign or cancerous. The sample can also show the benign changes called atypical hyperplasia, in which the cells of breast tissue are growing too rapidly and some are not normal.

TREATMENT

The purpose of surgery is to remove the original tumor so that it cannot send cancerous cells to other parts of the body. Depending on the size of the tumor or the stage of the cancer, a woman and her doctor must make several decisions regarding her treatment. The first is the amount of tissue to be removed: should it be just the tumor, the tumor and part of the surrounding breast, or the entire breast?

If the cancer is found while the tumor is quite small (3–4 cm, or 1–1.5 inches), then treatment options include lumpectomy, mastectomy with immediate breast reconstruction, delayed reconstruction, or no reconstruction.

▶ *What is a lumpectomy?*

A lumpectomy is a surgical procedure in which a cancerous breast lump with a rim of normal tissue is removed. In addition to taking out the cancerous tissue, the surgeon may remove one or more lymph nodes from the armpit on the side of the affected breast.

▶ *Why are lymph nodes analyzed?*

Lymph nodes are removed and biopsied to investigate whether the cancer has spread to other parts of the body. There are two methods for doing this. One, called lymph node dissection, involves removing a percentage of the lymph nodes and testing them to see whether cancer cells are found. The second technique, called sentinel lymph node biopsy, focuses on a single lymph node—the first one to receive drainage from the breast. This single lymph node is identified through a special technology. A dye is injected into the breast, and x-rays are taken to see which lymph node picks up the dye first. This node is most likely to be the first stopping site of any cancer cells as well. If the node is removed and found to be free of cancer, it is highly unlikely that the cancer has spread to other lymph nodes or anywhere outside the original tumor.

▶ What is a mastectomy?

A mastectomy is a surgical procedure in which the breast itself is removed. In a simple mastectomy, just the breast is removed. In more radical procedures, some of the muscles underneath are taken out as well.

▶ When is a lumpectomy a good choice?

A woman with a cancerous lump no larger than 3–4 cm who can tolerate radiation therapy has the choice of lumpectomy or mastectomy. About fifteen years ago a study called the National Surgical Adjuvant Breast Project showed that women who had lumpectomies for a single lump less than 3–4 cm in size had survival rates equal to those of women with similar tumors who had mastectomies. Since lumpectomy is less disfiguring, many women who have the option make that choice.

▶ What follow-up treatments are recommended for women with small tumors who have either lumpectomies or mastectomies?

Women who have lumpectomies usually have follow-up radiation therapy to destroy any cancerous cells in the breast that may not have been removed along with the lump. Radiation is quite effective in preventing recurrence of the cancer: about 40 percent of women who have lumpectomies but no radiation have recurrence of the cancer within five years, but only 10 percent of women who have follow-up radiation have recurrences in the same period.

Chemotherapy is often used as a follow-up treatment after a lumpectomy or a mastectomy. The purpose of the chemotherapy is to destroy any cells that may have escaped from the breast and been disseminated into the body.

▶ What is the treatment for inflammatory carcinoma?

Women with inflammatory carcinoma usually receive chemotherapy before surgery. After the tumor is reduced in size, most of these women undergo a mastectomy.

▶ *Are there any new ways of using chemotherapy or radiation therapies?*

Ongoing studies in Italy are examining the possibility of using chemotherapy before the removal of small cancers in women's breasts. The hope for the future is that perhaps women with such cancers will not need surgery; perhaps they can have a needle biopsy followed by chemotherapy or radiation that will destroy all the cancer cells. However, this kind of therapy is still experimental.

FIBROCYSTIC BREAST DISEASE

What is called fibrocystic breast disease (formerly called cystic mastitis) probably is not a disease at all; in ordinary terms it is just "lumpy bumpy breasts." In fact about 70 percent of women have fibrocystic breast changes. These lumps, which are fluid-filled sacs, may be large enough to feel or they may be microscopic in size. The breasts may be tender or sore, especially before menstrual periods.

▶ *Is fibrocystic breast disease dangerous?*

No, fibrocystic breast disease is not dangerous. It does not turn into cancer, although it can make cancer more difficult to discover, by making the breasts difficult for you or your caregiver to examine. Thus it may lead to unnecessary breast biopsies.

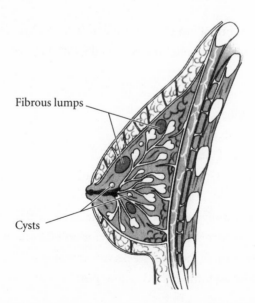

Fibrous lumps

Cysts

FIGURE 30. A fibrocystic breast feels bumpy because of small fibrous lumps and fluid-filled cysts.

▶ *Are there self-help measures for fibrocystic breasts?*

There are a few simple things that many women have found helpful. One is avoiding caffeine, which seems to stimulate fibrocystic changes. Caffeine is found in coffee, tea, chocolate, cola, some other soft drinks, and some painkillers.

Another measure is vitamin E, taken in a dosage no larger than 400–800 units daily. Vitamin E is beneficial to the body in many ways, but realize that it does not prevent breast cancer because it does not prevent the stimulation of breast tissue by a woman's own hormones. Vitamin B_6, taken in moderate or small doses of 100–200 mg daily, has been found helpful by some women, as has evening primrose oil, of which the usual dose is two 500-unit capsules daily (1,000 units total).

The published scientific literature on fibrocystic breast disease has not been convincing as to the effectiveness of these self-help remedies. Initial studies showed that they worked well, but later studies often said the opposite. All we know is that women do report them to be helpful, and these measures certainly have allowed many women to avoid unnecessary breast biopsies.

BOX 7.   Self-Help for Fibrocystic Breasts

The vast number of breast lumps are caused by benign fibrocystic changes. If you notice such changes in your breasts, your doctor may recommend the following:
1. Decaffeinate your diet: no coffee, tea, chocolate, cola drinks, or other caffeinated beverages.
2. Take 400–800 units of vitamin E daily.
3. Take 100–200 mg of vitamin B_6 daily.
4. Take two capsules of evening primrose oil daily.

Continue this plan through your next menstrual cycle. If at the end of that period the lump is no better, call your doctor for an evaluation. Nothing life-threatening can happen in the three weeks you are using self-help measures to see whether your breast lump or lumps disappear.

MASTITIS

Mastitis means infection of the breast. It can occur in women who are nursing a baby (or have recently finished nursing) or, occasionally, in women who are not breast-feeding. It is caused by bacteria, often *Staphylococcus aureus.*

Mastitis causes pain, swelling, and redness in the infected breast. Sometimes the swelling is in the form of a small, painful lump. Like many bacterial infections, mastitis can cause general symptoms, like chills, fever (sometimes quite high), and aches. If not treated, it can develop into an abscess, a pocket of pus beneath the skin.

▶ *What causes mastitis?*

In nursing mothers, the source of the bacteria is probably the baby's mouth. In women who are not breast-feeding, it is possible that bacteria can be introduced from the mouth of a sexual partner.

Insect bites can lead to mastitis. Once the skin is broken, bacteria can enter; and once into the breast tissue, an infection can smolder and then become full-blown mastitis. Any area of redness or change should be examined by a physician.

▶ *How is mastitis treated?*

Mastitis can be treated quite successfully with antibiotics. If it develops in a woman who is not breast-feeding, usually the course of antibiotics is quite long, to wipe out any bacteria that may be hiding within the breast tissues. Women who have one episode are likely to have recurrences, maybe several months or a year later. It is possible that these recurrences develop from bacteria "hiding" deep within the breast tissues.

As for self-help measures, warm soaks bring comfort. The heat from the compresses increases the dilation of the blood vessels, so that the blood cells that fight infection can more readily come into the infected area and do their work.

▶ *Are women who have had mastitis at increased risk for breast cancer?*

No, they are not. However, it is possible that the symptoms of mastitis can be mistaken for those of inflammatory carcinoma. That is why follow-up is important to make sure that any lump or lesion goes away or resolves itself completely.

▶ *If you've had several episodes of mastitis during breast-feeding, should you consider giving up nursing?*

It depends on the severity of the infection and on how important breast-feeding is to you, in terms of both your child's nutritional status and your own emotional and psychological priorities. Certainly you can nurse from one breast if the other is infected. Try to keep the infected breast as empty as possible. If it is too painful to nurse from the infected breast, you can hand pump that breast to empty it.

Many women are concerned about antibiotic use while breast-feeding. Most antibiotics are safe: the two principal categories you cannot use are tetracyclines and quinolones (cipro-type drugs).

BREAST AUGMENTATION AND REDUCTION

In a culture that emphasizes the way women look, many women feel dissatisfied with the faces or bodies nature gave them and choose to improve their appearance through plastic surgery. Cosmetic breast surgery—whether it is breast augmentation with implants or breast reduction—has implications for health as well as beauty.

▶ *Do breast implants cause disease?*

No scientific studies have shown that implants increase the risk for breast cancer. Furthermore, research has shown again and again that silicone breast implants do not increase the risk for any kind of systemic disease, including autoimmune diseases or connective tissue diseases.

Juries have in several instances awarded large settlements to women who claimed that they had autoimmune problems after their breast implants leaked. In this highly charged atmosphere, the Food and Drug Administration in 1992 banned the use of silicone in new implants until safety could be assured. The agency did not, however, demand that silicone implants already in place be removed unless they were leaking significantly. Later the agency amended the decision, allowing the use of silicone gel implants for reconstructive breast surgery after mastectomy.

▶ *What kind of breast implants are available today?*

Today the implants available are either filled with a saline solution or made from a woman's own tissues. Natural tissues can be removed from other parts of the body—the abdomen or the back. Along with the tissues, skin, fat, and muscle are taken to provide circulation for the living tissues. Silicone gel implants are currently being studied and are available from doctors participating in these clinical trials.

▶ *What kinds of problems can breast implants cause?*

The usual problems are leakage from the implant and scarring from the surgery, but in terms of causing medical diseases, transplants are safe.

▶ *If silicone gel breast implants are not causing problems, is there any reason to have them removed?*

I urge women with silicone gel breast implants to continue their monthly self-exams, mammograms, and yearly breast exams, but I see no reason to remove implants that are not causing problems.

▶ *When is breast reduction worth considering?*

Breast reduction is plastic surgery that decreases the size of one or both breasts. It is appropriate for women whose breasts are so large that their size interferes with upper-body function. Some women with very large breasts have problems with posture and back, neck, and shoulder pain. Other problems are skin rashes in the folds beneath the breasts and breathing problems. Large breasts can interfere with athletic activity, and they can cause social pain, particularly for young women and teenagers.

▶ *Will insurance pay for breast reduction surgery?*

If you are having the surgery to relieve neck, back, or shoulder pain, then your insurance should pay for it. If you want breast reduction surgery for psychological or social reasons, you certainly have the right to have the procedure, but your insurance will probably not cover it.

▶ *Can a woman breast-feed after she has had breast reduction surgery?*

It depends on how the plastic surgeon has done the reduction. Often, it *is* possible to nurse, but if you are considering this kind of procedure, you should discuss it very carefully with your surgeon ahead of time.

▶ *Can I have breast reduction or augmentation surgery if my breasts are different sizes?*

It is not uncommon for women to have asymmetrical breasts. The difference in size between the two breasts is not generally dramatic, although in some women it can be significant. The difference, especially noticeable during early puberty, may even out with age and hormonal changes.

Adolescent girls in particular find the asymmetry extremely distressing, because at this age they are very concerned about the appearance of their bodies. Often I can reassure a young woman that asymmetrical breasts are merely a variation on normal, and that with a little "tincture of time," her body will develop according to its own pattern. Only in rare cases is surgical intervention necessary.

Since asymmetry can be a sign of cancer, it is important that the change in size is not something new. If your breasts have always been asymmetrical, there is no problem; but if they have recently become so, you should consult your physician right away.

▶ *What are the risks of breast reduction surgery?*

Breast reduction is considered major surgery. It is done in a hospital, usually with a general anesthetic. The procedure may take as long as three or four hours. Any surgery carries with it the risks of infection, adverse reaction to the anesthesia, and bleeding—though these risks are slight.

The surgery will always leave scars on the breasts, which will be quite visible (though they are likely to fade somewhat with time). Some women have a risk of large, raised scars (keloid scars) from this or any other surgery. Before you have surgery, ask your surgeon to see examples of the results of the different procedures, so that your own expectations will be reasonable.

11 Planning for Pregnancy

▶ **MYTH** The best time to have a baby is when you have achieved your career goals.

FACT Women's fertility decreases with advancing age, fairly dramatically at about age 35. Although there may be no perfect moment to become pregnant, you should respect the consequences of decreasing fertility and consider becoming pregnant in your late 20s or early 30s, even though you may find the timing inconvenient.

DECIDING to have a baby is one of the most important decisions you will ever make. If you are like most women, you will cherish parenthood and your children will bring joy to your life, but there is no denying that having and raising children will require major adjustments from you and your partner. Ideally, pregnancy should be something you choose, not something that happens to you, for your life will change irrevocably from the moment your pregnancy test is positive.

Kara, a medical resident at the hospital where I teach, is intelligent, competent, energetic, and highly professional. As she was nearing the end of her residency program, she became pregnant. Knowing Kara, my guess is that she had planned the pregnancy to coincide with the end of her residency and the beginning of further graduate work in cardiology. She had booked flights to Boston and California a day apart to interview for training programs.

The day before her Boston flight, she had a miscarriage. The possibility of this sad event had not even occurred to her, since she was used to taking charge of her life and meeting her commitments. The miscarriage disrupted her job search and her carefully timed pregnancy. Eventually Kara did find a satisfying postdoctoral fellowship, but the experience made her realize that she was subject to the uncertainties of biology in ways she had not realized.

Although you cannot control every facet of your pregnancy, you can do some things to prepare for a healthy pregnancy and a healthy baby, and it is best to start before you become pregnant. If you have to make lifestyle changes (quit smoking, lose weight, start an exercise program, or cut down on caffeine or alcohol), you will need some lead time to deal with ingrained habits.

▶ When is the right time to get pregnant?

While this question does not have one right answer for everyone, there are several major issues to think about before you and your partner stop using contraception. First, because pregnancy will bring major and unpredictable changes to your life, wait a while if you and your partner have not been together long. Familiarity and communication are important. Before you decide to plunge into parenthood, you and your partner should have spent enough time together to be used to each other's desires, habits, and peculiarities and to have reached an understanding about long-range goals. You should have worked out ways to handle the stresses that pregnancy, childbirth, and parenthood will cause. Marriage itself is not the issue: if you have lived together for five years but got married last month, you have already had time to grow used to each other.

Second, I have discovered from patients and from having my own family that there is never an ideal time to become pregnant. There is always that promotion waiting for you if you just finish this or that project. Or there is a time when you will be more comfortable financially and better able to afford child care. Or your parents are moving closer (so they can help with the baby-sitting); or they are moving farther away (so they won't offer too much advice). Or your husband has health problems that demand your care and attention.

Once you have recognized that there is no perfect time, at a certain point you just have to bite the bullet and go for it. Years ago I counseled women to wait until they were sure that they wanted a baby before they tried to have one. Now I encourage couples to start trying earlier, even if everything in their life is not in order. The more cases of infertility I see, the more I encourage young people to get going while their fertility is at its peak. I would not advise anyone to wait until she is 45 or even 38 to start trying to have a baby.

If you are in a stable relationship by the time you are 32 or 33, think seriously about starting your family. Fertility diminishes with age, although not drastically until a woman is about 35. Thereafter we see a significant decline, which women should respect. Sometimes your partner's status may be a determining factor.

> When Marcy discovered that she was pregnant, she was concerned because her husband had severe back pain that required surgery. We discussed the timing of his operation knowing that Marcy would be his primary caregiver while he recuperated. Since she was getting along well during her first trimester, we decided that the surgery should take place early in her second trimester, when she would have more energy than during the first months of the pregnancy. This schedule gave him time to recuperate so he could help Marcy late in her pregnancy and after the baby was born.

The decision is an equation in which you balance your age against your psychological, financial, and professional situation. You should be ready to deal with the consequences of getting pregnant (though until you actually become pregnant, you do not really know what they will be), and then you should take the leap as soon as possible.

▶ What is the risk of birth defects?

The baseline statistical risk of birth defects in the general population is about 3 percent. So you can be about 97 percent sure of having a healthy, normal child, and there are things you can do or avoid doing to enhance your chances of being in that 97 percent.

LIFESTYLE HAZARDS

My list of do's and don't's before and during pregnancy starts with worst-case scenarios and works upward from there. In my opinion, the two worst things you can do if you intend to become pregnant are use cocaine and smoke cigarettes. I feel very strongly about these issues, so before I turn to the bright side of things, I would like to talk about them.

▶ *What is the effect of cocaine on pregnancy?*

Cocaine is a drug that should fall outside the acceptable boundaries of a healthy life by anyone's standards. Using cocaine during pregnancy can lead to premature separation of the placenta from the uterine wall (abruption), which leads to premature labor and delivery. Cocaine use causes so many cases of preterm labor that we almost automatically screen for it when a woman comes in to the hospital in early labor. If you are committed to having a child, you should also commit to staying away from cocaine. As an obstetrician-gynecologist, I categorically state that using cocaine during pregnancy can kill your newborn.

▶ *What is the effect of cigarette smoking on pregnancy?*

The second worst thing you can do is to smoke cigarettes, a habit that unfortunately is still too common. To continue smoking when you are pregnant is to willfully continue an action that can damage your baby. Smoking cigarettes is associated with low birth weight and although the statistical relationship is not so certain as with cocaine use, smoking is also associated with premature separation of the placenta, premature delivery, and occasional stillbirth. Babies of mothers who smoke are at greater risk for sudden infant death syndrome (SIDS), a tragedy with long-term psychological consequences.

> Sue, a brilliant college friend of mine, and her husband both have degrees in computer science. They are very rational people. Sue didn't smoke; she was far too sensible to jeopardize her own health or that of her family. After having two healthy children, she had a third child who inexplicably died from SIDS.
>
> Although this tragedy happened about twenty years ago and Sue's two children have grown to be fine young adults, Sue hasn't really recovered. She understands intellectually that she did nothing wrong, but wondering whether she could have somehow prevented her loss has caused her immeasurable pain. Imagine how much worse she would feel if she knew she had done something that contributed to the death of that child.

If you are even thinking about getting pregnant, stop smoking. It is difficult, but there are support groups and other resources to help. Try every avenue open to you. If you cannot totally stop, cut your smoking to less than half a pack a day.

▶ *Does your partner's smoking have any effect on your pregnancy?*

While no evidence links the father's smoking to birth defects, smoking may contribute to male infertility. Men who smoke heavily may have lowered sperm counts, though the evidence is not conclusive. Evidence does exist that men who use marijuana heavily have lowered sperm counts. If you are having difficulty getting pregnant and your partner is a heavy pot smoker, urge him to stop.

Some researchers believe that passive smoking can lead to an increased risk of SIDS. There is also firm evidence that smoking, even passive smoking, leads to premature ovarian failure, so that women who smoke have an earlier menopause than women who do not.

▶ *Is alcohol dangerous during pregnancy?*

Third on my personal list of things to avoid during pregnancy is alcohol. In the popular mind, alcohol may well constitute the greatest potential danger to an unborn child, but the literature on the subject is controversial. Several well-designed scientific studies have shown without question that two or more drinks a day on a regular basis can lead to fetal alcohol syndrome, which can cause low birth weight, smaller brain mass, intellectual impairment, and other problems. The effects are the same whether you drink early in the pregnancy or toward the end.

Will taking one drink a week hurt your baby? We don't know much about the consumption of alcohol in very small amounts during pregnancy. There are gynecologists in the United States who say that under no condition should you ever take any alcohol at all during pregnancy, perhaps feeling that if they sanction one drink, their patients will take several. No scientific studies show that one drink a week will harm you or your baby. It is quite likely that the French mother of the brilliant scientist Pierre Curie did not go all nine months of her pregnancy without a glass or two of wine. The same could be said of Enrico Fermi's Italian mother or even Albert Einstein's German mother, who may well have downed a glass or two of beer while pregnant with the future Nobel Prize winner.

▶ *Will a single episode of heavy drinking cause birth defects?*

Although it is unlikely that one episode of heavy drinking would cause birth defects, there are no data on this question. Over the years many women have come to my office upset because they discovered that they were pregnant and during the two weeks between conception and realization, they had had an episode of binge drinking. For the next nine months they would be racked with guilt and anxiety.

It is hard to live with guilt, especially guilt you can avoid. So if at all possible, take the advice of the French physicist, mathematician, and philosopher Blaise Pascal (1623–1662), which still holds today: live a moderate life "just in case." Pascal pointed out that it made sense to lead a morally virtuous life in case there was a heaven where your virtue would be rewarded. If there turned out to be no eternal reward, at least in this world you would reap the benefits of living virtuously. The same can be said of a physically virtuous lifestyle: it has its own rewards.

▶ What about marijuana use during pregnancy?

This is another area where we have no firm data, but if you are contemplating pregnancy, give yourself and your child the benefit of healthy living. If you don't have to, why use a substance that could be harmful?

▶ What about caffeine during pregnancy?

Although plenty of mothers-to-be drank plenty of coffee in the good old days of blissful ignorance, caffeine use during pregnancy has become controversial. Over the years several well-designed scientific studies showed that moderate caffeine consumption, the equivalent of two or even three cups of coffee a day, will not harm you, cause birth defects, or increase the risk of miscarriage. Then in late 1993 a study by Canadian researchers published in the *Journal of the American Medical Association* showed that the caffeine equivalent in three cups of coffee a day did indeed increase the risk of miscarriage.

My belief is that these studies are not cause for alarm. One variable the researchers failed to consider was the way the coffee was brewed. Both the American researchers, who found that moderate caffeine intake was safe, and the Canadians who found it dangerous, considered one cup of coffee to contain the equivalent of about 100 mg of caffeine, although of course they did not analyze the coffee the pregnant women were actually drinking; they simply asked how many cups. But in Montreal, where the culture is French Canadian, the coffee is French in style—very black and very strong. Three cups of coffee in Montreal probably contain the caffeine equivalent of five cups of ordinary American-style coffee. At any rate, moderation is the key.

MEDICATIONS DURING PREGNANCY

▶ *What prescription and over-the-counter drugs are dangerous during pregnancy?*

Fortunately, many medications are safe just before and during pregnancy. Life's common ailments go on even when you are pregnant. Is it safe to take antibiotics for a tooth abscess or Tylenol for a headache? Consult with your internist or gynecologist before taking anything, just to be sure, but the list of dangerous drugs is actually much shorter than most people think.

Certain categories of prescription drugs do need to be avoided if you are pregnant or trying to become pregnant. The ACE inhibitors, used to treat high blood pressure, belong to one such category. There are safe drugs for this condition, but your internist and your obstetrician should consult with each other and make sure that you are taking a safe medication.

Women who regularly take antiepileptic drugs like Dilantin should also check on appropriate medications. Some data in the scientific literature suggest that Dilantin may be associated with an increased risk of birth defects, so it is critical to check with your internist and your neurologist *before* you become pregnant.

The FDA has divided all medications into five general categories (A, B, C, D, or X) with respect to their safety during pregnancy. The category to which a drug belongs has been determined by human and animal testing. Still, many drugs, for example those whose very nature suggests risk, have not been tested even in laboratory animals.

Category A: no risk. These drugs have been tested in carefully controlled studies on pregnant women and have shown no risk to the fetus. Almost no drugs have been rated Category A, because the FDA will not go on record as stating that a drug is safe when there is even the remotest chance of harm to a developing fetus. Therefore many drugs that do not have A ratings are perfectly safe; there simply are no tests that *absolutely* prove their safety.

Category B: no proven risk in humans. Drugs in category B can receive their rating one of two ways. When tested on pregnant women, the drugs show no risk, even though studies using laboratory animals, which usually involve very large dosages, may have raised the possibility of problems. Or, if adequate studies have not been carried out in humans, animal studies have shown no risk. Remember, however, that just because a certain medication does not cause problems or birth defects in rats does not mean it will be absolutely safe in humans. Thalidomide, which had been found safe in rats and rated category B, was withdrawn from the market when it was shown to cause severe birth defects in humans. It was later re-released in the United States, but only for the treatment of certain diseases including HIV, leprosy, and some kinds of cancers. Stringent testing and monitoring of contraceptive methods ensure that the women who are using it are not pregnant.

The common antibiotic amoxicillin is in category B. Studies on mice and rats have shown no evidence of harm to the fetus. Nor has human experience with amoxicillin during pregnancy shown adverse effects, but there are no scientifically controlled studies on pregnant women that conclusively rule out any harmful effects.

Category C: possible risk. Drugs in this category have not been tested on pregnant women. They may have been tested in animals, usually in large doses, and the tests have shown evidence of fetal risk, or they may not have been tested in animals at all. These drugs are used only when their benefits outweigh the potential risks. The antimigraine beta-blocker Inderal (propranolol) is in Category C.

Category D: proven risk. Drugs rated D have demonstrated positive evidence of risk. They have not been tested in women and are used during pregnancy only when there is no safer alternative and when the benefits to the mother outweigh the risk to the fetus. Sometimes there is a safe alternative.

While most antibiotics are safe, tetracycline and its derivatives like doxycycline are rated category D. If you have Lyme disease, one of the common diseases for which doxycycline is used, talk to your doctor about substitute medication. If you are planning to get pregnant, you should probably take amoxicillin rather than tetracycline or doxycycline.

Category X: contraindicated in pregnancy; not to be used at all. The clear evidence of risk to the developing fetus outweighs any possible benefit to the mother. These are drugs you should avoid even if you merely think you might get pregnant. Accutane, used to treat severe acne, is rated X; women taking Accutane should not get pregnant.

POSSIBLE COMPLICATIONS

▶ *What diseases need special consideration during pregnancy?*

Diabetes and some collagen vascular diseases like lupus and rheumatoid arthritis fall into this category. If you have one of these conditions, tell your gynecologist.

If you are diabetic, consult the internist or endocrinologist who is treating your diabetes as well as your gynecologist before you become pregnant and throughout your pregnancy. Get your blood sugar completely under control, close to 100 mg/dl, before the pregnancy begins. It was formerly thought that a normal blood sugar was 100–200 mg/dl and that diabetics should aim for the 150–200 range, within which they seemed to feel and function well. Today that level is considered far too high during pregnancy. Keeping blood sugar as close to normal as possible (a state called euglycemia) markedly reduces the risk of birth defects in the babies of diabetic women.

Hemoglobin A1-C is a marker of long-term diabetes control, of whether your blood sugar stays in an appropriate range for a long time. If your hemoglobin A1-C is normal, then it is reasonable to try to get pregnant; if it is elevated, you should wait until you are under better control.

▶ What are the concerns for diseases like rheumatoid arthritis and lupus?

These diseases, which frequently affect young women, are commonly treated with steroids. There are two problems here: one is the impact of pregnancy on the disease itself; the second is steroid use during pregnancy.

Years ago, women with these diseases, particularly lupus, were counseled not to even think about getting pregnant. The pregnancy, in addition to being difficult, could make the disease worse. Recent studies have suggested that the risks are smaller than was formerly thought. If you are in reasonably good shape and your disease is under reasonable control, it is probably fine to become pregnant. Nevertheless, consult your internist and your gynecologist before you stop using contraception.

Your doctor will probably try to wean you from steroids during pregnancy. But even if you have to take them during a flare-up, their effect on the fetus will be minimal.

▶ What about pregnancy and multiple sclerosis?

Multiple sclerosis has such a variable course that it is hard to predict during pregnancy, but the general view is that the disease will not harm the mother or the fetus and the pregnancy will not worsen the disease. Keep in close touch with your neurologist before and during your pregnancy.

▶ Does pregnancy complicate asthma?

If you use inhalers to control your asthma, discuss this issue with your physician. The medications used to treat asthma are generally safe during pregnancy, but the physical conditions of pregnancy can worsen asthma. In the third trimester, when the baby pushes up against your diaphragm, you may feel short of breath even if you do not have asthma; there is less room for your lungs to expand, a situation that is aggravated by asthma.

▶ *Are there diseases that absolutely prohibit pregnancy?*

There are only one or two very rare diseases that contraindicate pregnancy. One is a congenital heart disease called pulmonary hypertension that involves the blood vessels of the lungs. Another is Marfan's syndrome, which is a connective tissue disorder. If you have one of these conditions, discuss the situation with your gynecologist and your internist.

▶ *Are there diseases for which your husband or sexual partner should be tested for before you try to become pregnant?*

This question raises problems that may result from the genetic makeup of both the man and the woman. Sickle-cell anemia, most commonly seen in blacks, was formerly considered dangerous for pregnancy and still needs to be closely monitored. Perhaps as many as 10 percent of blacks of African descent have the genetic trait, but many have no clinical symptoms. Still, it is prudent to know whether or not you carry the trait. The disease involves a change of only one amino acid in the entire hemoglobin protein, the component of red blood cells that transports oxygen to body tissues. The alteration causes blood cells to become sickle shaped instead of round. These sickle-shaped cells are poor carriers of oxygen and may clog small blood vessels, interfering with circulation.

> Tamika has sickle-cell anemia. When she became pregnant, she worried that her husband might carry the sickle trait. She knew that if he did, there would be a 50-percent chance that her baby would be born with sickle-cell anemia. Her husband was screened and did not have the trait, so her children will have the sickle trait, but not sickle-cell anemia.

The Tay-Sachs gene is carried by 3–4 percent of Jews of Central European ancestry and is also found in French Canadians. It causes degeneration of nerve cells within the brain and central nervous system. If you and your partner belong to one of these ethnic groups, think about being screened before becoming pregnant. The disease has symptoms only if the child inherits defective genes from both parents; people with only one defective gene are carriers and do not actually have the disease. Children of parents who are both carriers have a one-in-four chance of inheriting two defective genes and thus having the disease. A blood test before pregnancy occurs can determine whether you carry the defective gene. If both parents are carriers and you are pregnant, amniocentesis (a procedure for genetically screening the amniotic fluid surrounding the fetus in the uterus) can determine whether the fetus has the disease.

Another disease carried by 2–3 percent of Jews of Eastern European origin is Canavan disease, which results in neurological degeneration because of a defect in myelin (a protein that protects nerves and allows messages to be sent to and from the brain). For the child to have the disease the defective gene for Canavan disease must be inherited from both parents. Jewish couples or those with a family history of the disease can be screened for it.

Other genetic diseases for which testing is available include cystic fibrosis and certain blood diseases. Cystic fibrosis is a genetic disease in which abnormally thick mucus obstructs the pancreas and clogs the lungs, leading to chronic infections. It afflicts primarily Caucasians, of whom about 4 percent are carriers, but the disease appears only if defective genes are inherited from both parents. Physicians routinely offer screening for cystic fibrosis. If you have a family history of this disease, of hemophilia, or other genetic blood diseases, you should be tested.

▶ *Is it important to have certain immunizations before becoming pregnant?*

Certain infectious diseases can have a negative impact on a pregnancy, so check into your immunity for them. If you get married in Connecticut, you will be tested for syphilis and German measles. Most states require this testing, but if you and your partner are not married, do get tested for these diseases if you decide to have a child. Syphilis is not very common, but it does exist and should be ruled out before you become pregnant. Children nowadays are routinely immunized against German measles, but it is worthwhile making sure that you either have had the disease or were immunized against it.

Chicken pox can be dangerous for pregnant women. Children seldom get very sick with it, though occasionally it has serious complications. Adults can become quite ill with chicken pox, but pregnant women get even sicker and sometimes have serious pneumonia. There is minimal danger to the fetus. If you have had chicken pox, you are safe from getting it again; if you are not sure, have a lab test called a varicella titer to see whether you are immune. There is a vaccine that will protect you when, for example, your toddler comes home from day care with chicken pox. If one of our pregnant patients who has not had chicken pox is exposed to it, we treat her aggressively with immunoglobulin (a protein in the blood that fights infections).

Immunizations usually become effective in about three months. If you need to be immunized, wait about three months after your shots before you try for a pregnancy.

▶ *What about HIV testing?*

The other big question nowadays is prenatal HIV testing. I am one of many who believe that testing should be mandatory for everyone contemplating pregnancy. First of all, knowing that you are HIV positive can guide you in your decision on whether to have a child. Second, if you do decide to have a child, certain medications can substantially reduce the risk that the fetus will develop HIV.

My own feelings are that if you are HIV positive, you should seriously consider not becoming pregnant. You may choose not to become a mother because you do not wish to leave your child an orphan. Or you may elect not to have a child because even though AZT (zizovudine), the primary anti-HIV drug, can reduce the chances of infecting your unborn child, you do not want to take this risk at all.

▶ *How effective is AZT in preventing transmission of HIV to an unborn child?*

Before the development of AZT, 25–30 percent of HIV-positive mothers passed the disease on to the fetus. Today, aggressive therapy with AZT reduces that risk to about 8 percent. For this reason HIV testing during pregnancy is mandatory in Connecticut and many other states.

The Centers for Disease Control report that from 1996 to 1997 the number of children under age 13 diagnosed with AIDS declined 40 percent, reflecting the success of efforts to reduce transmission at birth through HIV testing and AZT therapy for pregnant HIV-infected women and their infants.

▶ *What about testing for STDs before pregnancy?*

If you are planning pregnancy and think you are at risk for a sexually transmitted disease like chlamydia and gonorrhea, it is worthwhile to be tested. Unlike German measles, for example, these diseases do not cause birth defects, but they can increase the chance of premature labor. Testing is a simple matter of swabbing the cervix. Furthermore, these diseases can be treated.

If you have been in a monogamous relationship for a long time and were tested previously, there is no need to be retested. But if you have had several sexual partners, it is definitely desirable.

▶ *What about pregnancy and anorexia?*

Women with anorexia often have difficulty becoming pregnant, because their body weight is so low that they stop ovulating. Pregnancy can cause significant psychological distress for women with bulimia or other problems with body image. Ideally, women gain 25–35 pounds during pregnancy, and women who are already conflicted about their bodies may find this healthy gain unacceptable.

▶ *Does obesity complicate pregnancy?*

You should be in top physical shape when you become pregnant. Pregnancy makes great physical demands on your body, and labor and delivery are more strenuous than running a half-marathon. No serious runner would consider starting a long-distance race without training, and I encourage women to train during pregnancy. Being in shape includes being as close to your ideal body weight as you can manage.

Why is that important? First, I have said that you will gain a good deal of weight during pregnancy. If you are already 20 pounds overweight, you will be carrying 45 extra pounds or so when you deliver—and even 25 pounds is a lot of excess weight to be carrying around all day long. Second, the more overweight you are, the more you are at risk for high blood pressure or diabetes during pregnancy.

Many women just cannot shed those extra pounds. If you have been trying for years to lose 30 pounds, at some point you are simply going to have to say to yourself, "Overweight or not, now's the time to try for a pregnancy." If you really want a child and cannot manage to lose weight, the problem can be managed. But be realistic in your expectations. The weight may make you uncomfortable. You may need a cesarean section, a higher statistical risk for overweight women than for those of normal weight. While the procedure is not pleasant for either the patient or the physician, many women have had C-sections and gone on with their lives. On the other hand, some women who have weight problems do not gain significant additional weight during their pregnancies.

> Danielle weighs 250 pounds despite her best efforts to control her weight. When she found herself pregnant, she worried about gaining another 35 pounds. I suggested she stick to a reasonable diet, exercise, and not think she was "eating for two." As a result she didn't gain weight at all, although her baby developed normally.

▶ *What nutritional guidelines should you follow if you are planning to become pregnant?*

Calcium, iron, and folic acid are especially important during a pregnancy. Babies steal from their mothers, which is how they get formed, and the specific nutrients they steal are calcium and iron. Often I prescribe prenatal vitamins for women who are planning pregnancy. Most of these vitamins contain 1 mg of folic acid, extra iron, and extra calcium.

Most American women are calcium deprived. If you are planning to become pregnant, start making sure that your diet contains at least 1,000 mg of calcium, the recommendation for pregnant women.

If you tend to be anemic, pump yourself full of iron. Iron, taken as dietary supplements, can have one unfortunate side effect: constipation. And pregnancy often has the same effect. If you are anemic before pregnancy, decide to take iron, and become constipated, you are still better off than you would be if you were both constipated and anemic during your pregnancy.

Increase your folic acid intake. This substance is critical in preventing neural tube defects such as spina bifida or anencephaly. The neural tube is an embryonic structure that appears between the fifth and sixth weeks of pregnancy; normally it closes and forms the brain and spinal cord. If the tube does not close completely, spina bifida or anencephaly result. Spina bifida ("divided" spine) is a condition in which the vertebrae do not form over the back of the spinal cord, leaving it unprotected; the severity of the defect depends on the location of the opening. Infants with anencephaly, in which the head and brain do not develop completely, usually are stillborn or die shortly after birth.

The relevant research on these diseases came from Great Britain, where neural tube defects seem more common than in this country, where their incidence is somewhere between 1 in 500 births and 1 in 1,000 births. The Centers for Disease Control encourage women to take folic acid prenatally, since studies suggest that the incidence of neural tube defects can then be brought down significantly. The standard recommendation for folic acid supplements is 0.4 mg (400 µg) daily. Women at high risk for producing children with neural tube defects should take larger doses, 4 mg daily. If you have previously been pregnant with a fetus that had a neural tube defect, you are in the high-risk category. You are also at increased risk if you have a strong family history of this problem: for example, your sister has had two children with these defects.

▶ *Does pregnancy worsen depression or other psychological problems?*

Women who have had psychological difficulties usually do well during pregnancy if they became pregnant because they want a child. If the pregnancy was unplanned or was entered into grudgingly (perhaps because someone else wants the child), then women who have been depressed may become more so. Some of the side effects of pregnancy can depress women with tendencies in that direction.

> Sharon struggled with depression in her daily life. When she was about two months pregnant, she came for a checkup and burst into tears, weeping uncontrollably. She felt nauseated and vomited in the mornings, which although unpleasant is not unexpected during the first trimester. Unlike many women in the same situation, Sharon did not cope well at all with the nausea. The last straw came when her mother-in-law, who helped care for Sharon's older child, got sick and couldn't babysit. Sharon was not taking antidepressants or other medication for her emotional state.
>
> I asked Sharon how I could help her. Basically, she said, she needed someone to watch her child so that she could nap during the afternoon (she was having difficulty sleeping at night). In my estimation she was on the brink of serious emotional difficulties, so I called her HMO and asked for home health care, describing her fragile state. The HMO refused, saying that if Sharon did get worse and needed hospitalization, they would think about skilled nursing care, but they could not possibly provide for home help unless she suffered a breakdown. Sharon continued to feel more and more depressed and anxious; I eventually did send her to the hospital, for which the HMO agreed to pay. It was a very expensive way to take care of Sharon's problems.

▶ *Are women who have had problems with depression likely to suffer from postpartum depression?*

Unfortunately, the answer is yes. No one knows why postpartum depression happens and who is at risk. Of the many theories, the one currently in favor stresses the changing levels of hormones. During pregnancy women have higher levels of steroids and estrogen, both natural antidepressants, which explains why most women feel pretty cheerful at this time. In fact, some women with depression actually feel better during pregnancy.

Once the child is born, all these hormones return to their prepregnancy levels and women can become severely depressed. If you have been treated for depression, even if you are totally off the medications, it is wise to stay in touch with your psychiatrist and be prepared for the possibility that you may be depressed after the birth. You may be perfectly fine, but if you should experience postpartum depression, you can get help quickly.

Try to be realistic about what will happen once your child is born. Of course he or she will be wonderful (maternal instinct takes care of that), but your wonderful child will still poop and pee and wake you at three in the morning. These stresses exist for every new mother, and if your hormones are not in balance and you are not getting a good night's sleep, you can expect to be less than completely cheerful.

▶ Can you take antidepressants if you are pregnant?

Most antidepressants currently in use, called SSRIs (selective serotonin reuptake inhibitors), are reasonably safe during pregnancy. Several studies show that seriously depressed women do better taking the medications than not taking them. SSRIs include Prozac and Zoloft.

▶ What about over-the-counter drugs just before or during pregnancy?

Most over-the-counter drugs are fine. Tylenol is probably better as a painkiller than ibuprofen or naprosyn and has the best track record as far as safety is concerned. If you have heartburn, you can take Maalox, Mylanta, or Tums, which are great because they contain the calcium you need in increased quantity during pregnancy. If you have a cold, the ordinary tried-and-true antihistamines and decongestants, including Benadryl and Sudafed, are safe.

▶ When should you stop using birth control if you want to get pregnant?

I encourage my patients on birth control pills to stop taking them about three months before they intend to become pregnant, because some women experience a slight delay in the return of ovulation after stopping the pill. My second reason for suggesting this buffer zone is that some studies show that women who conceive in the first cycle off birth control have a higher incidence of twins. So you might want to wait an extra cycle unless you are actively seeking twins.

With other forms of contraception, you can stop the month before you plan to become pregnant. If you use Depo-Provera, you may have to wait several months for your menstrual periods to resume, though many women resume ovulating the month they stop taking their Depo shots.

▶ *Should you take special measures, like planning the time of intercourse, when you do want to become pregnant?*

My advice is to relax, have fun, and enjoy your sex life and the freedom of the moment. Throw away your thermometer, and don't sit and look at your watch. For many women, this is probably the first time they have not had to worry about birth control.

Having stopped your birth control methods, don't be disappointed if you do not get pregnant immediately. Remember that your statistical odds of getting pregnant in any one month are only 15 percent. On the other hand, you may be one of the 15 percent—so you can't plan on its taking you six months to conceive.

If you stop using contraception and do not conceive during that first month, don't immediately conclude that you have an infertility problem. Try to maintain your perspective. It is far too early to get out the menstrual calendars, or to wake up at three in the morning and have sex because that seems to be the optimal moment. Try to avoid sex on demand, which lessens the enjoyment. Have fun!

▶ *If you don't succeed in becoming pregnant, when should you seek help?*

Years ago I saw patients who would try for as long as five years before investigating the problem. That is rare in this day and age. If you are in your mid-30s, about six months is an appropriate wait. Then give your gynecologist a call and you can start some simple testing to try to find out what is going on. If you are in your early 20s, you can try for a year before consulting your gynecologist. (Chapter 12 will tell you about rates of conception.)

PREGNANCY TESTING

▶ *How soon can a pregnancy be detected?*

Modern pregnancy testing is both sophisticated and sensitive. Gone are the days when a woman had to wait at least two weeks after a missed period to determine whether she was pregnant, weeks that were stressful whether she was hoping she was pregnant or praying she was not.

Nowadays ordinary blood tests can accurately diagnose pregnancy as early as one or two days after a missed period. Urine tests conducted in a doctor's office may be taken a day or so later. Home pregnancy test kits also are quite accurate as little as two days after a missed period.

▶ *How do pregnancy tests work?*

All pregnancy tests, whether of urine or blood, look for the presence of beta hCG, the beta subunit of human chorionic gonadotropin, a hormone produced by the dividing cells of the embryo even before it is implanted within the uterus—though hCG levels become detectable only after implantation. The hormone makes its way into the mother's blood (and thereafter into her urine) through the blood vessels of the placenta. The tests work by measuring antibodies to this hormone.

There are also special blood tests that use radioactively labeled hCG. These tests, called radio immunoassays or radio receptorassays, can detect pregnancy even before you miss a period. Because they are expensive, they are used only in special situations; for example, to check women at high risk for an ectopic pregnancy or those who have some medical condition (such as diabetes or kidney disease) that increases the risks of pregnancy.

▶ *Are some tests more accurate than others?*

Blood tests are a little more reliable than urine tests, but the urine tests, even the home kits, are quite accurate. The blood tests in general can detect as little as 25 units of hCG in the sample; the urine tests do not turn positive until the hCG level has risen to something like 50–100 units, which happens a day or so later, since in a normally developing pregnancy the level of hCG in the mother's blood doubles every forty-eight hours or so.

Urine tests and regular blood tests give qualitative results: they tell you whether or not you are pregnant. By repeatedly measuring the amount of hCG, more sophisticated quantitative tests can indicate how well the pregnancy is going.

▶ *Where can you get a pregnancy test, and how much does it cost?*

You can have a urine test at your doctor's office, a private laboratory, or a clinic. You can buy a home pregnancy test kit at a pharmacy. In some communities, women's health centers or family planning organizations like Planned Parenthood offer tests free or at minimal cost. Blood tests must be done in laboratories.

Urine tests done in your doctor's office cost about twenty-five dollars. Qualitative blood tests, which give a simple yes or no answer, are done by a laboratory and cost forty-five to fifty dollars. Your insurance may cover the costs.

▶ *How accurate are pregnancy tests?*

Modern pregnancy tests are generally reliable, though no test is 100 percent accurate. Occasionally false positives result (indicating that you are pregnant when you are not) or false negatives (indicating that you are not pregnant when you are). Sometimes a test is inconclusive and must be repeated.

False negatives can come about if the test is done too soon in the pregnancy or too late, since hCG levels fall again after the second month of pregnancy. Sometimes abnormal pregnancies or pregnancies on the verge of spontaneous abortion will give false negatives. If a urine sample has been contaminated or has sat too long without refrigeration, the test may yield a false negative.

False positives can come about if the test "mistakes" luteinizing hormone (LH) for hCG, to which it is chemically similar. LH levels spike at the time of ovulation and are also elevated in the urine of older women approaching menopause. Certain medications can skew the test: tranquilizers, antidepressants, methadone, and drugs for high blood pressure that contain methyldopa. Marijuana and even large quantities of aspirin can produce false positives. After you have a miscarriage or abortion, a pregnancy test will read positive for about ten additional days.

▶ *How accurate are home pregnancy testing kits? How expensive?*

Home pregnancy tests use the same techniques as the urine tests you take in a doctor's office. If you follow the directions correctly, they are just as sensitive as the office tests and will detect pregnancy as early as two days after a missed period. They are about 98 percent reliable, but do give occasional false positives and negatives.

They cost between ten and twenty-five dollars, a little less perhaps than the urine tests in a doctor's office; but you must pay for a home test kit out of pocket, while most insurance companies will pay for pregnancy testing in an office or lab setting.

12 Fertility and Infertility

▶ **MYTH** Women are responsible for almost all infertility.

FACT Female problems alone account for about 30–35 percent of cases, male problems alone cause infertility in another 30–35 percent of cases, and a combined problem of both partners causes another 20 percent. The remaining 10–15 percent of couples receive a diagnosis of unexplained infertility, which means that their infertility workup shows that everything is functioning normally.

MEDICALLY speaking, infertility is the inability to conceive a child after a year of unprotected intercourse. *Primary infertility* is the inability to conceive any children at all. *Secondary infertility* refers to infertility in someone who has at least one child.

Infertility can be a significant crisis in the marriage of any couple who have assumed, individually or together, that they would be parents. Despite the astounding biological complexity of the process of conception, somehow it seems that it should be simple to achieve, because so many couples do have children (some even when they would rather not). The failure to conceive can therefore be emotionally devastating at a very basic level.

FERTILITY FACTS AND FIGURES

Today in the United States, or so the media would have us believe, we are in the midst of a major infertility epidemic. Although statistics do not quite bear out that hypothesis, infertility is increasing. Surveys taken by the National Center for Health Statistics in 1995 suggest that 10.2 percent of American women of childbearing age (15–44 years) have impaired fertility. Of these women, 2.5 million have never had children and 3.4 million have had at least one child. Similar surveys in 1988 show only 8.4 percent of American women with infertility problems.

While only 15 percent of couples will succeed in their first month of trying, within six months about 50 percent will be pregnant. And by the end of the first year about 80 percent will be, which explains why physicians use the standard of one year of unsuccessful trying as the benchmark for infertility. During the second year another 5–10 percent will conceive a child, which leaves a core infertility rate in the range of 10–15 percent in the general population. These figures have not changed drastically over the past thirty years, though several factors have somewhat increased the infertility rate in both sexes.

THE CAUSES OF INFERTILITY

About 20 percent of women who have difficulty becoming pregnant have a problem with ovulation: the egg is not maturing and being released properly from the ovary. Another 25 percent have tubal problems: egg and sperm cannot get to their designated meeting place in the fallopian tube. About 5 percent of women have a problem with cervical mucus, which may kill the sperm or impede their progress. Another cause is endometriosis (see Chapter 8), a condition in which the kind of tissue that normally lines the uterus grows in the pelvis outside the uterus and continues to respond to hormonal stimulation. Endometriosis may not actually block a fallopian tube, but it may alter the tube's ability to push the egg toward the uterus. It may also have subtle hormonal effects that somehow interfere with the process.

Infertility in men may come from having too few sperm, sperm that are not active enough, or sperm that are abnormal in some other way. Men can have anatomical defects or abnormal chromosomes that cause infertility. And sexual dysfunction can contribute to infertility in both sexes.

▶ *What possible causes could there be for the 15 percent of infertile couples who are diagnosed with "unexplained" infertility?*

Although research in infertility has advanced a great deal in the last generation, there is still much that we do not understand. We do not know, to take one example, how a particular sperm penetrates a particular egg. You may be ovulating perfectly, and your husband or partner may be making plenty of very vigorous sperm, but for some reason the sperm do not penetrate the egg.

▶ *How many couples who are infertile for unexplained reasons eventually get pregnant?*

Half of these couples, and some couples whose infertility can be attributed to a known cause, eventually do become pregnant. I encourage people not to give up hope.

> Ann Marie and Richard adopted two children because they seemed unable to have their own. Richard's sperm count was extremely low and despite everyone's best efforts remained so, less than 1 million, when about 20 million is considered the lower level of fertility. After some discussion they decided to adopt rather than using donor sperm. Subsequently and unexpectedly, Ann Marie became pregnant, not once but twice.

Although this couple did conceive children after they adopted, the two events are unrelated: the success rate of couples who adopt is statistically the same as that of couples who do not.

INFERTILITY IN THE POPULATION

Several studies have suggested that during the past twenty years, men in the industrialized world have statistically experienced a decline in the quality, concentration, and vigor of sperm. Although no one knows for sure, occupational hazards and environmental pollution, medications, and sexually transmitted diseases may be risk factors.

The causes of lowered fertility among women are more apparent. The first factor is age. Women are much more fertile at 18 than they are at 38. As more women put off childbearing into their 30s and beyond, it stands to reason that the population will have lower fertility rates. Women in the 35–44 age group are about twice as likely to have fertility problems as women in the 30–34 bracket.

Another important issue for women is that the incidence of pelvic inflammatory disease (PID) has soared over the past generation in the United States, with 3 million to 4 million cases of chlamydia every year. Women may be unaware that they have this silent STD, even as it scars their fallopian tubes and makes them infertile. Years later many of these women, trying unsuccessfully to become pregnant, have a laparoscopy that suggests past PID and a blood test that reveals a past infection with chlamydia.

Although it is difficult to obtain exact statistics, researchers estimate that having one episode of PID lowers fertility in women by about 12 percent, two episodes by about 20 percent, and three episodes by about 50 percent. The increase in PID also seems to account for an increasing rate of pregnancy outside the uterus. Surveys formerly rated ectopic pregnancy at about 0.5 percent of all pregnancies; now the rate has climbed to somewhere between 1 and 2 percent. These statistics give a compelling reason for young women to protect themselves by using condoms, not only to avoid pregnancy but also to protect themselves from disease and preserve their fertility.

▶ Are there environmental causes of infertility?

Few reliable statistics are available, but we know some answers to this question. Cigarette smoking reduces fertility, for both men and women. In men, smoking appears to lower sperm count; in women, it may interfere with the function of the fallopian tubes. Caffeine has been implicated in decreased fertility in women, as have alcohol and illegal drugs, including cocaine and marijuana. Exposure to pesticides, chemical solvents, and other occupational hazards can affect fertility in both sexes.

TRYING ON YOUR OWN

In theory, you are not having fertility problems until you have tried for a year, so you should wait that long before you consult your gynecologist. However, I bend the rules according to the woman's age. If she is 24, I do counsel her to wait a year before having an infertility workup; if she is 37, I start testing after six months. I use age 35 as the cutoff point and counsel women younger than that to wait longer. Some doctors choose a different age.

The decision about when to start testing and what tests to do may also have something to do with your health insurance coverage. Some managed-care companies cover some tests, but not all; some cover none at all.

▶ When are your most fertile times of the month?

Your most fertile period is just before and around the time of ovulation. If you have fairly regular twenty-eight-day cycles, you are likely to ovulate on day 14 (counting the first day of your period as day 1). If your cycle is longer or shorter, the interval between ovulation

BOX 8.   Protecting Your Fertility

Many of the causes of infertility are beyond your control. There is little you can do to assure that you will not get endometriosis or have an incompatibility with your partner's sperm. But the factors within your control are certainly worth your attention.

- Consider having children in your 20s or early 30s, if your life situation permits this choice.
- Protect yourself from STDs. Use condoms during intercourse unless you and your partner are 100 percent mutually monogamous. The fewer different sexual partners you have, the less chance you have of meeting up with someone who carries an STD.
- If you have any symptoms that suggest infection (for example, pelvic pain), get treatment right away.
- Don't smoke. If you do smoke, quit. Smoking shortens your reproductive life; nicotine is toxic to the ovaries; and women who smoke often have early menopause.
- Limit your caffeine intake to two or three cups of coffee daily (or the equivalent).
- Decrease your alcohol intake or stop drinking altogether. In addition to causing possible problems with fertility, two or more alcoholic drinks per day during pregnancy can cause fetal alcohol syndrome.

and the beginning of the next period is still fourteen days, but the first part of the cycle is longer or shorter. If you have a thirty-two-day cycle, you will probably ovulate on day 18; if you have a twenty-six-day cycle, ovulation is likely to take place on day 12.

▶ *How often should you have intercourse to maximize your chances of getting pregnant?*

Frequency of intercourse is important. You should have intercourse at least every other day, especially around your fertile time of the month. Having sex once a month, even when you think you are ovulating that day, probably will be unsuccessful. In fact, the definition of infertility means that the couple is trying and not succeeding. "Trying" means having frequent intercourse.

Sometimes a woman will tell me that she knows exactly when she ovulates and can time her intercourse perfectly. If this is the only time that month that she has sex, she lowers her chances of getting pregnant, in that she may be a day or two early or late ovulating.

Another justification I have heard in recent years is that the woman and her husband are too busy to have intercourse frequently. To me this statement indicates less than total commitment to having a child. After all, it takes a great deal more time to care for a child than it does to have sexual intercourse. So when I hear this explanation, I ask the couple to reassess their motivation.

▶ *Does very frequent intercourse make conception less likely?*

Once a day is fine. Infertility specialists suggest that more than once a day may be too frequent if you are interested in becoming pregnant, since it lowers your partner's sperm count.

Some sexual practices advocated by certain religions seem to take into consideration the issue of sperm count. Orthodox Judaism says that a woman is "unclean" during her menstrual period and until the seventh day afterward. If a woman and her husband abstain from sex for the first twelve days of a twenty-eight-day cycle as their religion requires, and then have intercourse, the husband by then has a very high sperm count and the wife is quite likely to become pregnant. The practice certainly helps account for the large size of orthodox Jewish families.

Of course, these rules do not work as well for women with very short or very long cycles. Suppose a woman has a twenty-four-day cycle and a five-day menstrual period. She and her husband are not allowed to have intercourse on day 10, when she is likely to be ovulating. By day 12, when they resume intercourse and he is at his peak sperm count, she has already ovulated. Her egg is past its prime, and conception is much less likely to take place. We treat such women with Clomid, a drug that stimulates ovulation and can delay it until a better time, thereby changing her pattern of ovulation so that it fits the religious requirements.

Other religious conditions, for example the prohibition against masturbation, also work to increase the likelihood of conception.

▶ *How long should you remain lying down after intercourse?*

Somewhere between fifteen and twenty minutes should be sufficient. You should not jump up immediately after the act, though you can still become pregnant if you do.

PSYCHOLOGICAL ISSUES

No one who has experienced it doubts for a second that infertility puts stress on both husband and wife and on their relationship. I see intelligent, motivated, highly successful couples become frustrated, bewildered, and filled with self-doubt because they cannot conceive a child. Everyone likes to believe that the world is a fair and just place, and that we have some control over the important issues in our lives. So it can be devastating to discover that your fertility is not entirely within your control. In fact, once you decide to become pregnant (whether you end up dealing with infertility or with pregnancy and children), you can no longer control many aspects of your life.

Some women feel that infertility diminishes their femininity, but I think it is even more common for men to equate their infertility with lack of masculinity. Of course, fertility and masculinity are no more synonymous than are femininity and fertility. Some men who are great historical symbols of masculinity have not been able to father children. Think of George Washington, *father* of our country, a man known for his physical courage and qualities of leadership. (Modern medicine suggests that he had a disease called Klinefelter's syndrome, a chromosomal abnormality that may have made him sterile.) Some male athletes who take extra testosterone to bulk out look very virile but cannot father children.

From talking to couples undergoing fertility workups, it seems to me that often women want children more than men do. I don't think too many men blame their wives so strongly for infertility that the marriage falls apart—unless they belong to a religious group that believes in copious reproduction. I see very few cases where the husband is devastated by his wife's inability to conceive, but I see many brokenhearted women.

Because couples dealing with infertility must have intercourse on demand, sex necessarily loses its spontaneity and often its pleasurable qualities. Understandably, the anxiety builds through the month and if at the end of the month the wife has her period, she is disappointed and distressed. I get monthly calls from women in tears because of their frustration. Infertility can be an emotional roller coaster, with swooping highs and lows that continue for years.

It is certainly appropriate to have counseling at this stressful time. Any well-run assisted reproductive technology program should have a social worker who can help couples individually or together. Most often, I find, it is women who seek help. In addition to local support and self-help groups, RESOLVE, a national nonprofit organization, helps people cope with infertility, offering information and support for both the medical and emotional aspects.

▶ *Can anxiety on a woman's part cause infertility?*

It is certainly possible that for some women stress can interfere with ovulation, but most women being treated for infertility continue to ovulate, as fertility tests show. If the woman is ovulating, it is unlikely that fertilization would fail to take place simply because she is anxious. Although people may tell you that you are "trying too hard" and that you should "just relax and you will get pregnant," this well-meant advice is insensitive and lacks a basis in reality.

Stress *can* cause performance anxiety. The wife may become so tense that she and her husband cannot have intercourse, or the husband is so anxious that he cannot achieve or maintain an erection. More than once I have scheduled a postcoital test (the wife comes in after intercourse for an examination of her cervical mucus) that was canceled because the couple could not manage to have intercourse on demand.

THE INFERTILITY WORKUP

In recent years assisted reproductive technologies, including methods that use donor sperm and eggs, have been developed that help many people who in the past would not have been able to have a child. Unfortunately, infertility workups can be intrusive, costly, and emotionally exhausting. Many doctors (including myself) begin with the easiest, least expensive, least invasive tests, especially those that yield meaningful information. If these do not get at the cause, we can move to more difficult, invasive tests.

Most infertility tests can be done by an ordinary gynecologist. But if testing reveals a significant problem with ovulation or blockage of the fallopian tubes, your gynecologist may refer you to a reproductive endocrinologist. A specialist of this sort has had two or three years of training beyond regular gynecology training and can do complex surgery and manage the procedures of assisted reproductive technology.

▶ *What does a basic infertility workup include?*

An ordinary infertility workup, the kind your gynecologist can do (with the help of a laboratory), may include tests that will determine whether your partner's sperm are vigorous and capable of fertilizing an egg, whether your reproductive anatomy is generally healthy and normal, and whether your female hormones are doing their job adequately.

HISTORY AND PELVIC EXAM

The first step is a history and a pelvic examination. Your doctor will be interested in your general medical history and your menstrual history. Do you have regular periods? How heavy are they? How long is your cycle? Do you have cramps? Have you ever had pelvic inflammatory disease or another sexually transmitted disease? Your sexual history is also important. Are you currently monogamous? How many sexual partners have you had in the past? How many has your husband (or current partner) had?

The pelvic exam for an infertility workup is similar to the usual gynecological exam. Your caregiver will check to see if your uterus and ovaries are normal in size and "move well." Endometriosis and PID can cause scarring that "glues" down your reproductive organs, hindering their freedom to move slightly within your pelvis.

NONINVASIVE LABORATORY TESTS

If your pelvic exam does not turn up anything significant, then the infertility workup proceeds to some relatively inexpensive, noninvasive lab tests.

Semen Analysis

This test is easy to do, and it can rule out (or diagnose) certain causes of male infertility. You and your partner should not have intercourse for two or three days before the sample is collected. Your partner provides a sample of sperm by masturbating into a sterile cup or, if he has religious strictures against masturbation, a special condom can be used and the sample collected during intercourse.

Sometimes it is difficult to get the man to donate a sample. Even when I suggest that his partner take the specimen to the lab to spare him embarrassment, some men simply refuse. Presumably they fear being responsible for the infertility problem. In a way, this test also shows the man's commitment to having a child; if he is not willing to give a semen sample, the couple has problems other than those strictly related to infertility. If malefactor infertility does turn up, then the woman may be able to avoid or at least put off tests that are far more invasive than donating a sperm sample.

▶ *What does a semen analysis measure?*

For the simplest tests the lab looks at five things: volume, viscosity, sperm count, motility, and morphology. First the lab looks at how much semen there is. Most labs define as normal anything between 2 and 5 ml, though others look for as little as 1.5 and as much as 8 (a teaspoon is 5 ml). It is unusual to find less than 1 or more than 8 ml of fluid in the ejaculate. Less does not necessarily mean that the man cannot father a child, but it does indicate a possible problem. More is not always better, since concentration is important.

Viscosity, the thickness of the fluid, is important because sperm must be able to swim easily in this medium. If the semen is too thick, it impairs motility, the sperm's ability to move around.

One of the most telling tests is the sperm count. A normal sperm count is 60 million per milliliter of fluid; most fertility specialists consider something like 20 million per milliliter an acceptable minimum, and certainly a man with a count in that range can father a child.

The lab will also look at motility. How fast are the sperm swimming around? Are they moving forward? Are they still active an hour later? (We hope to see at least 60 percent continue to move around energetically, though probably the motility during the first hour is most important.) It is a bad sign if the sperm count is normal but only 10 percent of the sperm are mobile.

The test also looks at morphology, the shape of the sperm. How many are normal in appearance and how many abnormal? Do the abnormal ones have one head or, as occasionally happens, two heads? Are the tails normally formed?

▶ *What factors can affect sperm production?*

Illness, injury, infection, perhaps a drug reaction or exposure to pollutants can interfere with sperm production. Another potential problem, though this is controversial, is a varicocele, a cluster of varicose veins in the scrotum near the testes.

Since sperm take about two months to make, a low sperm count or other poor evaluation may reflect an illness two months previously. So it is worthwhile to do a repeat test a few weeks later. If the count improves with the second test, so much the better. If not, then the man should seek help.

▶ Does a varicocele interfere with sperm production?

It is possible that a varicocele interferes with sperm formation because its distended veins either cause a backward flow of hormones or allow more warm fluid to bathe the testes. The reason the testes are outside the body, of course, is that in order to thrive, sperm must live in an environment cooler than body temperature.

However, these theories are controversial. A varicocele can be corrected with surgery, and many researchers believe the procedure really helps; others are not so sure.

▶ What kind of doctor deals with male infertility?

A urologist specializes in urinary problems and male reproductive difficulties. There are a few gynecologists in this country who also specialize in male infertility, but for the most part the two specialties are segregated by the sex of the patient. Urologists are trained to help with physiological problems (for example, poor sperm production) as well as anatomical ones (for example, blocked tubes) that require surgery.

Tests to Pinpoint Ovulation

Another easy and inexpensive test is a month-long basal body temperature (BBT) check for ovulation. (For instructions about taking BBT, see Chapter 5.) I am not a great believer in basal body temperature charting as a way to determine ovulation; there are more sophisticated and accurate ways to find out the same thing. Furthermore, you can have a classic temperature pattern, with dips and rises in all the right places, and still not be ovulating. Conversely, your temperature pattern on the chart can look extremely doubtful, yet you can be ovulating perfectly.

▶ What are ovulation predictor kits?

More accurate than the BBT method (but not 100 percent foolproof) are kits that confirm ovulation by measuring the so-called LH surge. Luteinizing hormone (LH), which triggers ovulation, rises dramatically in the blood just before the egg is released; it is excreted in the urine, where it can be conveniently measured. These tests indicate the extent of the surge by color changes or other means. The kits are available over the counter at a pharmacy. Some common brands are First Response, Clear Plan, and Conceive. They cost less than thirty dollars, which you will probably have to pay out of pocket, since your insurance is unlikely to cover them.

Ovulation predictor kits will tell you whether you are ovulating and will give you a little advance notice to help you time intercourse for your most fertile days. But remember, even if you time the act perfectly, you still have only a 15–20 percent chance of getting pregnant in a given month.

▶ *Is it possible to have an LH surge and still not ovulate?*

Although possible, it is very rare. The condition is called luteal unruptured follicle (LUF) syndrome. It means that your hormones surge in the usual way and the follicle matures, but it does not burst out of the ovary. It remains inside and is gradually reabsorbed.

▶ *Are there other ways to test for ovulation?*

A blood test that looks for a high progesterone level can confirm ovulation. It should be taken toward the end of the menstrual cycle, day 23 or 24 of a twenty-eight-day cycle. A level below 3 nanograms per milliliter (a nanogram is one billionth of a gram) indicates that you are probably not ovulating at all. A level lower than 10 might indicate that you are ovulating but not ovulating well, which means that the egg leaves the ovary and can be fertilized, but does not implant solidly in the uterine wall and is not hormonally well supported during the early stages of pregnancy. The condition is known as inadequate luteal phase and is so controversial that some researchers do not even believe it exists. A progesterone level higher than 10 suggests that you are ovulating well.

▶ *What can you do if ovulation tests show that you are not ovulating?*

Fertility drugs can enhance ovulation, but if tests show that you are not ovulating or not ovulating well, then it is advisable to try to ascertain the cause before proceeding. Some of the reasons women fail to ovulate include problems with weight (being overweight or underweight), and certain diseases or conditions (including polycystic ovarian syndrome) that interfere with the normal cycle of hormone control.

▶ *What is polycystic ovarian syndrome (PCOS)?*

Polycystic ovarian syndrome is a noncancerous condition in which the ovaries contain many partially developed eggs (cysts) just beneath their outer walls, which become thickened and fibrous. Women with PCOS have abnormally high levels of androgens (male hormones, including testosterone) circulating in their blood, much higher than the small amounts all women normally produce.

The symptoms of the condition include loss of ovulation and of menstrual periods, unwanted hair growth in a masculine pattern, and sometimes obesity. Women with PCOS who do not ovulate can be treated with Clomid or Perganol.

▶ *How is body weight related to ovulation?*

Although researchers do not understand the exact mechanism, it is clear that body weight (or the ratio of fat to lean tissue) and ovulation are related. Girls do not begin to menstruate or ovulate until they have reached a certain critical body weight. Women who are extremely thin—whether because of anorexia, excessive dieting, or an extremely high level of exercise—often fail to ovulate and stop having menstrual periods. In terms of infertility treatment, women with anorexia and athletes are very different, though both have infertility problems because of low body weight.

Some women who are obese do not ovulate. Their fat tissue makes a kind of estrogen that circulates in the blood at a more or less constant level, unlike the usual monthly hormonal ebb and flow whose ups and downs rouse the pituitary gland to action. The constant level tricks the pituitary into "thinking" that ovulation has already occurred, and it does not start the hormonal process that results in ovulation. Sometimes obese women begin to ovulate once they have succeeded in losing weight.

▶ *Is there a way of knowing whether you are eating too little or exercising too much when normal ovulation doesn't occur?*

If low body weight seems to be inhibiting ovulation, it is worthwhile to determine the underlying causes of the problem before you start dealing with pregnancy. Is this woman underweight because she is anorectic or because she runs ten miles a day?

Women with anorexia do not handle pregnancy well because they have problems with body image, problems that are made worse by the weight gain and increasing girth of pregnancy. Because an anorectic woman is likely to starve both herself and her unborn child during pregnancy, it is vital that she resolve the issues underlying her anorexia before she becomes pregnant. We think of the body as wise, as capable of making subtle adjustments in its own interests. If a pregnant woman continues to starve herself, the fetus will also be malnourished. It seems that the body, sensing its own malnutrition, shuts down ovulation and eliminates the possibility of an unhealthy pregnancy.

Women who exercise a great deal, for example elite runners, have a different problem. Most of these women are not troubled psychologically; they just like to run. Sometimes changing their exercise habits a little, training a little less, and putting on a little weight will solve the problem. Or these women may need help starting a pregnancy, but they usually do very well once they conceive.

▶ *What can be done about failure to ovulate?*

It is quite easy to bring about ovulation in women who are underweight or have certain types of hormonal problems by using so-called fertility drugs, medications that imitate the natural hormones that prod the ovaries into action. One of these drugs is Clomid (generic name clomiphene citrate); the other is Perganol, a preparation of the actual hormones FSH and LH.

Clomid is less powerful and simpler to use because it comes as a pill, taken five days in a row, around days 4–8 of the cycle. Clomid seems to work by blocking estrogen receptors at the pituitary level. That is, it prevents the pituitary gland from recognizing that estrogen is circulating in the blood; the pituitary "believes" that there is no estrogen in the body, so it kicks into overdrive to stimulate the ovary to ripen follicles and head toward ovulation.

Perganol, given as an injection, stimulates the follicles to grow and mature, but does not actually cause the follicle to burst out of the ovary. It is sometimes used along with human chorionic gonadotropin to accomplish that purpose. It is more powerful than Clomid and needs more monitoring. Both these drugs are used in assisted reproduction technologies, such as in vitro fertilization.

▶ *Do these fertility-enhancing drugs have side effects?*

Clomid has relatively few serious side effects, and most of the drug has been released from the woman's system by the time she ovulates. A few women get headaches and have hot flashes. A few notice visual changes, for example spots and dots in front of their eyes. If any of these things happen to you, call your doctor.

Other women report that they have premenstrual symptoms. They may become irritable and have hormonal mood swings; some notice cramps, which may be focused on one side of the abdomen. These symptoms are indications that the woman is ovulating well, so they are good signs. Rarely, Clomid can cause ovarian cysts and ovarian enlargement. Pergonal can cause the same and other side effects, including ovarian cysts.

▶ *What is the likelihood of multiple births with these fertility-enhancing drugs?*

With Clomid, the rate of multiple births is fairly low, about 6–8 percent, and most of those births are twins. With Pergonal the risk is in the range of 20–30 percent, and the pregnancy is likelier to produce triplets or larger numbers of infants. Of the total births to women who took Pergonal, 5 percent involve three or more babies.

Since multiple births can be dangerous to both mother and infants (even without considering the difficulties of raising several children at once), you and your partner should understand and accept the risk before you agree to this therapy. The number of fertilized eggs can be reduced from several to two, but obviously this is a type of abortion and poses its own set of questions.

▶ *Do Clomid and Perganol increase the risk of ovarian cancer?*

No one knows. Early research was based on case reports of very few women, and to date there have been no rigorous studies on women who took either Clomid or Pergonal for certain numbers of months (see Chapter 9).

Miscellaneous Blood Tests

Easy and inexpensive blood tests for two other hormones, thyroid hormone and prolactin, can help rule out other causes for infertility. Women with abnormal thyroid function, either too much or too little, often have difficulty getting pregnant because proper ovulation depends on a normal level of thyroid hormone. The thyroid function test measures for a hormone called TSH (thyroid stimulating hormone) and for thyroid hormone itself. Abnormal thyroid function is easily corrected with medication.

Prolactin, a hormone made by the pituitary gland, stimulates the breast to produce milk after the birth of a child. When its levels in the blood are elevated, it can inhibit ovulation and interfere with the normal menstrual cycle without causing noticeable symptoms. Elevated prolactin levels are easy to remedy with medication.

OTHER DIAGNOSTIC TESTS

Endometrial Biopsy

An endometrial biopsy, a small sample of the lining of the uterus taken for diagnostic purposes, is the gold standard of fertility investigation. The procedure can show whether the uterine lining is thickening and maturing as menstruation approaches, a sure sign that ovulation has occurred and a necessity for supporting a fertilized egg. Because the biopsy shows the effect of progesterone on the lining of the uterus, it should be done toward the end of the menstrual cycle, when progesterone has had a week or so to work. Usually it is performed around days 23–25.

▶ How is an endometrial biopsy done?

The procedure can be done in about two minutes in an office setting without anesthesia. A sharp tool (a curette) or a suction device is slipped through the cervix into the uterus and used to scrape away or suck out little samples of the lining.

Over the years the tools have gotten more sophisticated. The pipelle, a relatively new gadget from France, is narrower than earlier tools and easier to insert through the cervix;

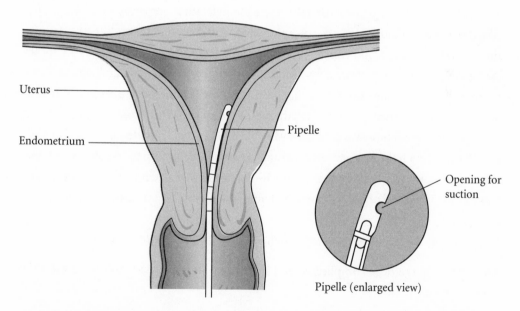

Uterus

Endometrium

Pipelle

Opening for suction

Pipelle (enlarged view)

FIGURE 31. An endometrial biopsy involves removing a sample of tissue from the lining of the uterus. A new tool, the pipelle, makes the procedure more comfortable.

it samples tissue by suction rather than by scraping. My patients tell me it is a real improvement over the older technology.

▶ *Does an endometrial biopsy hurt?*

While it is not painless, most women say it is manageable. Try taking an over-the-counter painkiller like Motrin or Aleve ahead of time to make the procedure less uncomfortable.

▶ *Can you have an endometrial biopsy during a cycle when you are attempting to get pregnant?*

Doctors have different policies on this issue. Some women are concerned that if they are pregnant, the physician might remove the fertilized egg along with the biopsy sample. There is no danger that the procedure will damage the fetus; either it will remove the whole fertilized egg or it will leave the pregnancy undisturbed. However, some women prefer not to conceive during the cycle when they are to have an endometrial biopsy.

▶ *What can an endometrial biopsy show?*

Your physician is hoping to see signs that the endometrium is preparing to receive the fertilized egg. If that is indeed the case, the microscope will show that the endometrial tissue is thicker and has more blood vessels, giving the tissue sample the classic appearance for the day of the cycle on which the test was done. If your cycle is normal, a pathologist (a doctor trained to look at tissue samples for diagnostic purposes) can look at a sample of the endometrium, even a small piece, and tell the day of the cycle—day 18, day 27, or whatever.

An endometrial biopsy is especially valuable for diagnosing inadequate luteal phase, a condition in which the egg gets fertilized and continues on its path to the uterus, but does not implant properly because the uterine lining does not thicken in time to accept and support it. (The luteal phase is the second half of the menstrual cycle, after ovulation.)

▶ *How does an endometrial biopsy help diagnose inadequate luteal phase?*

The procedure is a little complicated and involves counting backward from the day the woman gets her period.

> Sasha decides to go ahead with an endometrial biopsy after earlier testing shows that she is probably ovulating and that her husband has plenty of viable sperm.

Sasha has had thirty-two-day cycles since she was 15 years old, so we plan the test on day 28, four days before her period is due. By the criteria that pathologists use, that day is called day 24. Though Sasha thinks of herself as having thirty-two-day cycles, the pathologist evaluates her biopsy as if she (and every other woman who menstruates) has twenty-eight-day cycles. There are always fourteen days between ovulation and menstruation, though there may eighteen or twelve or some other number of days between menstruation and ovulation. Pathologists are only interested in the second half of the cycle.

So Sasha has a biopsy on day 24. The pathologist looks at the sample and decides that what he sees looks like a typical endometrial lining for day 24, or maybe day 23 or day 25. This is good news (pathologists are allowed to be wrong by a day or two): the assessment means that Sasha is ovulating well enough to produce the hormones that will cause her endometrium to build up and support a fertilized egg.

If Sasha's tissue sample looks as if it were taken on day 16 or day 17 (and her period arrives three days later), then something is wrong. Her endometrium will not be ready to accept a fertilized egg. We call this time a lag phase or delay, a time when her uterine lining should be building up but is not.

▶ *Are there other symptoms for inadequate luteal phase?*

Women with inadequate luteal phase are often in their mid-30s and beyond, when they probably are producing less progesterone than in younger days. Symptoms may include spotting or staining just before the menstrual period.

▶ *Can inadequate luteal phase be treated?*

If your endometrial biopsy suggests inadequate luteal phase, your physician may suggest a repeat biopsy a couple of months later, to determine whether the results of the first test were a fluke or whether this problem happens with some regularity. Some doctors do not ask for a second test, deciding that if you have the problem once you probably will have it again.

The two therapies for inadequate luteal phase are hormones to bring about ovulation and progesterone to support the endometrium in the second half of the cycle.

Usually Clomid is used to stimulate ovluation. The progesterone must be natural progesterone (not any of the synthetic kinds used in birth control pills or for other kinds of therapy). Natural progesterone is available in oral and vaginal forms.

The first person to describe inadequate luteal phase was Georgeanna Seegar Jones, a gynecologist trained at the Johns Hopkins University School of Medicine. She and her husband, Dr. Howard Jones, are perhaps better known for being the first in the United States to do in vitro fertilization, in 1981 creating "test tube babies." Together the couple founded the Jones Institute for Reproductive Medicine in Norfolk, Virginia.

(As an aside, I diagnosed myself with inadequate luteal phase when I was trying to get pregnant for the second time. I took Clomid, which worked on the second cycle and gave my husband and me our son. When I had the honor of meeting Dr. Jones, I thanked her for our darling Max.)

Hysterosalpingogram

Also called an HSG or hysterogram, this long name describes an imaging procedure for viewing the uterus (Greek, *hystero*) and the fallopian tubes (Greek, *salpingo*). The purpose of the test is to find out whether the fallopian tubes are open to the passage of egg and sperm, so that fertilization, which usually takes place in one of the tubes, can occur.

▶ How is a hysterogram done?

Usually the test is performed in a radiology department. You lie in the dorsal lithotomy position, on your back with your feet up in stirrups; the radiologist holds the cervix with a special instrument and injects radio-opaque dye into your uterus through a thin tube, using a fluoroscope to watch the results on a screen so that she can tell right away if something is wrong. The radiologist will also take an x-ray picture to document the procedure. If the tubes are open, your doctor can see the dye squirt out through the fallopian tubes; if not, the x-ray will show where the blockage is.

▶ What is the best time of the month to do a hysterogram?

With infertility testing, timing is important. The ideal time for a hysterogram is after the menstrual period and before ovulation, so that during the procedure none of the menstrual flow or a fertilized egg can be swept backward toward the open end of the tubes by the dye which is pushed into the tubes. The ideal time is around day 8, 9, or 10 of the cycle.

▶ Is a hysterogram painful?

The procedure sounds painful, and it can be uncomfortable. According to most of my patients it is not as distressing as an endometrial biopsy (though one patient told me it was the worst thing she ever endured). The entire test takes between two and five minutes. Most women get up and go home or back to work immediately afterward. You can certainly take Motrin or Advil or some other nonsteroidal anti-inflammatory painkiller before the procedure, just as you might for an endometrial biopsy.

▶ What are the advantages of a hysterogram?

The hysterogram is an important test because about 25 percent of female infertility involves a tubal problem. It gives instantaneous results, as opposed to an endometrial biopsy, where you wait several days while the pathologist looks at the tissue samples. Another benefit is that many women do get pregnant within two or three months after the procedure, perhaps because pushing the dye through the tubes clears them out, even though they are not blocked by tubal disease. Since this test seems to have therapeutic benefits as well as diagnostic ones, we do it fairly early in the infertility workup.

▶ Can a hysterogram give false results?

Yes, hysterograms can have false positive and false negative results. False positives come about because some women have a tubal spasm while the test is going on. There is no mechanical obstruction, but the tubes tighten up so that the dye will not pass through. Thus the test falsely suggests that the tubes are blocked when they are only in spasm.

Some physicians use a drug called Glucogon to relax the tubes. If the hysterogram shows obstruction, the tubes can be viewed directly with a laparoscope. But the procedure requires anesthesia and is more invasive. Laparoscopy will show whether the tubes are blocked or simply in spasm.

A second problem is that the dye can spill out the ends of the tubes, even if they are not functioning properly. Infection may have damaged the hair-like projections inside the tube that help move the egg along, but tube still looks open even though it does not function correctly. Nor can a hysterogram rule out endometriosis if the disease is not actually blocking the tube.

▶ Can hysterograms have complications?

There is about a 1-percent chance of infection. If you have had PID, a hysterogram can make the old infection flare up again and your risk rises to about 3.5 percent. If you do have a history of PID and your doctor recommends a hysterogram, remind her before you go for the test. She may advise preventive antibiotics. Women who have previously had an ectopic pregnancy, tubal surgery, or a ruptured appendix may also be at increased risk for infection and may benefit from preventive antibiotic therapy.

▶ What happens if the hysterogram shows blocked fallopian tubes?

If the test suggests that your tubes are blocked, your doctor may wish to have those results verified by a laparoscopy. If the laparoscopy confirms tubal blockage, you are a candidate for in vitro fertilization or tubal surgery.

▶ Can the x-rays and dye used during a hysterogram damage a fetus?

No, neither the minimal x-ray exposure nor the dye has been shown to cause any problems later. Because the hysterogram should be done before ovulation, women are unlikely to be pregnant during the procedure.

▶ Can blocked fallopian tubes be treated?

There is a surgical procedure called a tuboplasty, during which a surgeon cuts out the blocked portion of the tubes and then reattaches the ends. It has only about a 30-percent chance of success, so infertility specialists often prefer in vitro fertilization if they discover tubal blockage. The decision depends on the condition of the fallopian tubes, the location and extent of the blockage, and so on.

If the blockage is near the ovary, at the end of the tube where the fimbriae reach out and sweep the egg into the tube, unblocking the tube has a reasonable chance of success. This operation is called a fimbrioplasty. But if the blockage is near the uterus, tubal surgery is much more difficult. The surgeon can cut out the obstruction and then attempt to reimplant the narrow end of the tube into the main body of the uterus. This kind of very delicate surgery should only be undertaken by someone who has performed it many times.

Insurance companies will sometimes pay for tubal surgery but not for in vitro fertilization. In an ideal world, cost would not be a major consideration in such an important decision; in the real world, it is often a factor.

Postcoital Test

The next test I usually prescribe is a postcoital test, which checks the woman's cervical mucus and looks for incompatibilities between it and her partner's sperm. Although there is no magic order in which to do fertility tests, I tend to hold off on this one because it does not have a very high yield (only about 5 percent of couples have incompatibility problems). The test is not painful but it does put a direct demand on the couple and may be psychologically difficult.

Problems with cervical mucus can be physical: the mucus can be too thick for the sperm to swim upstream or there can be too little of it. Or there can be problems of incompatibility between this man's sperm and this woman's immune system, which may produce antibodies that kill the sperm.

▶ *How is a postcoital test done?*

The couple has intercourse two to twelve hours before the examination. The time depends on the physician's individual style of investigation: some doctors prefer to do the test only an hour after intercourse, others wait eight hours.

You go to your gynecologist's office and have a pelvic exam. The doctor takes a sample of your cervical mucus, puts it on a slide, and looks at it under the microscope. The sample will show immediately whether the mucus has the right consistency—thin, clear, and stretchy like egg white. It will also reveal how the sperm are progressing. Ideally, the test should show lots of active, forward-moving sperm. Sometimes it shows only a few sperm, suggesting a low sperm count. Sometimes it shows a great many dead sperm, killed by antibodies in the cervical mucus or possibly dead before they entered the vagina.

▶ *Can a postcoital test substitute for a semen analysis?*

If the man absolutely refuses to have a semen analysis (and I find that difficult to accept), a postcoital test will give some of the relevant information. If the postcoital test shows plenty of active, forward-moving sperm, then we know that sperm production is not a problem. However, if the postcoital test shows many sperm, but most or all are dead, then there is no way to tell whether the sperm was not viable to begin with or the cervical mucus has killed it. A semen analysis is necessary to get the vital information.

▶ *When during the cycle is a postcoital test done?*

This test should be performed right around the time of ovulation. If you have a twenty-eight-day cycle, we do the test around day 13 or 14. If the test is done at the wrong time and misses ovulation by as little as a day or two, it can give misleading results. Suppose you ovulated on day 17 instead of your customary day 14. Your cervical mucus looks as if it is far too thick for sperm to swim through it, but in fact there is no problem at all, just poor timing.

Sometimes I schedule a repeat visit the next month because I think I may have guessed wrong about ovulation, and the couple becomes pregnant in the interim. That is the optimal result of an infertility workup.

▶ *How is a sperm antibody problem treated?*

Years ago there were various approaches. One was to treat the woman and sometimes the man with anti-inflammatory medications, including steroids, which calm down the immune system's reactions to antibodies. Another (not very successful) way was to treat the problem as an allergy. The man wore condoms during intercourse for six months, allowing her allergic reaction to subside. Then when the couple tried again for a pregnancy, the allergic response would not kill the sperm. Today a cervical mucus problem is treated with intrauterine insemination.

▶ *How does intrauterine insemination work?*

Intrauterine insemination is a procedure whereby the sperm are placed up inside the uterus, bypassing the cervical mucus altogether. Although it sounds simple enough, the procedure has one complication. In the normal arrangement of things, semen does not reach the uterus: sperm do, but the seminal fluid does not. Seminal fluid contains prostaglandins, hormone-like substances that make the uterus contract. Therefore if ordinary semen is introduced into the uterus, it will cause uterine contractions, which can be very painful and even cause women to go into shock.

For the insemination to succeed, the sperm must be washed free of seminal fluid and then resuspended in a solution similar to salt water. This requires special laboratory equipment, so most physicians cannot do the procedure in an office setting.

▶ *Does ordinary artificial insemination work if there is a problem with cervical mucus?*

Artificial insemination (called AIH, artificial insemination with husband's sperm) does not usually succeed with this kind of problem, because the cervical mucus kills the sperm whether they get into the vagina through ordinary intercourse or through artificial means. It is useful occasionally when there is some physical or anatomical problem—for example, an oddly shaped uterus—that might impede the progress of sperm.

INVASIVE TESTS

Laparoscopy

Next on the agenda, and further along in terms of invasiveness, is laparoscopy, an investigative surgical procedure for observing the inside of the pelvis. A laparoscopy can provide information about scarring or adhesions around the fallopian tubes or growths of endometrial tissue outside the uterus, information not revealed by a hysterogram. Often it is the best way to diagnose endometriosis or assess the damage of pelvic inflammatory disease.

A laparoscope is a thin metal tube with light-transmitting fibers that permits your doctor to see inside your pelvis. It can be used in conjunction with small surgical tools to allow the physician to take little samples of the tissue if there is any question about the diagnosis.

▶ *Can a laparoscopy be done in an office setting?*

In the past, laparoscopy was performed under general anesthesia in a hospital setting with operating room personnel, including an anesthesiologist and a gynecological surgeon. In these present days of cost-conscious medicine, laparoscopies are sometimes performed in surgicenters or offices. Instead of a general anesthetic that puts you to sleep, your doctor will give Novocain to anesthetize your skin, plus some light sedation (perhaps Valium) to make you drowsy. Instead of a regular laparoscope, which is approximately 1 cm in diameter, your doctor may use a smaller instrument, only about 3 mm in diameter. This tiny laparoscope helps to show what is happening in the abdomen, but it is not as useful as the larger version for actually removing endometriosis or doing other procedures.

Laparoscopy generally takes less than an hour. If an operable problem such as scar tissue is discovered, it can be removed through the laparoscope and the procedure may take

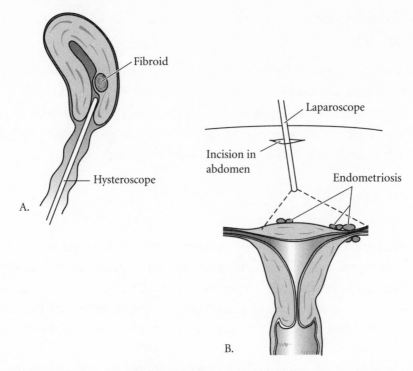

FIGURE 32. A, the hysteroscope can be used to view the inside of the uterus; B, the laparoscope shows the inside of the pelvis and can be used to reveal endometriosis, scarring, fibroids, or other conditions.

longer. Laparoscopy should be done by a surgeon trained and experienced in the procedure.

Hysteroscopy

Hysteroscopy is a procedure for looking at the inside of the uterus. A hysteroscope, like a laparoscope, is a long narrow tube with a light at the end; it is inserted through the vagina and cervix into the uterus and does not require an incision. Hysteroscopy is useful in diagnosing fibroids, benign tumors of the uterus, or scarring within the uterus, but is not usually done unless your caregiver has reason to suspect one of these conditions. It can be performed with or without anesthesia. You will be able to do sedentary work the next day and will probably be back to your full schedule a few days later.

▶ Do fibroids interfere with pregnancy?

Most women with fibroids do not have problems with infertility. Only rarely do fibroids prevent conception, for example by blocking the entrance to the fallopian tubes. If they do cause a problem with pregnancy, it is likely to be miscarriage.

▶ What is Asherman's syndrome?

Occasionally hysteroscopy will turn up a condition called Asherman's syndrome, which involves such extensive scarring of uterine lining that menstrual periods cease. It is a complication for women who have had several D&Cs, maybe after miscarriage. If one of my patients stops menstruating after a D&C, I suspect Asherman's syndrome. It can be treated by a combination of surgery and hormonal therapy.

ASSISTED REPRODUCTION TECHNIQUES

Although we think of assisted reproductive technology as relatively new, artificial insemination is an ancient technique, used in livestock as far back as the second century and in human beings as early as the eighteenth century. Although artificial insemination is still used, more sophisticated techniques are available. The three principal techniques of assisted reproduction are GIFT (gamete intrafallopian transfer), ZIFT (zygote intrafallopian transfer), and IVF (in vitro fertilization—fertilization "in glass," a petri dish or other laboratory glassware). These techniques involve harvesting eggs from the ovary. The woman is usually treated with medication to produce and mature more than one egg in a single cycle.

Unless donor eggs and sperm are used, all these techniques require that the woman be able to produce and mature eggs (possibly with hormonal help) and the man be able to produce healthy sperm. With the exception of artificial insemination (AIH and AID), these techniques are done by fertility specialists, often in major hospitals or fertility clinics.

ARTIFICIAL INSEMINATION

Artificial insemination simply means depositing sperm in the woman's reproductive tract without intercourse. The sperm can belong to her husband or partner, in which case the procedure is called AIH (artificial insemination with husband's sperm), or it can be from a donor, in which case the procedure is known as AID (artificial insemination with donor sperm).

▶ *How are donor sperm screened?*

Years ago, donor sperm were sometimes used live; today, because of HIV, sperm banks make sure the donor is disease free before his sperm are used. The donor is given blood tests for HIV, hepatitis, and syphilis at the time of donation. After a six-month wait, during which the sperm are frozen, he is tested again to make sure that his tests have not turned positive. If a donor was infected with HIV two weeks before he made his donation, his blood test might not yet have turned positive, but it will certainly do so during the waiting period. The down side is that frozen sperm are less potent than fresh and less likely to fertilize an egg. It is an acceptable negative, given the seriousness of sexually transmitted diseases.

Sometimes a lesbian couple will use donor sperm from a male friend, without medical supervision or screening. I strongly advise the couple to be sure that the sperm donor is not infected with hepatitis, syphilis, or HIV.

▶ *How does artificial insemination work?*

You go to your doctor's office at the time of ovulation, which you can determine with an ovulation predictor test. While you are on the examining table in position for a pelvic exam, your caregiver will dilate your vagina with a speculum to isolate your cervix and, with a syringe, place the sperm sample right in the cervical opening. You should remain lying down for fifteen or twenty minutes.

Some women try "home methods" of artificial insemination using donor sperm. They obtain a speculum, a syringe, and an intravenous catheter and inject the sperm through the tubing into the cervix. Women without access to medical devices have been known to use a turkey baster.

▶ *How are eggs gathered from the ovary for advanced reproductive technologies?*

Usually you start by taking a drug, Clomid or Pergonal, which stimulates the eggs in your ovaries to mature. The choice of drug depends on the physician. Usually Clomid is preferable because it is easier to use and can be taken orally. If Clomid does not succeed, Pergonal is a stronger and more expensive alternative. It must be injected and monitored with blood tests. With Pergonal as many as thirty eggs may ripen and all are harvested. Ultrasound imaging and tracking the blood levels of estradiol, the primary form of estrogen made in the body, can be used to check the progress of maturation.

Harvesting itself is a minor surgical procedure, usually done with intravenous sedation. The ovary, stimulated by the Clomid or Pergonal, becomes heavy with eggs and hangs down near the vagina. The surgeon, guided by ultrasound, puts a long thin needle through the vaginal wall into the ovary and aspirates the eggs into the needle. After the procedure, most women feel sedated by the medication and rest for the remainder of the day. Usually they are able to resume work the next day.

IN VITRO FERTILIZATION

▶ *How does IVF work?*

Once the eggs and sperm are collected, they are mixed together and placed in a glass dish containing a nutritive medium, in the hope that fertilization will take place and some of the eggs will begin to divide. If this happens, the embryo is placed in the uterus with a straw-like device. A pregnancy test two weeks later can determine whether the embryo has been implanted in the wall of the uterus.

▶ *Is in vitro fertilization right for you?*

In vitro fertilization is an appropriate technique if your tubes are blocked or impaired, perhaps by endometriosis or infection, and if you have had previous ectopic pregnancies. If you are ovulating well but your partner has a problem with sperm production, your eggs can be retrieved and mixed with the sperm of a donor, fertilized, and then replaced in your uterus. On the other hand, if your partner is producing viable sperm, but you do not ovulate at all or do not ovulate well, the option of donor eggs exists. You will need hormonal assistance in addition to the implantation, because your body has to be prepared to receive the fertilized egg.

Occasionally sperm may need help in penetrating an egg. This can be done in a petri dish; the technique is called intracytoplasmic sperm injection, or ICSI.

GIFT AND ZIFT

Not frequently used nowadays, GIFT (gamete intrafallopian transfer) is a technique whereby eggs and sperm are placed into the fallopian tubes in the hope that fertilization will take place there. (A gamete is a reproductive cell, either an egg or a sperm.) For this procedure, you must have healthy tubes, though you may have difficulty ovulating. Again, your partner must be able to produce healthy sperm.

The procedure starts off like IVF: your ovaries are stimulated with Clomid or Perg-onal; the eggs are harvested; the sperm are collected. Then both are placed in the open end of one of your fallopian tubes with the help of a laparoscope. GIFT is a more invasive pro-cedure than IVF because it involves an incision for inserting a laparoscope into the ab-domen to transfer the eggs into the fallopian tube. IVF simply involves transferring em-bryos into the uterus through the cervix without surgery.

ZIFT (zygote intrafallopian transfer) is similar to GIFT, except that it is the zygote, the fertilized egg, that is transferred to the fallopian tube, again with the help of a laparoscope. Fertilization takes place in a petri dish in a laboratory. The fertility specialist checks to be sure that the cell division that marks successful fertilization has actually taken place before the transfer is made. As in GIFT, an incision must be made to insert the laparoscope.

▶ *Do these assisted reproductive techniques increase the chances of multiple births?*

During IVF, usually several eggs are implanted in the uterus in the hope that one of them will take hold, so it is certainly possible to have twins, triplets, or even more births. Data gathered in the Centers for Disease Control and Prevention 1999 survey show that 37 per-cent of all births with assisted reproductive techniques were multiple births, compared with less than 3 percent of births in the general population. Twins accounted for 29 percent of these multiple births; triplets or larger numbers of infants accounted for 8 percent. Be-cause multiple births pose risks for both the mother (cesarean section) and the babies (preterm delivery, low birth weight, long-term disabilities) laws in some countries, in-cluding England, prohibit placing more than two embryos in the uterus.

▶ *How successful are assisted reproduction techniques?*

As the technology improves, so does the success rate. Some estimates reach 80 percent for couples who are willing to make repeated attempts—which are expensive, time consum-ing, and emotionally challenging. According to the 1999 data, 25.2 percent of IVF proce-dures using fresh nondonor eggs resulted in live births, with younger women having higher rates than older ones. Women younger than age 35 had a rate of 32.2 percent live births, while women 41 and older had a rate of only 9.7 percent.

▶ *How expensive are assisted reproductive techniques?*

Assisted reproductive technology comes at a high price and is not universally reimbursed by insurance. Costs differ from clinic to clinic, but it has been estimated that therapy with Clomid or Perganol costs about thirteen hundred dollars per cycle; the cost of intrauterine insemination (where donated semen is placed within the uterus) is about five hundred dollars per cycle. More sophisticated techniques such as IVF cost in the range of three thousand to ten thousand dollars per attempt and take as long as ten days.

SURROGACY AND OTHER TECHNIQUES

Women who cannot produce eggs even with the help of hormonal stimulation and men who cannot make viable sperm do have the option of donor eggs or sperm. This means that women in their late 40s who are nearing menopause can bear a child by using the eggs from a younger woman, fertilized by the older woman's partner. On occasion, an older mother has borne her own grandchild—her daughter's egg fertilized by her son-in-law's sperm—because the daughter had a uterine malformation.

13 Abortion, Miscarriage, and Ectopic Pregnancy

▶ **MYTH** Having an abortion means that it will be hard to get pregnant when you want to.

FACT When legal abortions were difficult to get, complications of botched illegal abortions did affect many women's fertility. Since abortion became legal in the United States, no scientific studies have upheld the notion that abortion leads to infertility.

A S we have seen, no contraceptive is perfectly reliable even if used correctly every single time, though in theory some are more than 99 percent safe. In real life, contraception can fail because you don't use it, or you don't use it correctly, or the method lets you down. Unintended pregnancies, whether they come about through carelessness or method failure, can be devastating because they will alter the course of your future. Pregnancies that come about through sexual assault or incest can be unbearably painful.

Before 1973, when *Roe* v. *Wade* made abortion legal in the United States, there were three choices for women who became pregnant and did not want or could not take care of the child: going through with the pregnancy and giving up the baby for adoption, having an illegal abortion, or going somewhere where abortion was legal.

Today the option of legal abortion does exist, and *should* exist for women as an adjunct to birth control. No physician likes to perform abortions: it is far better to prevent a pregnancy than to end one. Ideally, abortion should be limited to cases where contraception fails, where prenatal testing discovers some serious fetal abnormality, or where the pregnancy resulted from rape or incest. The issue of abortion can touch a woman's deepest feelings about herself, her relation to her partner, and the values that shape her life.

Once an unwanted pregnancy begins, women have several choices, but all have consequences. Pregnancy is not something that can be undone by wishful thinking or denial.

> One evening I answered a page from a patient I'll call Doris. She had discovered she was pregnant and desperately wanted not to be. I pointed out that she had two choices, to go through with the pregnancy or to have an abortion. "No," said Doris, "no baby, and no abortion either." Again I stated what seemed obvious, that in that case she had only three options: have the child and keep it, have the child and give it up for adoption, or have an abortion. Doris rejected all three.
>
> My husband, who had overheard my end of the conversation, said, "Ah, what that woman wants is an 'unscrewing pill.'" He meant a marvelous medication to undo what Doris and her partner had done, essentially a pill that would take her back in time to before conception had occurred.

Since such a magic pill does not exist, I believe that women (and men, too) should think about their risks before they become sexually active. I strongly encourage my teenage patients in particular to realize that from the moment they have intercourse, they expose themselves to the possibilities of STDs and unwanted pregnancy. Since no contraceptive short of a hysterectomy is 100 percent effective, the safest sex is abstinence from intercourse. Even having your fallopian tubes tied has a known rate of failure.

Give some serious thought to what you would do if the unforeseen happened: Would you keep the baby? Would you give up your child for adoption? Would you have an abortion? If none of these is a viable choice for you, then you should not have intercourse.

When I was a medical student, in the days before *Roe* v. *Wade,* many young women who became pregnant went through with their pregnancies and offered their babies for adoption. This does not happen often anymore, maybe once or twice among the five hundred babies my medical group delivers each year. The woman chooses abortion or she raises the child, possibly with the help of her family.

▶ When can an abortion be performed?

Ideally, abortions should be performed during the first trimester of pregnancy—the first three months, or thirteen weeks. Most gynecologists will not recommend doing them until four to five weeks after conception, two to three weeks after you have missed your period. A few abortions are done during the second trimester, the second three months.

These guidelines have been established because of fetal viability, the age at which the fetus can survive on its own outside the mother's body. No one can pinpoint when that moment arrives, but it is quite certain that the fetus cannot live independently before twenty-two weeks of gestation. It is very rare to save a baby born prematurely at twenty-four weeks gestational age, but it is not uncommon to save one at twenty-six weeks. So the lower limits of viability are somewhere between twenty-two and twenty-six weeks of gestation.

Unusual circumstances may cause variations of these guidelines. If, for example, ultrasound reveals that the fetus has a severe deformity that would prevent its ever living outside the mother's body, then viability takes on a different meaning even though the fetus may be older than twenty-six weeks. I do not consider the termination of this kind of pregnancy an abortion at all, since the fetus could not survive independently.

ABORTION

An abortion is the termination of a pregnancy before the fetus can live independently of the mother. Abortion can occur spontaneously, without intervention, in which case it may be called miscarriage, though physicians often use the term "abortion" to describe this event. People outside the medical profession use the word to describe the deliberate, intentional ending of a pregnancy.

ABORTION VERSUS ADOPTION

When someone, particularly a teenager, comes to me with an unwanted pregnancy, we first discuss the possibility of adoption. If she chooses this route, I assure her that in this day and age she can find parents who are quite desperate to have a child and will give her baby the love and care that all children need and deserve. She may grieve that she has given up her child, and she may continue to think about that child for the rest of her life, but she will know that the child is provided for.

A second choice is to raise the child herself, with or without the help of her parents. I have seen 15-year-old girls responsible for infants; more frequently, I see mothers helping their daughters by taking on these responsibilities. Neither scenario is easy. Teenagers with a baby to care for find themselves with all the burdens of adulthood. They love their babies, but see their friends going to college, getting the education necessary to better their

---

BOX 9. A Few Facts About Abortion

Since the landmark Supreme Court decision *Roe* v. *Wade* struck down restrictive laws in 1973, abortion has been legal in the United States.

According to the Centers for Disease Control, about 2.7 million unintended pregnancies occur in the United States each year. Family planning experts estimate that about half of these end in abortion.

There is no evidence that making abortion illegal would reduce the number of abortions performed; it would only make them more dangerous.

Almost half of American women have had an abortion by the time they reach the age of 45.

About two thirds of women who have one abortion never have another.

---

lives, or simply having a good time. Many of these young mothers say they love their children—but I can see that they resent them also, because they refer to them as "rugrats" or "little brats." Children are sensitive and smart; they pick up on parental resentment.

Some of my older patients, women in their 40s, 50s, and even 60s, help their daughters by raising the grandchildren, in part because they want to save their daughters from being trapped in a downward economic spiral. While the grandmothers do love their grandchildren, they express sorrow at losing the freedom they thought would be theirs when their own child rearing was done.

Liz, now 50, works as a nurse in the labor and delivery unit at the hospital. Her daughter, who never married, has three children between the ages of 10 and 13. After giving birth to these three, the daughter simply left town, unhappy with the responsibilities of mothering. Liz and her husband felt they had no choice but to take on the children and care for them.

One of the boys, now 12, has attention deficit disorder and is a difficult child. Liz must work hard to support her grandchildren. While she is facing the stresses of menopause, she is also trying to cope with three children on the brink of adolescence. She is discouraged but determined to succeed.

I do not believe that most women in the United States use abortion as a substitute for birth control. Rather, they choose it because something has gone wrong with contraception. This is not the case in, for example, Eastern Europe, where women formerly had an average of five abortions during their reproductive lives.

The reasons women seek to end unwanted pregnancies can be medical, financial, personal, or a combination of these factors. Among the medical reasons are genetic abnormalities or serious malformations of the fetus, which have been uncovered by prenatal testing. Fetal abnormality is one of the major motives for second-trimester abortions, and as testing becomes increasingly prevalent and sophisticated, more abortions will probably be performed for medical reasons.

Women who are the victims of incest or rape frequently seek abortion. Some women, especially the younger ones, seek abortions because they are unmarried, because they have no financial means of caring for a child, because they are still pursuing their education or furthering their careers, or because they know they are not mature enough to care for a child. Older women seek abortions because they have completed their families, or feel they are physically too old to care for a child (or another child). Still others seek abortions because they recognize that they are emotionally unable to care for a child, perhaps because of depression or instability.

▶ Do abortions scar women emotionally?

Studies on the psychological aftermath of abortion have had conflicting results. Because abortion is so politicized in this country, people with strong opinions tend to interpret study results in ways that support their own points of view. Conservative groups, who believe that abortion should be legally banned, generally discover that the long-term emotional impact on women is harmful. Groups who uphold women's legal right to terminate a pregnancy emphasize data suggesting that most women feel significant relief at not having to bear and raise an unwanted child, and that the emotional effects are less significant.

We must also realize that the issue of abortion comes with considerable baggage in a society that is ambivalent about sex. Although it is legal, abortion still carries a stigma; so even if women feel relief at not having to go through with an unwanted pregnancy, some still feel the burden of stigmatization.

Although some women have multiple abortions, most women do not terminate a pregnancy lightly. For many the decision is painful even though the child is not wanted. However, most women do deal successfully with the emotional consequences: they feel overwhelming relief, even as they acknowledge a sense of loss.

In my practice I have met women who later in life regretted an abortion, especially if infertility problems arose. I have also met women who suffered long-term psychological consequences because they did not have an abortion and raised an unwanted child. And I have met women who endured a profound lack of self-esteem because they knew their own mothers did not want them.

▶ Are abortions likely to cause later physical problems?

Now that abortion is legal and is performed by trained practitioners in sterile settings, usually during the first trimester, abortion is unlikely to result in complications that will reduce fertility later on. There is no evidence that having a first-trimester abortion increases risk for future ectopic pregnancies. One study raised the possibility that having an abortion increases risk for breast cancer, but subsequent work has shown no connection.

▶ Do abortions often have complications?

While abortions are not high risk, any surgical procedure has its dangers. Even when performed by a board-certified gynecologist or obstetrician who has had special training beyond the usual medical school work, surgical abortions can occasionally have complications. Because the walls of the uterus are softer during a pregnancy, there is a greater chance of perforating the uterus during the procedure than there is during a D&C, which is essentially similar. Uterine perforation happens in about 1 or 2 of every 1,000 abortions (a rate of 0.1–0.2 percent).

The other risks of this and any surgery are infection and bleeding. The earlier the abortion is performed, the less the chance of complications. Abortions performed in the second trimester are riskier than those done in the first.

▶ Do women die of abortions?

The death rate in the United States is 2–3 of every 100,000 legal abortions, much lower than the death rate from childbirth, which is in the range of 15 per 100,000 deliveries. Again, later abortions are riskier than those done in the first trimester.

FIRST-TRIMESTER ABORTIONS

There are two primary methods for early abortions: medical (drug-induced) abortions and surgical abortions. The choice depends on your preference, the length of time you have been pregnant, and the availability of medical abortion. The nearest Planned Parenthood chapter is the best source of information on what is available in your area.

A surgical abortion is similar to a D&C, with vacuum or suction aspiration of the contents of the uterus. Some physicians perform menstrual extractions, which also use vacuum or suction aspiration but take place very early in the pregnancy. Mifepristone, a drug originally used in Europe and Canada for medical abortions, has recently become available in this country. Medical abortion with methotrexate is a little-known procedure that uses a readily available drug to produce much the same results as mifepristone.

Menstrual Extraction

A menstrual extraction, sometimes also called a miniabortion or a minisuction, is a procedure for suctioning out the contents of the uterus without dilating the cervix. It was quite popular a number of years ago and was often performed by midwives.

Menstrual extractions, often done before a test has established the fact of pregnancy (between four and five weeks gestational age), must be performed when there is very little fetal tissue. Requesting this procedure, it seems to me, involves self-deception and denial, since the woman asking for menstrual extracting is seeking a way of terminating a possible pregnancy "without having an abortion."

▶ How is menstrual extraction performed?

Menstrual extractions are just like suction D&Cs performed slightly later in the pregnancy, except that there is no need to dilate the cervix. A thin tube, or cannula, maybe 3–4 mm wide (about as thick as a piece of spaghetti), is inserted through the cervix. The contents of the uterus are suctioned out with a small pump or a bulb syringe. The procedure takes only a few minutes and may not require any anesthesia.

▶ What are its advantages and disadvantages?

The advantages are several: it is easy to perform and does not usually require anesthesia. It is very low risk and low cost. But it also has a high failure rate. Because the dividing egg is so small, it is easy to miss during the suction procedure.

Sherry, the girlfriend of a medical student I was teaching some years back, asked whether I would do a menstrual extraction for her. When I asked Sherry how long it had been since she had missed her period, she said that she was only a week late but she just "knew" she was pregnant and was very anxious to have an abortion.

This was early in my career and I agreed to do the procedure, though I explained that there was a risk I might not end the pregnancy. My concern was well founded. Three weeks later Sherry had to have a D&C, a repeat of an uncomfortable procedure.

Medical Abortion with Methotrexate

Methotrexate is a drug used for treating cancer, especially tumors of the placenta. Like other chemotherapeutic agents, methotrexate attacks cells that are dividing rapidly, which includes not only cancer cells but also the cells of the placenta.

Because it kills rapidly dividing cells and destroys the placenta, methotrexate terminates a pregnancy, whether it is in the uterus or in the fallopian tube. Methotrexate has also been used quite frequently in this country during the past five years to terminate ectopic pregnancies without surgery, and similar drugs have been used in China for many years for the same purpose. In addition, methotrexate is sometimes prescribed for treating psoriasis and rheumatoid arthritis.

▶ *How is methotrexate given for purposes of abortion?*

This is a treatment that requires a doctor's care and supervision. First, you are given a quantitative pregnancy test to measure the amount of hCG in your blood. When this baseline level is established, you are given methotrexate as an injection in the muscles of the arm or the buttocks. A week later, another quantitative blood test will show whether the amount of hCG is decreasing. If it is, then the placenta is degenerating and the fetus will miscarry. If not, a second shot can be given. Some physicians will follow up the methotrexate with a prostaglandin, which stimulates uterine contractions. If the methotrexate still does not work, a D&C can serve as a backup procedure.

▶ *How effective is methotrexate in inducing an abortion?*

Since the drug has not been widely used in this country, reliable statistics have not been gathered. In one experimental study where methotrexate was followed by a prostaglandin to stimulate uterine contractions, 96 percent of the women in the study group did have successful abortions.

▶ Does methotrexate have side effects?

If taken in large doses and for extended periods, as it is for people with arthritis or psoriasis, methotrexate can be toxic to the liver. This does not seem to be a danger for women getting a one- or two-shot dose of the drug for abortion purposes.

Medical Abortion with Mifepristone

The drug mifepristone (formerly known as RU-486, the "French abortion pill") is widely used in Canada, the United Kingdom, and Sweden as well as France, where it has been shown to be generally safe and effective. For many years it was used only experimentally in the United States, because the antichoice lobby effectively prevented any pharmaceutical company from marketing it for the purpose of abortion.

Clinical trials began here in 1994 and lasted about a year. The drug received FDA approval in 2000, and today is manufactured under the trade name Mifeprex.

▶ How does mifepristone work?

It blocks the production of progesterone, the hormone necessary for sustaining early pregnancy. It can be used for abortions before the ninth week of pregnancy, but is most effective when used during the first forty-nine days or seven weeks of pregnancy (counting from the beginning of the last menstrual period).

▶ What are the advantages and disadvantages of this procedure?

Mifepristone offers more privacy than other methods because it requires visits only to a doctor's office, not to a surgicenter or abortion clinic. In parts of the country where it is difficult to get a surgical abortion, women may be able to find physicians close to their homes who are able to provide this procedure. It is less invasive than a surgical abortion. Women who took part in the clinical trials suggested that it was more "natural," because it resembled a spontaneous miscarriage, and therefore was less frightening.

Disadvantages include the fact that a medical abortion lengthens the period of cramping while the fetus is expelled. There is a period of waiting and uncertainty before the abortion takes place. The abortion happens at home (or at work or somewhere else), where there is no immediate access to professional help or intravenous pain control. Although mifepristone is relatively safe and has been used by millions of European women, no long-term safety statistics are available for the United States. The method must be used before the ninth week of pregnancy and preferably before the seventh, which means within the first month after you have missed a period. Mifepristone is said to be dangerous for smokers.

▶ *What is the regimen for taking mifepristone?*

Using mifepristone effectively is a multistep process, requiring three or more visits to a doctor's office. The first step is a dose of mifepristone, taken orally. The second step, three days later, is the administration of a prostaglandin, either as an injection or as a vaginal suppository. The prostaglandin causes the uterus to contract and expel the fetus, which has been weakened by depriving the uterus of progesterone. After the miscarriage has taken place, a follow-up exam is scheduled to make sure that all the fetal tissue has been expelled.

▶ *How effective is mifepristone?*

European studies have suggested that it is 95 percent effective when used in conjunction with a prostaglandin. Clinical studies in the United States returned a figure of 92 percent, with the success rate declining as pregnancy advanced.

▶ *What are its side effects?*

The side effects, common to almost all women who use mifepristone, are like those of a natural miscarriage—cramping and bleeding. The actual amount of blood lost is about the same as for other kinds of early abortions, whether medical or surgical. Bleeding or spotting lasted an average of thirteen days. A few women, roughly 2 in 1,000, have heavy bleeding and require transfusion. About 5 percent of women need a D&C to complete the procedure because their bleeding continues. Other side effects include nausea, diarrhea, and vomiting, but these take place mostly within four hours of taking the second drug, the prostaglandin.

Dilation and Curettage

This kind of first-trimester abortion is not very different from a D&C performed for other purposes, for example to help with heavy menstrual bleeding. The contents of the uterus can be removed via a vacuum procedure, curettage (scraping with a sharp tool, called a curette), or both. Most doctors do the vacuum procedure first and follow it with curettage.

This procedure is usually performed after the sixth or seventh week of pregnancy and before the thirteenth. Most doctors do not advocate a D&C earlier than about seven weeks after your last menstrual period (five weeks after conception); before that the fetal sac is so tiny that there is a significant chance of missing it.

▶ How long does a D&C take?

This depends on several factors, the most important being the duration of the pregnancy: the more advanced the pregnancy the more difficult, and therefore the longer, the procedure. The actual D&C takes somewhere between five and fifteen minutes. After resting for about an hour in a setting where you can be observed for pain or bleeding, you can usually go home.

▶ Is a D&C done with anesthesia?

Again, this depends on how far the pregnancy is advanced. Dilating the cervix can be painful, so sometimes you will have intravenous tranquilizers that make you sleepy and reduce anxiety. D&Cs can be done with either local anesthesia or with a general anesthetic, which puts you to sleep. Many women prefer this for emotional as well as physical reasons. Even with general anesthesia, the procedure can be done in a surgicenter or other outpatient facility.

▶ How is the actual D&C performed?

Because the length of the pregnancy will determine how far the cervix must be dilated, your doctor may use an ultrasound image to check duration of the pregnancy. The D&C is done while you are in the dorsal lithotomy position—on your back with your feet elevated in stirrups, the same position as for a pelvic exam. Your vagina is washed out with an antiseptic solution, perhaps iodine. When the anesthetic has taken hold, the physician gradually stretches your cervix using dilators, tapered metal rods of increasing diameter: the smallest are as narrow as a piece of wire, the later ones are considerably thicker.

Once the cervix has been dilated, the doctor introduces a little tube or hose called a cannula into your uterus. The cannula is attached to a pump that makes enough vacuum pressure to suction out the embryo, the placental tissue, and the lining of the uterine cavity. Most, though not all, doctors will follow the suction procedure by scraping the uterine lining with a sharp curette. This helps to ensure that no fetal tissue remains inside the uterus to cause infection or bleeding later on.

▶ *How painful is a D&C?*

This varies from woman to woman, depending on how far the pregnancy has advanced, her anxiety about the procedure, and her pain threshold. During the suction phase some women feel only mild cramping, something similar to a menstrual period; others feel more intense pain. The same variation is true of the scraping procedure, if the surgeon chooses to use it.

▶ *Are there any medical conditions that would rule out an outpatient D&C during the first trimester of pregnancy?*

Women with heart disease, high blood pressure, asthma, lupus, fibroids, clotting disorders, diabetes, or epilepsy that are not well under control may have to be hospitalized and take special precautions. Most women tolerate the procedure well.

▶ *How much does a D&C cost?*

Depending on where you live, where the procedure takes place, whether or not you have anesthesia, a first-trimester D&C can cost anywhere from two hundred to eight hundred dollars. Your insurance may pay for it, but this varies from company to company. Check with your carrier.

SECOND-TRIMESTER ABORTIONS

Although abortions should be done when they are safest and easiest, during the first trimester (and about 95 percent of them are), sometimes circumstances make that impossible. A primary reason for a second-trimester abortion is the discovery through prenatal testing that the fetus has a serious abnormality. Other reasons include late realization of pregnancy: some women, especially those with irregular or widely spaced menstrual periods, may not recognize that they are pregnant until many weeks have passed. Or women may not realize that a generally reliable method of birth control, for example oral contraceptives, has failed. Or women, especially teenagers, may psychologically deny that they are pregnant until the second trimester is upon them. Sometimes financial problems prevent women from seeking abortion in the early weeks.

▶ How are second-trimester abortions done?

During the second trimester, there are the same two general options, medical and surgical. The surgical procedure is similar to the D&C, though beyond thirteen weeks of pregnancy it is often called a D&E (dilation and evacuation). A second-trimester medical abortion, comparable to an early abortion using methotrexate or mifepristone, means inducing labor with drugs and letting the process continue until the fetus is expelled through the vagina.

▶ What are the advantages and disadvantages of each approach?

A D&E, which can be done with general anesthesia, is less painful than induced labor and the procedure takes less time, usually under an hour.

Induced labor can take a long time, a day or occasionally even longer. It poses the risks of bleeding and infection, even though there is less surgical interference with the uterus than with a D&E. Despite its greater pain and longer duration, some women prefer for psychological reasons to have labor induced. For example, some women who have chosen to terminate a pregnancy because the fetus is abnormal find that going through labor gives them closure. The baby, though it is not perfect, is born whole. The mother can see it and hold it, and this act can help with the healing process. Also, from a medical point of view, it is useful to have a pathologist examine fetal abnormalities that might impact a later pregnancy.

Talk frankly with your health care provider to see which option is best for you. Often, I find, women who ask to terminate a pregnancy involving an abnormal fetus have thought through the issue beforehand, at least in theoretical terms, and know which procedure they want.

Second-Trimester D&E

A surgical abortion after thirteen weeks of gestational age is more complex and somewhat riskier than a D&C done earlier. The uterus has stretched more and is softer, so there is greater danger of perforation. The procedure takes longer and may require more anesthesia.

▶ How is the procedure performed?

Basically it is performed the same way as a first-trimester D&C, but because there is more fetal tissue to remove, the cervix needs to be more fully dilated. Some physicians will stretch it a day or two before the procedure, using laminaria, which are small strips of dried seaweed (about 2 inches long and 1/8 inch wide). The vagina is held open with a speculum and the laminaria are inserted in the cervix. The seaweed absorbs moisture from the vagina and from the cervix, which then gradually dilates. During this procedure the patient may feel cramping as the cervix stretches, but the procedure is not usually painful. Some physicians use laminaria even for first-trimester abortions. Synthetic agents, like Lamisil and Dilapan, can also soften the cervix and help it dilate.

After the cervix has dilated, the D&E takes place in much the same sequence as a first-trimester D&C. Usually a D&E involves anesthesia, either a local injection of something like Novocain to numb the cervix, or regional anesthesia injected into the spinal column to deaden feeling from the waist down. Some physicians also supplement local or regional anesthesia with intravenous sedation, which causes grogginess and eases anxiety. Many women prefer general anesthesia, during which they are entirely unconscious, but it does relax the uterus and make it slightly more susceptible to perforation. Once the cervix has been dilated, the surgeon uses vacuum suction and/or curettage to remove the contents of the uterus.

▶ How long does a second-trimester D&E take?

The operation itself usually requires between fifteen and forty-five minutes, but counting the time for preoperative testing and cervical dilation with laminaria, which are often done the day before, the procedure lasts more than twenty-four hours.

▶ What happens if the surgeon perforates the uterus during an abortion?

Usually the hole heals by itself, but occasionally a second operation is needed to sew it up. Very rarely, the injury is severe enough that a hysterectomy is required. When abortions were illegal and therefore performed by less competently trained people or people who did not do the procedure frequently (and were therefore less skillful), perforation and infection were much more common than they are today. Still, even in the most skilled hands, a perforation can happen.

Induced Labor

A medical abortion during the second trimester makes use of prostaglandins or other drugs to cause the uterus to contract. The usual agent is a prostaglandin, though sometimes saline (a salt solution) or urea is used. Prostaglandins work more quickly than saline or urea, but also have some side effects, including nausea, vomiting, and diarrhea, which can usually be controlled with medication. The agent that will start contractions can either be injected directly into the uterus or be given as a vaginal suppository every three hours.

▶ Which is preferable, a medical or a surgical abortion?

Although the time frame or the availability of specific procedures at certain clinics or from certain physicians may determine which kind of abortion is possible at a given time and place, the answer to this question varies from woman to woman.

Some women dislike the invasiveness of a surgical abortion. They would much rather have a drug-induced miscarriage, which proceeds naturally once the process has been set in motion by drugs. Some women who have labor induced for second-trimester abortions want the sense of closure we have mentioned.

Medical abortions, even those undertaken early in pregnancy, involve spending a certain amount of time at the doctor's office: for the initial visit, for tests, for follow-up visits. Surgical abortions are quick. Some women do not want to wait for a drug to take its course, not knowing when or if the abortion will happen. They wish to get the abortion over with and put it behind them.

After an Abortion

Some physicians routinely give methergine or another medication to help the uterus return to its normal size; others give it if the occasion seems to demand it, or send it home for the patient to have in case bleeding starts in the next twenty-four hours. If the patient has had gonorrhea or chlamydia, her caregiver will give antibiotics. If she is Rh negative, she will get Rhogam, an agent that will prevent her being a candidate for Rh disease in future pregnancies.

After an abortion the patient should rest that day, resuming most normal activities the following day. She should avoid rigorous aerobic exercise, heavy lifting, and sexual intercourse for at least a week. Some physicians suggest waiting two weeks before intercourse or strenuous activity. For at least the first few days after the procedure, she should use pads, not tampons, for bleeding; the cervix is still somewhat open and the uterus is vulnerable to bacteria climbing up through the open cervix. Spotting or bleeding may continue, either continuously or intermittently, for two or three weeks, though some women do not have bleeding after the first day or so. You can take a shower immediately, but because of the possibility of infection it is better not to take a tub bath (or go swimming) for the first several days.

Motrin or another over-the-counter painkiller can help with the cramping, which may go on for several days. If the cramps get severe, call your caregiver, as they could be a sign of infection.

▶ When will the signs of pregnancy go away?

Usually breast tenderness will disappear after two or three days, as will any discharge.

▶ What are the signs of complication after an abortion?

The complications of abortion include incomplete abortion, in which some of the fetal or placental tissue is retained. This happens especially often in abortions performed very early in pregnancy, before six weeks of gestation. Fever over 100 degrees Fahrenheit, heavy bleeding (soaking a pad every hour or two), bleeding that gets heavier for two successive days, foul vaginal discharge, persistent and severe abdominal pain, swollen tender abdomen, and vomiting are all signs of complication. Call your physician if you have any of these symptoms or if you continue to have symptoms of pregnancy more than a week after the abortion.

▶ What happens at the postabortion checkup?

Usually your caregiver will schedule a checkup about two weeks after an abortion to be certain that the uterus has returned to its normal size, to make sure there are no complications, and to discuss contraception.

▶ Is there a "safe" period after an abortion when contraception is not necessary?

No, there is no safe period. If you have used a diaphragm or a cervical cap, you need to have it refitted, though the size will probably not have changed. If you take birth control pills, you should start taking them right away; use condoms and a spermicide or some other backup measure for the first month, until a full cycle has occurred.

▶ How long after an abortion do menstrual periods resume?

A normal menstrual period generally occurs within four to eight weeks after the abortion. If you have not had one by six weeks, call your doctor.

▶ What emotions do women feel after an abortion?

At the very beginning, almost everyone feels relief that the procedure is finished and the pregnancy is over. After that, feelings vary. Women who terminated planned pregnancies because of fetal abnormalities often feel the same grief and loss as women who have lost pregnancies through natural causes. Women who terminated unintended pregnancies may feel guilt and/or loss even though they chose not to continue the pregnancy.

MISCARRIAGE

Miscarriage is the common, everyday term for what physicians call spontaneous abortion or sometimes merely abortion. It means the unintentional loss, without human intervention, of a pregnancy during the first twenty weeks (counting from the first day of the last menstrual period).

▶ How common is spontaneous abortion during the first trimester?

Spontaneous abortion during the early stages of pregnancy is quite common. Estimates range from 15 to 20 percent of pregnancies, and those figures refer to recognized pregnancies—those that have been confirmed through a test or strongly suspected because of a missed menstrual period. There are probably many more instances where an egg and a sperm get together but the fertilized egg does not implant properly in the uterus, and the miscarriage occurs before a menstrual period is missed.

The very commonness of spontaneous abortion shows that even in this age of great technological advances, some very basic things remain beyond our control. It is a hard lesson. I consider it something of a miracle that miscarriage does not happen more often. So many things must go right once fertilization takes place: the fertilized egg must correctly make its initial divisions and begin to develop, it must travel down the fallopian tube into the uterus, and it must implant appropriately in the uterine lining and continue to grow there. It is amazing that 80–85 percent of pregnancies do result in the birth of a child and that only 15–20 percent end in miscarriage.

In the majority of miscarriages, the pregnancy would not have produced a healthy

> BOX 10. Medical Terms for Miscarriage

Threatened abortion: A miscarriage that may or may not happen. It is characterized by vaginal bleeding, with or without cramps, but the cervix remains closed.

Inevitable abortion: A miscarriage that is sure to happen because the fetus is no longer viable. Symptoms include vaginal bleeding, with or without cramps; the cervix opens.

Incomplete abortion: A miscarriage in which not all of the fetal tissue is expelled from the uterus. Symptoms include vaginal bleeding, sometimes heavy, for several days and continued cramping.

Complete abortion: A miscarriage during which all the fetal tissue is expelled from the uterus. Bleeding and cramping will gradually decrease and cease on their own.

Missed abortion: The fetus is not viable but has not yet been expelled.

child because the fetus was genetically abnormal. This may seem cold comfort when you are dealing with the loss, but many women find some consolation in realizing that a child with severe genetic abnormalities would have no normal life, or perhaps no life at all—unable to survive outside the uterus. It is crucial, I think, to focus on the potential quality of life.

▶ *If I have a miscarriage, should a genetic study be done on the tissue?*

About 99 percent of the time there is no valid reason to do so. Learning that the fetus was genetically abnormal has no bearing on subsequent pregnancies. The tests are very expensive and the results will not influence your future health care. Basically what your caregiver can say to you is, Try again; you had bad luck.

▶ *Who is at risk for miscarriage?*

Older women are at higher risk than younger ones; an older woman has older eggs, which are more likely to have some genetic abnormality. Some women do not produce adequate progesterone to support a pregnancy and are at increased risk for miscarriage: they become pregnant but miscarry early on.

A woman whose mother took DES (diethylstilbestrol) while she was pregnant is at increased risk. Some conditions of the uterus (multiple polyps or fibroids, or structural abnormalities) can cause spontaneous abortions, but many women with these conditions go on to have successful pregnancies. Some research has suggested that, in rare instances, immune factors play a role in spontaneous abortion.

Certain diseases or chronic illnesses may increase risk, but the details are not fully known. Nor is the role of environmental toxins, radiation, or drugs.

▶ *Does a genetically abnormal pregnancy happen because one or both parents are genetically abnormal?*

Sometimes, but quite rarely, parental genetic abnormalities can cause repeated miscarriages, but in my career I have only taken care of three patients with this kind of problem. Usually a specific egg and a specific sperm meet up and do not develop properly.

The most frequent genetic abnormality in the parents is something called a balanced translocation. People who have this condition have all the right chromosomes, but one of the chromosomes is "backward"—in the sense that when the chromosomes duplicate themselves, which they do when eggs and sperm are being produced, they produce genetically defective cells. People who have balanced translocations look perfectly normal, and they *are* perfectly normal except that their eggs or sperm can be defective. However, about one quarter of these eggs or sperm are not abnormal and can produce a normal pregnancy.

> Cassie had her first baby when she was 27. Everything went well and she had a healthy, normal child. Then Cassie had two spontaneous losses, so we decided to do a workup to see what was wrong. Her genetic tests showed that she had a balanced translocation. There was absolutely nothing I could tell her except, "Don't give up. The odds are that at some point things will work out well." Cassie was fortunate, because her next two pregnancies were perfectly normal and she had two more healthy children.

► *Are you at increased risk for miscarriage if your mother had one (or several) miscarriages?*

Unless your mother had some genetic problem, like a balanced translocation (which is statistically very rare), you are not at increased risk.

► *What are the symptoms of miscarriage?*

Ordinarily, the first symptom is vaginal bleeding. It can be light—just spotting or staining. Or it can be quite heavy. It may occur with or without uterine cramps and may go on for several days.

Bleeding and abdominal pain can also be signs of an ectopic pregnancy (a pregnancy that is developing in the fallopian tubes or elsewhere outside the uterus). Since such a pregnancy is dangerous, you should report bleeding to your caregiver so that the possibility can be ruled out.

► *Can your doctor tell whether you are miscarrying?*

Sometimes it is very difficult to tell whether a miscarriage is in progress, because women often spot or bleed during the first weeks of pregnancy without actually having a miscarriage. Many women bleed at the time the embryo implants in the uterine lining, which normally takes place at about the time of the first missed menstrual period, and some women continue to bleed on the monthly "anniversaries" of their regular periods (though no one knows why). Bleeding may be a sign of a threatened miscarriage or of one of these other events.

You cannot hear a fetal heartbeat with a Doppler stethoscope until nine or ten weeks of gestational life (four or five weeks after your missed period), so if the bleeding starts earlier, it is difficult to determine from a physical exam whether the fetus is still viable. The size of the uterus is not much help, since during the first and second months of pregnancy it is still quite small. If a woman has a great deal of body fat, it is especially difficult to assess the size of the uterus by a physical examination. About the only thing your caregiver can tell is whether or not your cervix is open.

For this reason, and because there is very little either you or your doctor can do to prevent a miscarriage that is about to happen, a threatened abortion is not a medical emergency—though understandably it may seem so if you are going through it.

BOX 11. Ultrasound Technology

Ultrasound is one of the tools used to assess the condition of a pregnancy. It can show the size of the uterus and the health of the pregnancy, help confirm a due date, reveal the presence of twins (or a larger multiple pregnancy) or an ectopic pregnancy, and disclose certain fetal abnormalities.

Ultrasound bounces high-frequency sound waves off internal body tissues. A sensor (transducer) produces the sound waves, which bounce back according to the different densities of the tissues they encounter. The transducer senses the patterns of these reflections or echoes, which are then processed by a computer to create a moving image. The image can be projected onto a monitor and photographed to create a permanent record.

▶ *How can your caregiver find out whether your pregnancy is going well?*

Although a physical exam in the early weeks of pregnancy will not give much information, there are two ways of testing to see how things are going. One is ultrasound imaging, which can be done either abdominally, by placing the sensor on the abdomen above the uterus, or vaginally, by inserting into the vagina a probe containing the sensor.

With either type of ultrasound procedure, your doctor is looking for the size of the fetus and the development of a fetal heart. Early in the pregnancy the vaginal probe will probably give more information, but by the seventh or eighth week of gestational life an abdominal ultrasound will supply the information you need. At about seven weeks an abdominal ultrasound will reveal a little sac and possibly a fetal heart. A vaginal ultrasound probe may give the same information as early as six weeks. If a heart is beating in the sac, the odds are in your favor. Only occasionally does a fetus develop far enough to have a heart and then cease growing.

A second test, a blood test that can be used earlier in pregnancy, is called quantitative beta preg levels—or just quants or beta preg testing. This test, which was a research tool in the mid-1970s and became available for clinicians later in that decade, measures blood levels of the beta subunit of hCG, the same substance used in a simple test for pregnancy. In fact, this test is very similar to a pregnancy test, except that it measures the amount of hCG instead of merely looking for its presence.

We do the quants test by taking blood samples every couple of days. If we get a level of 200 one day and two or three days later get a 400 level, and then 800, it looks as if things are going well. If the levels of hCG do not double every few days during the first trimester, it does not necessarily mean that something is terribly wrong, but a steadily rising level is encouraging. Once the pregnancy has developed far enough, we can do an ultrasound and see how the visual image correlates with the beta preg quants.

▶ *Is there any foolproof method to tell exactly when you became pregnant?*

Every pregnancy is different, even different pregnancies in the same woman. Urine testing will reveal that you are pregnant when the quantitative level of hCG is only about 50. Most women reach this level at about the time they miss their menstrual period. But women vary. Some may reach that detectable level a few days earlier, some a few days later. You cannot automatically say that when your quant is 1,500 you are five weeks and two days pregnant.

Suppose you measure your quant the day you miss your period (which is day 28 of your pregnancy, if you have twenty-eight-day cycles) and your level is 50; then you measure it three days later and it is 200, and in another two days it comes in at 400. At this rate by the time you are five weeks pregnant you will be at a level of about 800 and in five and a half weeks at 1,600. Now, five and a half weeks is about when something starts showing up on ultrasound: not necessarily a fetus with a heartbeat, but a gestational sac with a fetus forming. So beta quant testing in conjunction with ultrasound can give you a general idea of the date of conception, but it will not give you an exact date.

Nor can you yourself tell, unless you only had sex one time that month—or maybe only one time in two months, since occasional women have bleeding around the time of their expected period when the fertilized egg is being implanted. Perhaps what you thought was a period was actually bleeding at implantation.

Some women believe that they know intuitively when they get pregnant, and perhaps they do. I cannot vouch for the value of intuition one way or the other, since sometimes my patients' intuitive knowledge has turned out to be wrong.

▶ *Is it worthwhile to do an ultrasound three or four days after a missed menstrual period?*

No, an ultrasound done that early will not reveal anything useful. Before six weeks gestational age (about a month after conception) an ultrasound would, except in special circumstances, be a waste of time and money.

▶ *If an ultrasound does not reveal a heart or other fetal parts by seven weeks, does that mean that there is no pregnancy?*

Not necessarily. Remember that it is very difficult to determine exactly when conception occurred, and often it is worth waiting another week and doing another test. More than once I have had a patient ready to despair at not being pregnant, when a test a week later showed a fetal sac. The woman just got pregnant a week later than she thought. If the ultrasound does not show a fetal sac, there is nothing medically that your caregiver can do to improve the pregnancy.

▶ *What can you do to stop a threatened miscarriage?*

There really is not much that you can do, nor is there much that your caregiver can do for you. While this is distressing, it does make some sense. First of all, since many of the fetuses that spontaneously abort have serious genetic defects, miscarriage is nature's way of recognizing that the fetus is not healthy.

Second, we have learned from experience that it is dangerous to try to deal hormonally with threatened miscarriage. Forty or fifty years ago, if you had gone to your physician with vaginal bleeding during early pregnancy, he or she might have prescribed DES, a synthetic estrogen that was frequently given to prevent miscarriage, premature labor, and other complications of pregnancy, even though there was not much evidence that it was effective. Unfortunately, DES turned out to cause birth defects and reproductive disorders in the daughters of women who had taken it during pregnancy. The medical profession learned through that tragedy that it is a mistake to give hormonal medications (unless they have been thoroughly tested) during the first months of pregnancy.

For that reason there is not much your doctor can do to prevent a spontaneous abortion. If your cervix has opened, the miscarriage is inevitable. If your cervix has not opened and the miscarriage is only threatened, there still is not much that can be done.

▶ Will bed rest help prevent a miscarriage?

Bed rest is often prescribed for women later in pregnancy who have a condition in which the cervix threatens to dilate too soon, but bed rest will not help prevent a first-trimester miscarriage. There is no posture, even standing on your head, that will prevent it.

▶ Will stress, sexual activity, dietary habits, or environmental factors cause a miscarriage?

Ordinary activities, even emotionally stressful ones, cannot bring about a miscarriage. Fighting with your mother-in-law or worrying about your work will not cause a miscarriage. Nor will normal exercise, though common sense suggests that you probably should not run or do rigorous aerobics. At least if you go on to miscarry, you will not need to say to yourself, "Oh, if only I hadn't done kickboxing last week, I wouldn't be miscarrying."

Some women worry about having intercourse when they are spotting or having vaginal bleeding. Although I generally advise patients who are threatening to miscarry that they should abstain from sex, the reasons are again psychological. I don't want anyone to blame herself for losing a baby because she had sex.

Some women who are threatening to miscarry wonder whether changes in diet and environment will keep the miscarriage from happening. While it is a good idea to lead a healthy life, clean air and a diet rich in vegetables will not prevent a miscarriage. Nor is there evidence that exposure to video display terminals (computers and TV sets) or microwave ovens will cause a miscarriage.

▶ Does vaginal bleeding in the first trimester mean you won't be able to carry the pregnancy to completion?

Actually about one third of women bleed during the first three months of pregnancy, although we are not always sure why it happens. More than half of these women continue to carry perfectly normal pregnancies. We do know that some women bleed a little at the time of implantation and that other women become pregnant with two eggs, fraternal twins, and miscarry one.

If you start to bleed, don't panic; talk to your caregiver. If the bleeding is heavy, say heavier than a normal menstrual period, it is likely that you will have a miscarriage. On the other hand, occasionally even heavy bleeding does not result in a miscarriage.

Kelly came in to the emergency room bleeding so heavily that she had a towel between her legs. We used ultrasound to try to determine what was happening. We could see a fetus developing with a normal heartbeat, but we couldn't see any reason why she would be bleeding so heavily. One or two days later the bleeding stopped and Kelly continued her pregnancy. Her baby was completely normal.

▶ What is an incomplete abortion?

If the miscarriage takes place early in the pregnancy, before six or seven weeks gestation, chances are that the miscarriage will be complete. Nothing will be left behind in the uterus. However, if you are nine or ten weeks pregnant, a little piece of placenta or other tissue may be left behind.

The appropriate therapy is to scrape out the lining of the uterus in a procedure similar to a D&C, except that the cervix is probably already dilated because of the miscarriage. If there is even a fragment of placental tissue left in the uterus, it will not contract effectively, and it is the contraction of the uterus that stops the bleeding.

If possible, we do the procedure with a general anesthetic. But sometimes circumstances allow only local anesthesia, which numbs the cervix but does not deaden feeling in the uterus itself. If someone comes in to the office bleeding very heavily, we do not have general anesthesia available. Some women even request that they *not* have general anesthesia. The procedure is painful, but it only lasts a few minutes.

▶ What is a missed abortion?

A missed abortion is one in which the fetus dies but is not expelled for as long as several months. Women become aware of the possibility because after the symptoms of early pregnancy have been present for a while, perhaps confirmed by a pregnancy test, the signs diminish or go away.

A missed abortion can be diagnosed by a lack of the signs of a continuing, healthy pregnancy. If the uterus is not enlarging (or has shrunk since the last examination), if there is no fetal heartbeat by eight to ten weeks of gestational age, then missed abortion is a possibility.

▶ What is the treatment for a missed abortion?

The treatment can be watchful waiting, allowing the body to expel the fetus in its own good time, or the contents of the uterus can be removed through a suction D&C.

Lianne missed a period two months ago and had a blood pregnancy test that was positive. In the meantime, she had a little vaginal bleeding and some cramping, but did not actually have a miscarriage. Perhaps she had a threatened abortion that never actually happened.

We did some quantitative blood pregnancy tests and the results were not encouraging. Her hCG levels were not rising rapidly. An ultrasound did not showed a fetus forming in her uterus. We repeated the quants and did a backup ultrasound at about eight or nine weeks from the time Lianne thought she had conceived. The backup ultrasound still did not show a fetal heartbeat.

Testing showed she no longer had a viable fetus and sooner or later would miscarry on her own. One of her choices was to wait and let her body deal with the situation in its own way. She decided instead to schedule a D&C and have the fetal tissue removed from her uterus.

The advantage of a D&C is that the procedure can be done under controlled conditions. The patient can go to an operating room, have a general anesthetic, and have her own physician there to perform the procedure. If she comes in to the emergency room at 10:00 P.M. hemorrhaging heavily, she may be unable to have a general anesthetic because she had dinner only two hours earlier. Her own doctor may not be available. Or she may come in at 2:00 A.M. and find that the emergency room is crowded with patients who have been waiting all day.

Some women react to an ultrasound showing that the fetus has ceased to develop by wanting an immediate D&C. They know that a miscarriage will occur sooner or later and are very unhappy with the idea of harboring dead tissue until that time comes. Other women want to let nature take care of the problem in its own way and feel uncomfortable with the idea of a D&C even though the fetus is no longer viable.

▶ What are the risks of a D&C to resolve a missed abortion?

The risks of a D&C for *any* purpose are bleeding and infection. There is also a remote chance that the uterus will be perforated during the surgery. Women who have several miscarriages and subsequent D&Cs have the risk of scarring the lining of the uterus, a condition called Asherman's syndrome. Even though the risk is small, infertility can result later on.

▶ *What is the recuperation time after a miscarriage and D&C?*

I tell my patients to rest and take it easy the day of the procedure. You can go back to work in a day or so if you feel like it. I recommend that you not have intercourse for a week, though some physicians advise waiting two weeks. Take it easy on aerobic activity for a week or two.

▶ *Is there any risk to waiting for the body to expel a fetus that has died?*

There is a slight risk of infection, because the tissue inside the uterus is no longer living and can be infected by the bacteria that normally live in the vagina. But this is a very small risk and is limited by time.

▶ *How long should I wait before trying to get pregnant again?*

The most conservative physicians say two months. There is certainly no reason to wait longer.

▶ *If I have one miscarriage, am I more likely to have another?*

When someone has a miscarriage, the first thing I say, before we discuss any other issues, is that it will not impact her future reproductive life. Women who have had one miscarriage often feel very nervous when they become pregnant subsequently, because they fear another miscarriage. Having had one miscarriage does not increase your risk for having another. Large statistical studies have shown you have the same risk of miscarrying that you did the first time, somewhere around 15 percent.

▶ *If I've had several miscarriages, do I still have a chance to have a healthy child?*

If you have one, two, or even three miscarriages, your chances of carrying a pregnancy to term are almost the same as those of a woman who has not had a miscarriage. If you have had two spontaneous abortions, your statistical chances of having a third are not much higher than a woman who has had none, somewhere in the range of 20–25 percent.

Women who have had three or more consecutive abortions are called habitual aborters. That is a term I really dislike, and I hope it will drop from use. If you have had three consecutive miscarriages, your caregiver should recommend a workup to attempt to determine the reason.

▶ *What are the causes of repeated miscarriages?*

Sometimes, but not always, a workup will reveal a cause for repeated miscarriage. Nowadays there are clinics that specialize in testing and treating women who have repeated miscarriages.

Occasional women have a problem with inadequate luteal phase: they do not produce enough progesterone during the second half of the menstrual cycle to ensure that the fertilized egg will implant properly and be nurtured. There are also occasional anatomical causes, for example a uterine septum that divides the uterus into two parts and causes difficulties with implantation. This can be detected with a hysterogram (see Chapter 11). A uterus with a septum can usually be surgically corrected, and women with this problem sometimes have successful pregnancies. A fibroid that sticks out into the wall of the uterus can act similarly to a uterine septum. It too can be removed surgically, which may facilitate a successful pregnancy.

Once in a while, women have antibodies to the embryo. The miscarriage is caused by an autoimmune reaction, something like the process that goes on with lupus, in which the body's immune system produces antibodies that attack its own tissues. Steroid drugs that help block antibody production can be useful.

On rare occasions we find that chronic infections are causing the repeated miscarriages. These infections can be treated with antibiotics, so that a successful pregnancy is possible.

▶ *How soon after a miscarriage will the body go back to its prepregnant state?*

Bleeding or spotting may continue for several days after the miscarriage, and other signs of pregnancy, for example breast tenderness and abdominal swelling, may continue as long as a week. It is possible that hormonal changes may bring about mood swings, but since the miscarriage itself is usually a depressing event, it is hard to determine whether mood changes are hormonally caused or simply expressions of normal sadness.

▶ *What is the psychological impact of miscarriage?*

To many women a miscarriage, whether it occurs late or early, means the loss not just of a pregnancy—a potential child—but of a real and complete human being. The intensity of grief varies from woman to woman. Many feel isolation and loneliness, anger, and depression including inability to concentrate, comprehend, or remember. Many women blame themselves, believing if only they had done something differently, the miscarriage would not have happened. Guilt and loss of self-esteem are not uncommon. Nor is anxiety about future pregnancies. Many women feel anger toward their friends who do have children and whose pregnancies seemed easy and happy.

The impact of grief on a marriage can be difficult, since men and women are likely to express loss in different ways. They may have different reactions to sexual intimacy after such a loss and may find that sex is no longer the expression of love and hopefulness that it was before the miscarriage.

Well-meaning but tactless friends and relatives who have not experienced this kind of loss themselves, and do not really know the depth of your feelings, can say painful things intended as comfort. Among these is the suggestion that you have another baby. Women who have had miscarriages know that there is no such thing as a "replacement baby," and it may help to tell family and friends how important this baby was for you, and to ask them to support you by listening rather than by offering advice.

I expect women to be saddened when miscarriage happens. I expect them to cry. I expect them to have a bad day on their child's due date, at holidays, and other times. But I hope they will not cry indefinitely. Knowing the clinical cause of the miscarriage (if this is possible) helps some women. Others find solace through support groups, often made up of women who have experienced the same kind of bereavement and know what it is like. If these kinds of assistance are not adequate, professional therapy is also available.

ECTOPIC PREGNANCY

An ectopic pregnancy is one that happens outside the uterus. The vast majority take place in a fallopian tube, where fertilization occurs, so the terms ectopic pregnancy and tubal pregnancy are often used interchangeably. An ectopic pregnancy can also occur, though rarely, in an ovary, the abdominal cavity, or the cervical canal. Ectopic pregnancy is a dangerous condition that must be dealt with, because the fallopian tube (or other site) cannot accommodate the growing embryo and sooner or later will tear or rupture. The internal bleeding that follows can be life threatening.

Before the days of ultrasound and quantitative blood pregnancy testing, ectopic pregnancy was one of the three most common causes of maternal mortality in the United States. Now we have sophisticated tests that can detect an ectopic pregnancy early on; we also have better ways to treat the condition.

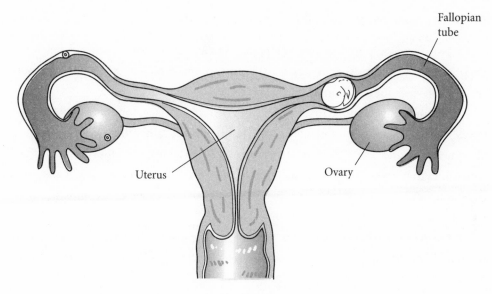

Fallopian tube

Uterus

Ovary

FIGURE 33. Ectopic pregnancies occur outside the uterus, usually in the fallopian tubes.

▶ *How common is ectopic pregnancy?*

In the United States the frequency of ectopic pregnancy is about one or two cases per hundred pregnancies. Some observers believe the rate is likely to rise because of the success of antibiotics in treating pelvic inflammatory disease. Before we had these drugs, women who had pelvic infections would often become totally infertile. With antibiotic treatment they may become pregnant, but their tubes may be scarred from infection and damaged, so that the fertilized egg remains stuck in the tube.

▶ *Who is at risk for an ectopic pregnancy?*

Any woman who becomes pregnant has a 1–2 percent risk for an ectopic pregnancy. Beyond that basic level, the women at greatest risk are those who have had a previous ectopic pregnancy. Once you have had one ectopic pregnancy, your odds of having a second go from 1–2 percent to about 10 percent.

If you have had pelvic inflammatory disease, endometriosis, or tubal or pelvic surgery (anything from removal of the adhesions caused by endometriosis, to a ruptured appendix), you are at increased risk. The common factor is scarring or damage to the fallopian tubes, which prevents the fertilized egg from completing its journey to the uterus.

▶ *What are the symptoms of tubal pregnancy?*

The classic symptoms are bleeding and pain. Usually, but not always, women know they are pregnant by the time they experience these symptoms, which frequently occur around six or seven weeks of gestational life.

The symptoms resemble those of a threatened miscarriage, but there may be differences. The pain of an ectopic pregnancy may be on one side rather than in the center of the abdomen, but since the ovaries or tubes are not far away from the uterus, it is difficult sometimes to pinpoint the precise location of the pain. Sometimes the pain is sharp and constant. Some women feel shoulder pain. The vaginal bleeding that accompanies an ectopic pregnancy is apt to be just spotting or staining.

If the pregnancy has ruptured a fallopian tube, the woman may pass out, because she has been hemorrhaging internally. This is a true emergency and must be treated immediately.

▶ *How is an ectopic pregnancy detected?*

When someone comes in with pain and/or bleeding and we suspect an ectopic pregnancy, we use the same tests that evaluate the health of a pregnancy: ultrasound and quantitative blood pregnancy testing.

In an ectopic pregnancy, as with a miscarriage, the blood levels of human chorionic gonadotropin do not rise rapidly as they do in a healthy pregnancy. In order to differentiate between the two, we can do an ultrasound scan. Usually when a miscarriage is threatened, we will see something in the uterus—not necessarily a well-formed fetus, but perhaps a sac or a little placenta. With an ectopic pregnancy, there is nothing in the uterus, but occasionally something visible in the fallopian tube. Ultrasound tests in this case seldom show a fetal heartbeat; by the time the fetus is large enough to have a heart, the tube would probably have ruptured.

Sometimes it is not possible to tell with certainty that there is an ectopic pregnancy. Perhaps the ultrasound and blood pregnancy testing are not definitive. Perhaps no ultrasound technology is available, as in some small towns far from major medical centers. In that case a diagnostic laparoscopy can help. During this surgical procedure the laparoscope is inserted into the abdomen through a small incision. The doctor can then look around and try to determine whether the fallopian tube has a bump in it, which would suggest the presence of a tubal pregnancy.

▶ *When do the symptoms of an ectopic pregnancy occur?*

Symptoms of an ectopic pregnancy usually make themselves known quite early in the pregnancy. The fallopian tube is narrow and as the embryo distends it, pain begins. Often symptoms begin at six to seven weeks of gestational life. When women call in because they are two days late for their period and feel abdominal pain, an ectopic pregnancy is probably not the reason for their discomfort. While it is not at all unusual for women to feel cramping when they are pregnant, it is rare to start having symptoms of an ectopic pregnancy that early.

▶ *Can an ectopic pregnancy be replanted in the uterus?*

The current state of technological advancement does not allow this; perhaps sometime in the future it may be possible.

▶ *Is it possible to tell whether an ectopic pregnancy has ruptured?*

Most tubal pregnancies are diagnosed early and treated before rupture is a threat. However, there is a procedure called a culdocentesis, which can be used to determine whether the pregnancy has ruptured. A needle is inserted behind the cervix into a pouch called the cul-de-sac, which lies between the back of the vagina and the rectum. Fluid is withdrawn from the abdominal cavity through the needle and examined to see whether blood is present. If there is blood, we know the pregnancy has ruptured and we treat the patient accordingly. Culdocentesis is painful and fortunately is not needed very often.

▶ *What is the treatment for an ectopic pregnancy?*

Basically the approach is to remove the fetus either surgically or medically. Since the laparoscope has become available as a surgical aid, it is often possible to make a small incision in the tube and lift out the embryo, scrape out the tube, and stop any bleeding. The tube will usually heal by itself, so stitches are not necessary. The procedure is called a salpingostomy.

Twenty-five years ago the standard procedure was to remove the entire fallopian tube through an abdominal incision. Nowadays we take out the whole tube only when we are unable to stop the bleeding. If a fallopian tube has ruptured, it may be better, for example, to make a small abdominal incision and remove the ectopic pregnancy that way, rather than to work through the laparoscope.

A recent nonsurgical approach uses methotrexate, a drug used for cancer therapy. Methotrexate kills cells that are dividing rapidly, whether they are in a cancerous tumor or an ectopic pregnancy. The tissue in the ectopic pregnancy dies and is passed out the end of the fallopian tube into the peritoneal cavity, where it is reabsorbed. Methotrexate therapy has a high rate of success, though it must be used early in the pregnancy *before* the situation becomes acute. If someone is having severe pain and bleeding, she cannot wait for the methotrexate to work and is a candidate for immediate surgery.

Interestingly enough, Chinese herbal medicine has long used a similar technique. One of my colleagues visiting China more than fifteen years ago was shown fifty women who had had documented ectopic pregnancies and had been treated with herbal medicines. Only two eventually needed surgery. The success of the Chinese technique is not surprising, especially since many of our chemotherapeutic medications come from plants. Vincristine, for example, which is used to kill rapidly dividing cancer cells, is obtained from the common flowering herb periwinkle (*Vinca rosea*).

▶ *Does treatment with methotrexate have serious side effects?*

Methotrexate for ectopic pregnancy is given in a single injection, in a much smaller amount than that used in chemotherapy, so the side effects are not severe. Women do not lose their hair or suffer severe nausea.

▶ *If you've had an ectopic pregnancy, will you have trouble conceiving again?*

As long as the underlying cause is not tubal disease, you will probably have no trouble. When you do conceive, however, ask your doctor about having early ultrasound to rule out ectopic pregnancy.

▶ *If your tubes have been damaged by ectopic pregnancies, can you ever have children?*

Women who have had tubal pregnancies are excellent candidates for in vitro fertilization, in which egg and sperm are mixed outside the woman's body and then implanted in the uterus. All that is needed is an ovary and a uterus.

> Dana, an art teacher, had an ectopic pregnancy, which we were able to treat conservatively, saving the fallopian tube. Later she had another ectopic in that same tube, and that time we did have to remove the tube. She went on to have a third ectopic pregnancy in her other tube. Since that time she has had two healthy children by in vitro fertilization.

14 Sex and Society

▶ **MYTH** Gays and lesbians choose their sexual orientation. If they really tried, they could change and become heterosexual.

FACT Most people discover their sexual preference in early adolescence, without previous sexual experience. While people can choose whether or not to act on their feelings, mental health professionals do not consider sexual orientation to be a conscious choice that can be altered by willpower or counseling.

A gynecologist's practice overlaps social issues in a way that an ophthalmologist's or a dentist's does not. Women's eyes and teeth do not carry the heavy symbolic moral or social meaning that their reproductive systems do. And so some of the issues that gynecologists deal with are not strictly medical. Because our society is ambivalent about sex, some of these issues are nebulous and difficult.

This chapter covers an assortment of topics where social and sexual issues converge. I have tried to outline the main concerns of each and to suggest reasonable courses of action or offer further resources. I have expressed my own opinions where it seemed appropriate to do so. On the one hand, I do not want to be preachy and moralistic, but on the other, I want women to protect their own physical and emotional health. I also want them to find mutually satisfying relationships that will enrich their lives in many ways.

BECOMING SEXUALLY ACTIVE

▶ *How do you know you are ready to start being sexually active?*

There are many factors to weigh as you make this important decision. First of all, it seems to me, age is a consideration, both biologically and emotionally.

Let me say at the outset, even though I may sound judgmental or straitlaced, that I think it best not to have sex until you are in a long-term, mutually supportive, monogamous relationship. At the same time, my twenty-five years of medical practice have constantly reminded me that people are going to have sex because human beings are sexual by nature. I cannot stop my patients from becoming involved in sexual relationships that may not be desirable for their physical or emotional health, but I can do my best to teach them how to avoid serious consequences, at least physically.

Experience with my patients has taught me that women do best becoming sexually active when they really want to begin. With women this tends to mean wanting to have intercourse with a particular person, someone they care about, someone with whom they have an ongoing relationship in emotional and other ways. A successful sexual relationship involves trust and communication. Your sexual partner should be someone with whom you have already established these qualities.

You should not feel pressured by your partner or by some vague societal notions that you "should" be doing it. Many young women have heard the argument, "If you love me, you'll have sex with me." If your partner loves you and cares about you as a person, not just as a sexual companion, then he (or she) should respect your values and decisions. You should not be having sex because you were bullied into it.

Nor should you do anything that conflicts with your moral or religious principles. If you do, you will probably feel guilty—possibly during the act and certainly afterward. Acting in ways that contradict your deeply held beliefs can saddle you with unnecessary emotional baggage.

You should be willing to be sexually responsible. Many young women fail to use birth control when they first become sexually active, perhaps because they are unaware of what is available, perhaps because they want sex to be romantic and spontaneous. Unwanted pregnancy and sexually transmitted diseases can have consequences that last a lifetime. Being unwilling to protect yourself shows a lack of responsibility to your own body and your own future.

In this day and age, many young women buy their own condoms. If your date shows up without one and you decide to have sex, it is a good idea to have some on hand—in your purse, in your dresser drawer, wherever you are likely to encounter this situation. You want to protect yourself against infection. Birth control pills will protect you against pregnancy, but they will not save you from herpes or any other sexually transmitted disease, including AIDS. Young people tend to believe they are immortal and invulnerable; learning to protect yourself from sexually transmitted infection may save your life.

In addition to being willing to protect yourself against disease or pregnancy, both you and your partner should be able to handle the emotional responsibilities of a sexual relationship. If an unplanned pregnancy would devastate you, conflict with your beliefs about abortion or adoption, negatively impact your relationship with your parents, or jeopardize either your plans for the future or your relationship with your sexual partner, then you should think carefully about the step you are taking. The surest method of contraception is abstinence; there is always a slight risk of unwanted pregnancy with even the most reliable contraceptive.

Give yourself breathing space to decide what you really want to do. Remember that when your feelings are intense, you are emotionally vulnerable. Sex cannot cure a failing relationship. If your relationship is stressed because your partner wants sex and you do not, sex alone won't solve the problem, at least not for both of you. Sex is not a substitute for self-esteem. It won't ward off loneliness or change you as a human being. However, if you are in a satisfying, mature relationship, sex can make it even better.

▶ *Are there any health consequences to becoming sexually active early in life?*

Yes, and they can be serious. Biologically, women are able to function sexually from the time they pass through puberty. But if they begin sexual activity early, they increase their risk for cervical cancer later in life. Although researchers are unsure exactly what agent triggers the gradual changes in the cells of the cervix that can eventually become cancerous, we do know that the agent has something to do with sexual intercourse. The leading candidate right now is the human papilloma virus (HPV, also called the human condyloma virus), the same microorganism that gives you genital warts.

Because the cervical cells are undergoing developmental changes during a young woman's teen years, her cervix is more vulnerable at that time. If she waits until she is 20 years old to become sexually active, most of these changes will have already taken place and she will be at lower risk than someone who has intercourse at 15 or 16.

The answer to the question "Can sex give you cancer?" is "Yes, absolutely." It matters how many different partners you have had and how early you began having intercourse, unless you have protected yourself *each time* with condoms.

An epidemiological study a few years ago focused on assessing the frequency of the condyloma virus among college women. The women were tested for the virus during their first week as freshmen and then again as seniors. The conversion rate from negative (no exposure to the virus) to positive was 70–80 percent. This does not mean that 70–80 percent of these women came down with genital warts or that the same percentage will have cervical cancer sometime down the road. Although only a few of the many varieties of the condyloma virus can cause cancer, the fact that it is so very widespread should give rise to caution, if not to alarm.

▶ *Does the number of a woman's sexual partners have any health consequences?*

Yes, it does. If you have unprotected intercourse, you increase your risk for disease or pregnancy with each new partner you encounter.

> Lindsay is a senior in high school. She came to me for birth control pills because she needed protection from pregnancy. Like some of my other teenage patients, Lindsay tends toward serial monogamy. She has one boyfriend at a time, but these relationships don't last very long. She went out with Jason for a month or two and then they broke up; then she went out with Pete for a while and broke up with him; now she is going out with Kevin.

It is worthwhile for Lindsay to date different people to find out what qualities she finds important in a man, but this benefit does not extend to sexual intercourse. From the point of view of her health, having sex with three or four boyfriends one after the other is no safer or better than having sex with all three during the same period. Her present pattern of behavior may make her feel more secure because she is not "sleeping around." At the time of each relationship, she is deeply in love with the young man of the moment. But whenever she has intercourse with anyone, she is being exposed to whatever bacteria, viruses, or other organisms the young man has in his reproductive tract, which include the bacteria, viruses, or other organisms of anyone with whom he has had intercourse in the past.

Usually I say something like: "Yes, I know you love Kevin (or Jason, or Pete) very much. I know that he is a wonderful person who would never do anything to harm you.

But we both know that before he went out with you, Jason went out with someone else, and you don't know what she was like. Or maybe you do, and you don't have much respect for her. Or maybe you even think she was a fine person. In the long run it doesn't matter what you think, because when you have unprotected intercourse with Jason, you are exposed to whatever he has and whatever his previous girlfriends may have had."

When I was describing this scenario to some of the female medical students I teach, they became irritated with me, because I was implying bad things about women, about Jason's previous girlfriends. But STDs are not gender biased. Both men and women get them. Both men and women can infect their sexual partners.

▶ *Are there differences between men and women in terms of sex drive?*

As recently as forty years ago, when the birth control pill was first introduced, it was thought that women were not interested in sex. But in the years since the sexual revolution of the 1960s, brought about in part because oral contraceptives put women in control of their own fertility, our understanding of female sexuality and our attitudes toward it have changed. Women do have a sexual nature.

The differences between men and women seem to be differences of intensity and focus. Women tend to think about an individual with whom they would like to see themselves in a loving relationship. Men, and particularly young men, are less directed toward a particular woman and tend to want sex for its own sake rather than as an expression of affection.

Young men produce high levels of testosterone, which enhances their sex drive to the point that many of them seem to be interested in having sex anytime, anywhere, with anyone. Young women, who produce less testosterone (but do produce some), are usually less sexually aggressive and more specific in their desires. I am not sure whether hormones or societal training causes this difference, but it does exist.

▶ *Does intercourse hurt the first time?*

First intercourse can be uncomfortable for women for one of two reasons. The first is the hymen or hymeneal plate, the band of tissue that surrounds the opening of the vagina. The hymen can have a small opening and be difficult to penetrate. On the other hand, many women do not have pain on their first experience of intercourse, because their hymeneal ring has a larger opening. It may have been stretched by tampon use or eroded through physical activity, including athletics.

Lack of lubrication can also be a problem, especially if the woman is nervous the first time she has intercourse. Lubricating agents, such as Aqua-Lube or Astroglide, can ease this problem. If you cannot communicate to your partner that you are not lubricated and are therefore uncomfortable, and if he does not care, then I have to wonder why you are having sex with him.

▶ Do most women have an orgasm the first time they have intercourse?

Although no one knows what proportion of women achieve orgasm the first time they have intercourse, I would imagine that it is a fairly low percentage. Sex is an acquired skill; we get better with practice. The fear and anxiety that surround the first event are likely to interfere with sexual pleasure.

Both men and women should also realize that many women do not achieve orgasm from intercourse alone. They require other stimulation, particularly clitoral stimulation, to get there. So plain old garden-variety intercourse, which often is what people are focused on the first time they have sex, is unlikely to result in an orgasm for the woman.

▶ Should you worry if you don't have an orgasm the first time?

If you do not have an orgasm the first time you have intercourse, or the second time or the third, you should not worry that anything is wrong with you. In fact, you are pretty normal. The chances of there being something anatomically wrong are very slight. Since this book is not intended as a handbook of sexual performance, the Resources section lists several helpful books on the subject of sexuality and sexual response.

▶ Do women have the same sex drive throughout the month?

Many women tell me that they have more libido, more interest in sex, around the time of ovulation. At this time women have high levels of the two hormones FSH (follicle-stimulating hormone) and LH (luteinizing hormone). They have a relatively high testosterone level as well—that is, in comparison to their level at other times of the month. Of course, women who are taking oral contraceptives do not experience these hormonal surges.

Therefore, women are most likely to want sex at the time that it is biologically desirable for them to do so. If you feel more eager for sex around the time of ovulation and do not want to get pregnant, you must be doubly careful, particularly if you use a barrier method of contraception. Be sure to use your diaphragm and spermicidal jelly; be sure to use a condom.

▶ *Do birth control pills depress sexual desire?*

Because women taking birth control pills do not have the hormonal surges that accompany ovulation (in fact, they do not ovulate), they do not seem to have a surge of interest in intercourse around the midpoint of their cycle.

Researchers believe that testosterone, which women produce in small amounts all month and especially at midcycle, is one of the forces that drive sexual desire. Some birth control pills contain a progesterone that is derived from testosterone-like compounds and can be helpful to women whose libido is lowered. In particular, pills that contain types of progesterone called levonorgestrel or norgestrel are direct testosterone descendants. Other pills, which contain derivatives of norethindrone, are less androgenic and do less to heighten your libido.

If you notice that you have decreased sex drive when you are on birth control pills, talk it over with your doctor. You may not have to go off the pill. You might be helped by one of the more androgenic pills (see Table 2).

▶ *Does norgestrel have any side effects, besides increasing sexual desire?*

Young women often tell me that they want the kind of oral contraceptive that will make them sexy. Unfortunately the pills that boost your sex drive probably do not help your skin. Skin problems such as acne and oiliness may be increased by androgenic contraceptives.

▶ *Does Viagra enhance sexual desire in women?*

This question comes up practically every day in my office, particularly with older women. These women say that they still enjoy sex, but have no desire to initiate it. They wonder whether Viagra would help them regain the level of sexual interest they had when they were younger. But Viagra is not an aphrodisiac; it enhances performance, not desire, which is the issue for these women.

Studies of the effects of Viagra in women are under way, but whether it will benefit women is unknown. We do know that it enhances male sexual response. Viagra is prescribed for men who want to have intercourse but have problems maintaining an erection. The politically correct term for this condition is now erectile dysfunction (sometimes abbreviated ED); it used to be called impotence.

Viagra can be dangerous for some men. Those who have certain types of cardiac disease should not take it, and their physicians should advise them of the dangers. But since

Viagra is available illegally or can be gotten under false pretenses (by not telling the doctor about pre-existing cardiac disease), many men are taking this drug who should not be. Several men with heart problems such as angina have died after taking Viagra, which shows that some men will risk their lives for potency. The future of Viagra is not clear to me. Product liability suits may be brought against the company that developed and markets this drug, even though the men who died taking it should not have done so in the first place.

▶ What can women use to increase their desire for sex?

Testosterone may enhance libido in women whose levels are known to be low. I often prescribe it for women of any age to see whether it intensifies their sex drive.

▶ Is masturbation a useful sexual outlet?

Despite what your mother or grandmother may have told you, masturbation is a very good way to deal with your sexual tensions. If you feel aroused and do not have a sexual partner, masturbation is a perfectly valid alternative. It will not make you blind or give you warts on your hands, as Victorians used to threaten their children. It does allow you to experience sexual pleasure with your one constant partner, yourself.

SAFE (OR SAFER) SEX
▶ What is safe sex?

We hear a great deal today about "safe" sex, sometimes called "safer" sex, which implies that no sex is ever safe. In the past, the dangers of sexual intercourse were unwanted pregnancy and certain sexually transmitted diseases (notably syphilis and gonorrhea); but when antibiotics became widely available in the 1940s, the threat of these diseases diminished, at least for a while. Twenty years later, the availability of oral contraceptives significantly lowered the risk of unwanted pregnancy. Everything seemed to be under control. Then, with the arrival of chlamydia, HPV, and HIV, the dangers increased and the discussion of what constitutes safe sex became more intense.

In its strictest form, safe sex requires that unless you are in a mutually monogamous long-term relationship, you should always use a condom, and both you and your partner should be tested for HIV. You should be aware that even a relationship that seems to be mutually monogamous can be dangerous, because your partner may have been infected years earlier or may not be entirely faithful. Furthermore, tests for STDs are not 100 percent reliable, though they are generally accurate.

The keys to safe sex are common sense and communication. Some kinds of sexual behavior defy common sense in terms of their safety: people who inject themselves with drugs and especially those who share needles are at very high risk. People who abuse alcohol or use recreational drugs and have sex while under the influence raise their risk levels, because alcohol and drugs impair judgment. People who have multiple sexual partners also raise their risk.

Certain forms of sexual activity carry higher risk than others. Abstinence, of course, carries no risk whatsoever. Masturbation is also risk free, though mutual masturbation may carry some risk if there are cuts or other breaks in the skin of the hands. There is no evidence that HIV can be spread by kissing, even deep kissing.

No one is certain about the chances of getting or spreading HIV through unprotected oral intercourse (on either a man or a woman). It is believed that the risk exists, even though it is fairly low and can certainly be made even lower by using a condom, latex square, or dental dam. Other STDs, for example herpes and gonorrhea, can be spread through oral intercourse. Both anal and vaginal intercourse carry potential risk: vaginal intercourse is riskier for women than for men; anal intercourse is risky for both parties.

SEXUAL ORIENTATION

Sexual orientation is an issue that some women deal with in their teens, 20s, and sometimes later in their lives. It is not uncommon for young women to be involved in sexual relationships with other women. This does not mean that their orientation is completely gay and will remain gay for the rest of their lives. Many women later become attracted to men. Other women continue to be involved exclusively with women. Sometimes older women, even those who have been married and had families, discover that they are attracted to women.

Research on sexual behavior suggests that like height, handedness, and other features, sexual preference is a continuum. It ranges from exclusive heterosexuality to exclusive homosexuality, with a large middle ground. People attracted only to members of their own sex are called homosexuals (lesbians, if they are women) and are believed to constitute about 10 percent of the population in this country. Individuals attracted only to members of the opposite sex are heterosexual. Those whose preference is more or less equally divided—between members of their own sex and the opposite sex—may call themselves bisexual.

Although times have changed since the end of the nineteenth century when the writer Oscar Wilde was sent to jail for his homosexuality, there is still a pervasive stigma against homosexuality, whether in men or in women. Although there are laws upholding the basic rights of homosexuals, discrimination abounds. Lesbians still have difficulty getting custody of their children; they may have trouble with employment. Homosexuals of both sexes are often ridiculed, condemned, or ostracized even by their own family members. Gay men in particular are at increased risk for physical violence, as a number of tragic incidents have shown.

For obvious reasons this kind of treatment by colleagues, family members, or society at large stresses homosexuals. Feelings of isolation and loneliness are not uncommon for undeclared homosexuals. Any group targeted for hatred or condemnation is likely to feel lowered self-esteem or depression. There are many lesbian support groups, active at colleges and universities and in the larger world. There are also homophobia workshops for friends and allies, and coming-out groups.

▶ Is homosexuality a disease?

In the past, it was believed that something was seriously wrong with anyone who was not exclusively heterosexual. Homosexuality was considered a form of disease, either physical or mental, from which people could and should be cured. In 1973, however, the American Psychiatric Association changed its opinion and stated that a sexual preference for people of one's own sex is not a form of mental illness but falls within the range of normal sexual behavior. Nor does the larger medical community define homosexuality as a physical disease.

While homosexuality has been dropped from the roster of physical or mental illness, there is still considerable debate on the causes of sexual orientation. Is it nature or nurture? And if it is nature (biology), is it determined genetically or by prenatal influences? Few authorities on human sexuality believe that people consciously choose their sexual orientation.

ABUSIVE RELATIONSHIPS

It is a sad fact of life that many women live with men—husbands, fathers, boyfriends—who abuse them physically and/or emotionally. The abuse can be psychological, sexual, or economic as well as physical. It can include verbal abuse, harassment, sexual coercion, excessive possessiveness, or social isolation. Sometimes it includes destruction of personal property. Whatever form it takes, it is a pattern of behavior used to establish power and control through fear and intimidation, and it often includes the threat or use of violence.

Although only a small proportion of incidents of domestic violence (also called intimate partner violence) are reported, the statistics are most readily available on physical violence. By very conservative estimates, each year 1 million women suffer nonfatal violence at the hands of an intimate. Less cautious estimates place the number at 4 million. Nearly one in three women experiences at least one physical assault by a partner during her lifetime. According to a U.S. Department of Justice survey, 28 percent of all violence against women is perpetrated by people with whom they are intimate, compared to only 5 percent of the violence against men.

Domestic violence happens in all locations, from the most affluent suburbs to the poorest inner-city neighborhoods to the remotest rural towns. It happens to women of all educational and income levels. No nationality, religious preference, race, or age group is exempt, though women between the ages of 19 and 24 are at greatest risk, as are women in households whose annual income is less than ten thousand dollars. Gay couples experience domestic violence at about the same rate as heterosexual couples.

Feminist organizations began raising awareness about domestic violence in the 1970s, and in the 1980s their efforts began to bear fruit. In 1984 the attorney general of the United States established a Task Force on Family Violence to study the scope of the problem; that same year, the Family Violence Prevention and Services Act allocated federal funds for programs helping victims. A year later, Surgeon General C. Everett Koop issued a report recognizing domestic violence as one of the nation's most serious health issues.

The problem tends to be repetitive. According to the Bureau of Justice Statistics, during the six months following an episode of domestic violence, 32 percent of battered women are victimized again; the American Medical Association, in its guidelines for diagnosis and treatment, suggests that 47 percent of men who beat their wives do so at least three times a year.

▶ *How do you know that your relationship is abusive?*

Many women are so abused or so conditioned to abuse that they fail to recognize it for what it is—perhaps because they were involved in controlling, if not abusive, relationships as children.

The National Coalition Against Domestic Violence has issued a set of questions for women to ask themselves if they think their relationship might be abusive. These questions can serve as guidelines for defining domestic abuse:

Does your partner shove, hit, shake, or slap you?

Does your partner make light of the abuse, insist that it did not happen, or shift the responsibility for his abusive behavior to you?

Does your partner continually put you down, call you names, humiliate you?

Does your partner intimidate you through looks or actions, destroy your property, or display weapons?

Does your partner control what you do, whom you see and talk to, and where you go, limiting your involvement outside the relationship?

Are you made to feel guilty about the children, or has your partner threatened to take the children away?

▶ Why don't women leave abusive relationships?

Often this question is answered in a way that blames the victim: Women who stay with abusive men are "women who love too much," or they suffer from low self-esteem, or (worst of all) at some level they feel they deserve such treatment.

Many women continue in relationships that they recognize as abusive, and there are complex reasons why they do so. One is that they believe the abuser's repeated promises to reform and change his behavior, or hope that some problem like alcohol or drug abuse can be overcome and the violence will disappear. Others are tied to the relationship through children and fear that they will lose custody if they leave. Some women have no resources of their own; all the economic and social status belongs to the man. Sometimes women dwell on the positive as well as the negative times in their relationship.

> Roxanne is a teacher, well respected in her profession. Her husband is a very successful businessman. She has several grown children, including a daughter who also is a patient of mine.
>
> Several years ago Roxanne came in with bruises on her arms and legs and a black eye, which she wanted me to document for her. She intended to use this documentation as evidence in a court case. Later she changed her mind, saying that she is still in love with her husband and that he is "better" and doesn't hit her any more. I still wonder whether she couldn't leave him because of socioeconomic considerations.

▶ *What are the consequences of domestic violence or abuse?*

The damage inflicted by abuse is both physical and psychological. Most obvious are the physical injuries from the abuse itself. But studies show that women who have been physically or sexually abused are more likely than other women to have a variety of physical ailments including headaches, abdominal pain, insomnia, fatigue, and irritable bowel syndrome. They also have higher rates of psychological and emotional problems, including depression, alcohol and drug abuse, and eating disorders. Because the problem of domestic abuse has come under serious attention only in the past couple of decades, studies of its physical and psychological effects are in their early stages.

If you are the victim of domestic abuse, your caregiver should be able to steer you to local resources. Your town may have a domestic violence hotline listed in the phone book, sometimes in a special section of community services or in the yellow pages (try "Domestic Violence" or "Social Services"). There is a national domestic hotline at 800-799-SAFE (7233). Many communities have support groups, emergency shelters, and child care facilities. Some support groups can help abused women with the legal aspects of their problems. They can advise on child custody issues or provide a court advocate to a woman seeking a restraining order against her abuser. Some will provide you with a cell phone for emergencies.

Remember that the longer you stay in an abusive relationship, the more difficult it becomes to get out of it. You have the right to live without threats or abuse. You are entitled to police protection and medical attention, as well as to legal help.

RAPE

Rape is a crime of violence that happens to be sexual in nature. It can involve sexual intercourse but is not limited to the sexual act. It is accompanied by force or the threat of force and is intended to intimidate, humiliate, and exercise control over the victim. The motive for rape is not sexual desire but aggression.

Some years back, women were often accused of provoking rape by their behavior, by their clothing, by allowing themselves to be in the wrong place at the wrong time. Sometimes women were even accused of desiring rape. Fortunately these attitudes, while still around, are dying out.

Victims of rape or sexual abuse can be of any age—from babies to elderly women. They can be male as well as female, but statistically the largest group is young urban women. Because rape is the violent crime least frequently reported to police, accurate statistics are difficult to obtain. According to the Bureau of Justice Statistics, 261,000 crimes of

rape and sexual assault were reported in 2000, but the bureau estimates that only 28 percent of such crimes are reported. If that is the case, the total number would rise to 929,000.
The most pessimistic estimates suggest that only about 10 percent of rapes committed by
strangers are reported, and even fewer of those committed by someone the victim knows.

REPORTING RAPE

According to bureau statistics, about 70 percent of rapes are committed by men known to
their victims. This suggests two reasons why many women do not report rape: they are unwilling to turn in someone they know, or they fear retribution. In addition, women may
blame themselves.

Between the mid-1970s and the mid-1990s the number of rapes reported rose significantly. (Since 1994 the total number of violent crimes has decreased and, along with it, the
number of reported rapes.) Victims may be more willing to report an attack because the
women's movement and the victims' rights movement have succeeded somewhat in di-
minishing the stigma attached to rape.

Other benefits have come from our increased awareness of the prevalence of rape,
which have made it easier for women to decide to report the crime. In the past two decades
many emergency room and other health care professionals as well as law enforcement offi-
cers have been trained to understand and respect the rights and feelings of rape victims.
Many communities have organized programs to provide women with medical care, emotional support, and follow-up counseling.

Some women hesitate to report rape because they do not want public exposure and
do not want to endure a trial. Although public support for victims is changing, and defense attorneys are no longer allowed to call in question a woman's character, past sexual
behavior, or personal history, many women do not want to make their private lives public.
Other women hesitate because the odds are that the alleged rapist will not actually be
brought to justice.

Nevertheless, if you have been raped, I encourage you to report it as soon as possible.
Awareness of the prevalence of rape and understanding of its nature have brought more
resources to bear on the problem and in the long run can benefit other women who are
victimized.

Reporting the rape is not the same as seeking prosecution. When you have had time to
explore your feelings, you may or may not decide to prosecute; but even if you ultimately
decide not to take legal action, there are real reasons for acting quickly. First of all, if there
is any chance that you might be pregnant, you can have the appropriate morning-after

contraception, which works well up to about seventy-two hours. If there is a danger that you have been exposed to a sexually transmitted disease, you can have immediate preventive therapy. You can receive help, practical information, and support from a counselor at a time when you may feel isolated, confused, and uncertain.

All gynecologists and many other physicians receive training in rape crisis intervention. If you have a gynecologist or another physician whom you regularly see and trust, call that person immediately. He or she should know what facilities are available in your town or city. If you do not have a private physician, the doctors on duty in your local emergency room are likely to have received appropriate instruction in crisis intervention.

Most emergency rooms have streamlined the procedure for dealing with rape victims, so that the hours formerly spent waiting can be avoided. At the hospital where I practice, a twenty-four-hour crisis team is available, including a social worker and a staff gynecologist. If you are a college student, you can report the assault to the college health services.

Many communities have organized rape crisis centers for support. These centers can provide advocates to be with you at the hospital and the police station during the crisis period; they can later provide assistance with legal, psychological, and other issues as they arise.

▶ What happens when you report a rape?

If you want to document the intercourse, you will have to have a physical exam, as soon after the event as possible. Because legal evidence will be collected, you should not shower or change your clothes. Ideally you should not even urinate, though that may be an unrealistic expectation. Since your clothing may be part of the forensic evidence, you might take extra clothes to the doctor's office or emergency room.

You will be the best witness when the assault is fresh in your mind and the samples that are collected are still viable. Even if you have not yet decided whether to press charges, you can give samples and the hospital will keep them for a couple of days while you make up your mind. Although the likelihood of providing evidence that will convict the rapist is better if you have a checkup right away, some evidence may be helpful even two days later. By the time a week has elapsed, although medical attention will help you, the chances of collecting valid forensic material will have decreased drastically.

At the hospital any physical injuries you may have will be attended to. The physician examining you will record those injuries in detail. If you give permission, you will undergo a pelvic exam and specimens will be collected for forensic evidence. If any other type of assault took place, appropriate specimens will be taken (blood, hair samples, swabs of fluids). A laboratory test can detect a substance called acid phosphatase, which indicates the presence of seminal fluid. Other lab tests can reveal the assailant's blood type and DNA "fingerprint."

You will be checked for STDs , which unfortunately can be transmitted as a result of rape. Since some tests for sexually transmitted diseases may not be definitive right away, you may have to have repeat tests for syphilis, gonorrhea, or HIV, but you will probably be given preventive antibiotics or other medications in the meantime.

THE EMOTIONAL CONSEQUENCES OF RAPE

Rape is a crime of violence, and women respond to it psychologically in the same way people of both sexes respond to other forms of trauma, including the devastation of war and natural disasters. Rape is also a crime in which a woman's deepest self is violated. The overwhelming experience of being victimized can lead to lasting emotional distress, self-destructive behavior, interpersonal problems, and behavioral disorders.

Researchers have identified what they call the rape trauma syndrome, and although various studies categorize the recovery process in different ways, there are several general stages in the healing process. Not everyone goes through the process in the same way, but certain feelings and patterns of behavior are common to most survivors.

The first stage is the crisis stage. Health care workers who interview rape victims notice two kinds of general reactions. About half of the women express their distress by crying, trembling, or other signs of anxiety. The other half hide their feelings, perhaps from themselves as well as from people around them; numb and shocked, they may appear detached from the event. Many women experience tension headaches, fatigue, and severe nausea right after the event.

During the crisis stage, the overwhelming reaction is fear: fear the attacker will return, fear of people who remind the victim of the attacker, and fear of being alone or in places similar to the one where the attack occurred. The victim may feel angry, depressed, confused, and irritable—or guilty and "dirty" because she wrongfully blames herself for the assault.

The next stage, according to many counselors, is a period of denial. During this time many women make changes in their lifestyle, move to a new residence, change jobs, switch phone numbers, or travel, often to visit relatives and reestablish connections with family members who live at a distance. The woman may tell friends that everything is "fine," in an effort to put the pain behind her. Or she may turn to destructive behavior like alcohol or drug abuse, overeating, or overworking, to help her forget.

The next stage begins when the reality of the attack sinks in. Most women experience depression and feelings of loss. The victim's sense of security and control over her life have been destroyed. Many women have nightmares or phobias, often focused on being alone; physical aches and pains; difficulty concentrating; and loss of interest in usual activities. They may have vivid and painful flashbacks, during which it seems that the attack is happening all over again. These symptoms can continue for a long time or suddenly recur long after the rape has apparently been put in the past. Sometimes they are stimulated by an event that recalls the attack, or even by an event or situation that suggests the victim lacks control over her life.

Problems frequently arise between the woman and her sexual partner, and a large percentage of these relationships are disrupted. Many men are conditioned by their social backgrounds to believe the myth that women are at fault for being raped and are therefore somehow tainted by being victimized. Others are unable to express their feelings and try to ignore an event that is deeply disturbing to the woman. Women may misdirect their anger at their partners or other loved ones, or turn it inward on themselves. Some men feel guilty, responsible, or betrayed.

The final stage in the healing process is resolution, which begins when the victim starts to reconcile her feelings about the assault, the attacker, and herself. The goal of this stage is to move from "victim" to "survivor" and to accept the assault as one event, though a very painful one, in her life.

Women follow their own timetables in the healing process and the passage may not be smooth or direct. They may go forward and then fall back, or remain mired in one stage. Some women continue to isolate themselves, withdraw from reality, or become seriously depressed and need psychiatric help as well as counseling.

▶ *Is counseling necessary or helpful after a sexual assault?*

Although for centuries women have recovered from the trauma of rape without the help of counseling, emotional support can be very helpful at any time during the healing process, not just immediately after the attack. Counselors can also work with other family members and sexual partners, who often increase the burden of the victim by blaming her, thus loading her with more guilt than she already feels.

Your caregiver should be able to refer you to a counselor trained in this area. If not, a community or state rape crisis, domestic violence, or victims' advocate program should be able to direct you.

15 Lifestyle Issues

▶ **MYTH** Your genetic makeup determines your general health and your physical makeup.

FACT While your parents' genes may predispose you to certain diseases and determine your hair color and foot size, you can influence both your general health and the actual physical attributes you see in the mirror. A lifelong plan of exercise and appropriate eating can make a vast difference in your health throughout your life.

I N these times of information overload, it is easy to find out what you should do to take care of your general health and well-being. As a reminder, here are some absolutely basic, bottom-line recommendations, which you can refer to when you are tempted to become a chocoholic couch potato. Two of the most important things you can do for yourself are eat a healthy diet and get enough exercise.

DIET AND NUTRITION

The science of nutrition is complicated, uncertain, and controversial, yet every day you must make decisions about what you are going to eat and what you are going to avoid. There seem to be as many nutritional plans as there are human ailments. There are diets to boost your energy, to make you stay young, to reverse heart disease, to prevent cancer, to help you win at sports, and of course to shed pounds. There are plans based on your blood type, your body type, and your ethnic background.

Yet many nutritional theories seem to have the longevity of New Year's resolutions. Today's "miracle food" can quickly become tomorrow's hoax, and supposed dangers can turn out to be harmless. A few years ago oat bran seemed to be a cancer preventive; then it proved to be worthless in this respect. Caffeine was said to stunt children's growth and give adult women breast cancer. Today scientists believe that it may make you nervous and give you bumpy breasts, but probably not give you cancer.

CONCEPTS OF BODY WEIGHT

One of the purposes of good nutrition is to maintain a healthy weight. As far as female body weight is concerned, our society is torn between an unreachable, unrealistic ideal and a less-than-healthy reality. Beauty as reflected in the media requires twig-like slenderness. Most of the models in fashion magazines appear to be barely postpubescent women, with prominent cheekbones, protruding collarbones, and thin coltish legs.

In reality, many Americans are overweight and they are becoming more so as time goes on. The National Health and Nutrition Examination Survey for 1999–2000 found an estimated 64 percent of adult Americans either overweight or obese. Of this group, 31 percent—nearly 59 million people—are obese. (An adult with a body mass index of 30 or greater is considered obese; for a woman five feet four inches tall, this means being more than 30 pounds above her healthy weight.) While the number of overweight individuals has increased 17 percent since the 1976–1980 survey, the obese population has more than doubled, with young adults 18 to 29 years old showing the greatest rate of increase of any age group. Obesity has reached epidemic proportions.

The more overweight you are, the greater your risk of premature death. Obese people are at increased risk for diabetes, heart disease, high blood pressure, cancer, back pain, gallbladder disease, and even chronic degenerative arthritis. In addition to the increased health risks of obesity, enormous social consequences begin in adolescence and continue throughout life. According to a study published in 1993 in the *New England Journal of Medicine,* young women who are overweight are less likely to marry and will have lower household incomes and higher rates of poverty than women of normal weight. These consequences, which hold true regardless of socioeconomic origin and ability as measured by aptitude tests, are only magnified over a lifetime. Since there is a strong cultural bias against overweight people, heavy women are discriminated against in the job market. But at least our notion of what is defined as overweight has been revised.

Because being overweight increases health risks and lowers life expectancies, some life insurance companies publish charts suggesting appropriate body weights. The Metropolitan Life Insurance Company, whose statistics were standard throughout the industry, recently revised its tables to reflect a broader interpretation of appropriate weight for a given height. Back in 1968, a woman 5′4″ tall with a small frame could weigh between 108 and 116 pounds and fall within the guidelines established by the actuarial tables. Today, that same woman can weigh between 114 and 127 and still fit within the suggested range. If you are 5′8″ and have a large frame, nowadays life insurance companies consider you a good risk, other factors aside, if you weigh between 146 and 167 pounds; in 1968, you would have had to shed 8 or 9 pounds and get down to between 137 and 154 pounds to meet the requirements.

Individual differences in bone diameter and in the relative proportions of muscle and fat account for the wide range of acceptability on the chart. If you are a strapping, heavy-boned woman of 5′6″, you can weigh more than a delicately boned woman of the same height and still be close to your desirable body weight. Since muscle weighs more than fat, you will weigh more inch for inch if you are muscular and athletically trained than if you are sedentary.

Today many health professionals use body mass index to determine whether you are overweight. The National Heart, Lung, and Blood Institute publishes a body mass index table. In addition to the general guidelines established by this table, there are other tests for overweight. Physicians specializing in weight control sometimes use calipers to measure the thickness of skinfolds on various parts of your body. Another method is to immerse you in a tank of water to find the volume of your body and, relating it to your weight, calculate your percentage of body fat. A newer method is called bioelectrical impedance analysis (BIA). It measures the body's ability to conduct an electrical current, which increases with the total amount of water in the body; more body water suggests more muscle and lean tissue. Mathematical formulas are used to convert percentage of body water into an estimate of fat and lean body mass.

If, in fact, you are overweight, you probably already know it and feel bad about it. A National Institutes of Health study on obesity suggests that its worst effect is the psychological suffering it causes.

FAT DISTRIBUTION AND DISEASE RISK

Scientists have suggested that fat distribution as well as its total amount affects the risk of disease, particularly of coronary artery disease. Researchers have described two general silhouettes in overweight people: the pear and the apple. Pear-shaped people carry their extra weight low, around the hips, buttocks, and thighs; apple-shaped people carry the

TABLE 4. Body Mass Index

Body Weight (pounds)

Height (inches)	NORMAL						OVERWEIGHT					OBESE										EXTREMELY OBESE														
BMI	19	20	21	22	23	24	25	26	27	28	29	30	31	32	33	34	35	36	37	38	39	40	41	42	43	44	45	46	47	48	49	50	51	52	53	54
58	91	96	100	105	110	115	119	124	129	134	138	143	148	153	158	162	167	172	177	181	186	191	196	201	205	210	215	220	224	229	234	239	244	248	253	258
59	94	99	104	109	114	119	124	128	133	138	143	148	153	158	163	168	173	178	183	188	193	198	203	208	212	217	222	227	232	237	242	247	252	257	262	267
60	97	102	107	112	118	123	128	133	138	143	148	153	158	163	168	174	179	184	189	194	199	204	209	215	220	225	230	235	240	245	250	255	261	266	271	276
61	100	106	111	116	122	127	132	137	143	148	153	158	164	169	174	180	185	190	195	201	206	211	217	222	227	232	238	243	248	254	259	264	269	275	280	285
62	104	109	115	120	126	131	136	142	147	153	158	164	169	175	180	186	191	196	202	207	213	218	224	229	235	240	246	251	256	262	267	273	278	284	289	295
63	107	113	118	124	130	135	141	146	152	158	163	169	175	180	186	191	197	203	208	214	220	225	231	237	242	248	254	259	265	270	278	282	287	293	299	304
64	110	116	122	128	134	140	145	151	157	163	169	174	180	186	192	197	204	209	215	221	227	232	238	244	250	256	262	267	273	279	285	291	296	302	308	314
65	114	120	126	132	138	144	150	156	162	168	174	180	186	192	198	204	210	216	222	228	234	240	246	252	258	264	270	276	282	288	294	300	306	312	318	324
66	118	124	130	136	142	148	155	161	167	173	179	186	192	198	204	210	216	223	229	235	241	247	253	260	266	272	278	284	291	297	303	309	315	322	328	334
67	121	127	134	140	146	153	159	166	172	178	185	191	198	204	211	217	223	230	236	242	249	255	261	268	274	280	287	293	299	306	312	319	325	331	338	344
68	125	131	138	144	151	158	164	171	177	184	190	197	203	210	216	223	230	236	243	249	256	262	269	276	282	289	295	302	308	315	322	328	335	341	348	354
69	128	135	142	149	155	162	169	176	182	189	196	203	209	216	223	230	236	243	250	257	263	270	277	284	291	297	304	311	318	324	331	338	345	351	358	365
70	132	139	146	153	160	167	174	181	188	195	202	209	216	222	229	236	243	250	257	264	271	278	285	292	299	306	313	320	327	334	341	348	355	362	369	376
71	136	143	150	157	165	172	179	186	193	200	208	215	222	229	236	243	250	257	265	272	279	286	293	301	308	315	322	329	338	343	351	358	365	372	379	386
72	140	147	154	162	169	177	184	191	199	206	213	221	228	235	242	250	258	265	272	279	287	294	302	309	316	324	331	338	346	353	361	368	375	383	390	397
73	144	151	159	166	174	182	189	197	204	212	219	227	235	242	250	257	265	272	280	288	295	302	310	318	325	333	340	348	355	363	371	378	386	393	401	408
74	148	155	163	171	179	186	194	202	210	218	225	233	241	249	256	264	272	280	287	295	303	311	319	326	334	342	350	358	365	373	381	389	396	404	412	420
75	152	160	168	176	184	192	200	208	216	224	232	240	248	256	264	272	279	287	295	303	311	319	327	335	343	351	359	367	375	383	391	399	407	415	423	431
76	156	164	172	180	189	197	205	213	221	230	238	246	254	263	271	279	287	295	304	312	320	328	336	344	353	361	369	377	385	394	402	410	418	426	435	443

Source: Adapted from Clinical Guidelines on the Identification, Evaluation, and Treatment of Overweight and Obesity in Adults: The Evidence Report.

weight around their waists. Typically, young women who are overweight are pear shaped, while overweight men (the sagging belly syndrome) and postmenopausal women (the potbelly syndrome) are apple shaped.

How do you know if you are an apple or a pear? Measure your waist at the navel. Then measure your hips at their fullest point. If you divide your waist measurement by your hip measurement and the result is less than 1.0, you are a pear. If it is greater than 1.0, you are an apple. For women, if your waist-to-hip ratio is greater than 0.8, you are at increased risk of heart disease.

▶ What is the best way to lose weight?

Although genetic inheritance has a great deal to do with body shape and you can do nothing to change the tendency to heavy thighs that you inherited from your grandmother, you *can* maintain something close to your ideal body weight, though it may take a lot of effort.

There are two basic ways to lose weight, and to succeed you have to pursue both: follow a moderate diet with not too many calories, and increase the amount you exercise. While it may be possible to lose weight by doing one without the other, it certainly is very difficult. Restricting calories without exercise usually results in frustration and failure, because the body in its wisdom turns down its metabolic regulator when it senses lowered caloric intake, trying to save you from what it interprets as threatened starvation. If you exist on, say, a thousand calories a day for a week or so, your body begins to believe that a thousand calories is all it is going to get. It readjusts its metabolic set point to maintain itself on a thousand calories.

Nor does exercise alone seem to do the trick. It is generally believed that just as the body shuts down its metabolic regulator if it becomes accustomed to a low caloric intake, so will the body boost its metabolic thermostat if it gets accustomed to a high-energy output, for example, needing to supply extra calories for regular exercise. However, in a 1989 study published in the *International Journal of Sports Medicine,* researchers followed a group of male and female novices who were training for their first marathon. The athletes trained for a period of eighty weeks, with no control over diet. During the training regimen, the men lost weight and fat but the women, alas, did not. A study in 1992 reported in the *Journal of Applied Physiology* showed similar results among female runners whose weight was tracked for a year. In a 1984 study in the *Journal of Obesity and Weight Regulation,* both men and women were monitored in a continuous exercise program for twenty weeks, again with no control over diet. The men showed significant decreases in body weight and percentage of fat mass, but the women experienced no change. Apparently exercise alone may result in decreased body weight for men, but not for women.

So the only answer has to be the two-pronged attack, controlling caloric intake while increasing exercise. More exercise helps counter the diet doldrums and, we hope, resets the metabolic regulator, helping you to burn more calories for the same amount of physical activity.

Aim for only a pound or two of loss per week. After all, your goal is a new set of habits that will keep you where you want to be for the rest of your life. If you are losing weight, even though you are doing it slowly and steadily, you will eventually reach your goal if you maintain your improved habits.

▶ What constitutes a healthy diet?

A healthy diet is one that will protect your heart (which means controlling fat intake), strengthen your bones (which means getting plenty of calcium), and help keep your weight in a healthy range. A generation or two ago, a healthy diet consisted of a lot of meat and plenty of milk, cheese, and dairy products, plus fruit and vegetables. Protein was "in." Starches, as complex carbohydrates were called, were "out" because they were thought to be fattening. Potatoes and pasta were regarded with suspicion. There were seven basic food groups and you were told to eat a certain number of servings of each one.

In 1989 the American Nutrition Society came out with totally new guidelines. The general structure of the ideal diet is a pyramid, and people are urged to eat more carbohydrates, less fat, and less protein than formerly. In general, the guidelines suggest the following daily intake:

One or two servings of lean meat, skinless poultry, or fish; or, if you prefer a
vegetarian diet, nuts, dried beans, peas or lentils, or peanut butter
Two to four servings of fruit
Three to five servings of vegetables, including at least one leafy green vegetable
and one orange or yellow vegetable
Two servings of skim or 1-percent low-fat milk, or low-fat dairy products (pregnant and postmenopausal women should have three servings)
Five to eight servings of polyunsaturated or monounsaturated oils, or margarine
Six to eleven servings of bread, cereals, pasta, rice, popcorn, or dried beans or
peas

This nutritional plan is low in cholesterol, low in saturated fats, relatively low in protein, and high in complex carbohydrates and calcium. It is a diet healthy for your heart and bones, and one on which it is relatively easy to lose weight if you control portion size and supplement your diet with exercise. It offers a variety of foods and emphasizes fruits, vegetables, and whole grains.

▶ How many calories do you need?

The average woman at age 25 needs about 2,000 calories to maintain her body weight and keep up her energy. Then caloric needs decline by about 100 calories per day for each ten years of age over 25. So at 35, you need only 1,900 calories for the same activities. By the time you are in your mid-50s, you will need only about 1,700 calories daily, unless you increase your exercise level. If you are trying to lose weight, remember that you are working toward slow loss, which is brought about by a change in your eating and exercise habits.

▶ How much calcium should you get?

The current recommendation is 1,000 mg daily for women before menopause. Women who have passed through menopause and are taking estrogen also require 1,000 mg daily, but postmenopausal women who are not taking estrogen should get 1,500 mg.

While dairy foods are the main sources of calcium, some other foods are rich in this mineral. Certain green and leafy vegetables, such as broccoli, collard greens, and kale (which may not be a part of your regular menus), are fine sources of calcium. Canned fish such as sardines and salmon (which is canned with the bones) is another source. Any vegetable with high oxalic acid is less desirable as a source of calcium, because the acid interferes with calcium absorption; among the culprits are spinach, beet greens, rhubarb, parsley, and chard. In case you had hoped to get your calcium from chocolate, you should know that it too is high in oxalic acid. If you dislike milk and dairy products, some orange juice now comes with added calcium, as do some cereal products. Remember, however, that although fortified products are high in calcium, all of this calcium is not available to your body. You have to be very conscientious if you are going to get adequate calcium from your diet: two cups of milk, a cup of yogurt, and a cup of fortified orange juice will give you a baseline 1,320 mg of calcium.

▶ *What about calcium supplements?*

Since the average calcium intake in the United States is something like 400 to 500 mg daily, only about half of what you need, many women who do not like milk and other dairy products find it difficult to get enough calcium in their diet.

Fortunately calcium supplements are available. A single chewable tablet of calcium carbonate or calcium citrate will supply an additional 200–300 mg of calcium beyond what you have in your diet. Some physicians recommend extra-strength Tums, the over-the-counter antacid used by many people to counteract heartburn and indigestion. A single one of these tablets contains 300 mg of calcium, so if you have one after each meal you will get 900 mg of calcium.

DIET AND CHOLESTEROL

Cholesterol is a fatty substance manufactured by the body. It is present in red meat and high-fat dairy products and has been linked to coronary artery disease. Cholesterol in itself is not harmful. It is used by the body to make certain hormones; it helps in digestion; and it is an important building block of bodily tissues. However, cholesterol in the wrong amounts or in the wrong places *is* dangerous. Coronary heart disease, also called coronary artery disease (CAD), arises when cholesterol is deposited inside the wall of the arteries that bring the heart its blood supply. These deposits contribute to buildup of a fatty blockage called plaque. Deposits of plaque inside the blood vessels are known as arteriosclerosis, or atherosclerosis, or hardening of the arteries.

Young women are protected by estrogen and do not have to worry as much as older women do about cholesterol and the diseases that result from cholesterol deposits. But it is worthwhile to start a heart-healthy diet while you are young. As research has provided new data, beliefs about cholesterol have changed. Fifteen years ago it was considered all right to have a serum cholesterol of 240 mg/dl (that is, 240 milligrams of cholesterol per deciliter of blood); ten years ago, 220 mg/dl was acceptable; in recent years, physicians and researchers have started looking at a cholesterol level of 200 mg/dl or lower as the desired goal.

GOOD AND BAD CHOLESTEROL

It is not merely your total serum cholesterol, the amount of cholesterol in your blood, that counts. Because cholesterol is a fatty substance, it does not mix easily with blood. In order to be moved around the body via the bloodstream, cholesterol gets packaged into molecules called lipoproteins. Researchers have identified a number of types of lipoproteins, of which two have received a lot of attention: LDL (low-density lipoprotein, "bad" cholesterol) and HDL (high-density lipoprotein, "good" cholesterol).

Bad cholesterol is bad because it seems to play a significant role in depositing cholesterol on the inside of the artery walls. Good cholesterol is good because it seems to help clean out the cholesterol deposits that have already begun to line the artery walls. Therefore it is the relative quantities of HDL and LDL that are important to the health of your arteries and your heart. These days an LDL level of up to 130 mg/dl is considered fine, 130–160 mg/dl is in a gray zone, and anything over 160 mg/dl is anxiety provoking. So if your total cholesterol is 220 but your HDL is 100, you are in good shape because your LDL is very low.

To further complicate this subject, levels of HDL and LDL must be taken as relative quantities. It is their ratio that is important. Suppose your HDL is 100 and your LDL is 160, which puts your total cholesterol at something higher than 260 and your LDL at the outer edge of the gray zone. But compare that person to someone whose total cholesterol is 190 mg/dl, but with an HDL of 20 and an LDL of 170. These people are few and far between, but they are at significant risk for cholesterol problems.

▶ *What can you do if your cholesterol levels are high?*

Suppose you have your cholesterol checked, maybe at a health fair, and find that your total serum cholesterol is high. If it is over 300, you should talk soon to your doctor—probably your internist, since most gynecologists in this country do not feel totally comfortable prescribing drugs to lower blood cholesterol. Various medicines on the market will lower blood cholesterol levels, but all have side effects and all have some toxicity. If your cholesterol is borderline, the two most helpful things you can do are start exercising and adjust your diet, especially if you are overweight.

Fortunately, you can have a significant impact on your cholesterol levels by controlling your diet. The main factor here, if you are overweight, seems to be not what you eat but the weight loss that follows a well-designed and controlled diet. The body is able to manufacture cholesterol and can produce it even though there is no cholesterol at all in your diet. If you live on a diet of 100 percent lettuce (which of course you should not) and have an intake of zero cholesterol, your body will still manufacture it for you.

Nevertheless, a diet low in fat and low in cholesterol kills two birds with one stone: it contributes to weight loss and it restricts intake of highly saturated fats, which worsen your blood lipid profile (that is, they increase the relative amounts of bad cholesterol).

A sensible low-cholesterol, low-fat diet includes less than 30 percent of total calories from fat and less than 10 percent from saturated fat, which is the kind found in animal products (meat, poultry, fish) and a few vegetable oils (notably palm oil and coconut oil). Adopting this kind of diet will, on average, reduce total cholesterol 5–10 percent.

One important feature of this kind of dietary restriction is that it reduces total calories. Proteins and carbohydrates have 4 calories per gram, whereas fats have 9 calories per gram, more than twice as much. By concentrating on carbohydrates (for example, fruits, vegetables, and grains), you can eat more food while ingesting fewer calories.

The second critical factor both in cholesterol control and in weight reduction is exercise. An appropriate aerobic exercise regimen can increase your HDL as much as 20 percent. If you come into my office with a cholesterol level of 260, I will not automatically send you to your internist for cholesterol-lowering drugs. Particularly if you are overweight, I will try to get you on a suitable diet and strongly encourage you to get involved in a good exercise program.

EXERCISE AS A LIFESTYLE CHOICE

As you probably already know, physical activity has many benefits. Exercise improves muscle strength, muscle tone, and flexibility. It promotes a sense of well-being and enhances self-esteem. Weight-bearing exercise helps develop and preserve bone. Aerobic exercise helps stave off cardiovascular disease.

If you are trying to lose weight, exercise depresses your appetite, which makes it easier to keep your caloric intake low. Exercise along with cutting back on calories encourages the loss of fat rather than muscle, so that you look trimmer, fitter, and healthier as you slim down. Exercise boosts metabolism, enabling you to burn calories faster. Why, then, don't people exercise? Most women say the problem is time, but you can make time to exercise if you really are determined.

Basically there are three kinds of exercise, which are important all through life and especially as you get older. The first is aerobic exercise, in which the muscles burn oxygen as fuel. Aerobic exercise, which includes fast walking, jogging, running, aerobic dance, and other forms of rhythmic exertion over fairly long periods, is important to cardiovascular health and weight control.

The second type, anaerobic or isometric exercise, involves using particular muscle groups in strenuous bursts for fairly short periods. As you age, your muscle mass turns to fat and you get weaker. Very elderly people, both men and women, often have difficulty getting up from chairs or lifting bags of groceries. Anaerobic exercise will help maintain muscle strength throughout life. Calisthenics, tai chi chuan, yoga, weight lifting, and working out on Nautilus machines are examples of this kind of exercise. The benefits of anaerobic exercise include strength, muscle tone, and stamina. If you play golf or tennis, windsurf, hike, or skate, improved muscle strength will transfer to these activities. Like aerobic exercise, strength training boosts your metabolic rate, which helps you lose weight, since a trained, muscular body uses more calories than a flabby one, even when sitting still. Furthermore, muscle takes up less space than fat, pound for pound, so if you are more muscular, you will be trimmer.

The third type is exercise for flexibility, which is critical to maintaining balance and agility as you go through life. Stretching before and after aerobic or anaerobic exercise helps avoid sore muscles and muscle injuries. Yoga and Pilates, which involve both mind and body, encourage flexibility, muscle stretching, and balance.

Although the ideal exercise program includes all three types, two goals are crucial: getting enough exercise to maintain ideal body weight and keep up cardiovascular fitness, and doing the kind of exercise that promotes healthy bone. One commonly used guideline for cardiovascular fitness suggests raising your heart rate into a target zone, which is somewhere between 60 and 75 percent of its maximum, and keeping it there for thirty minutes at least three times a week. To discover your target zone, subtract your age from 220 and take 60 percent and then 75 percent of that number. Your target zone lies between these percentages.

Another way to approach exercise, suggested by the American Heart Association, is to expend at least two thousand calories weekly in exercise. The American College of Sports Medicine offers guidelines, which suggest that you alternate aerobic and anaerobic types of exercise, doing strength training (anaerobic exercise) for two or three thirty-minute sessions each week, and on alternate days doing aerobic exercise such as walking, jogging, aerobic dancing, or swimming.

Establishing healthy habits takes time and patience, but in the long run they will make your life more enjoyable. Be persistent and patient. Take care of your body now, and you will reap benefits throughout your life.

BODY IMAGE

Body image is how you feel about how you look. The two are not necessarily related. Surveys repeatedly reveal that most American women (and some men) dislike their overall appearance. Overweight, real or imagined, is one of the main causes of negative body image, but many women fall within their normal weight range and yet consider themselves grossly fat. Or they think their noses are too big, or their hair too curly, or their ankles too thick. In the face of this pressure, maintaining a positive body image is a challenge for many women.

> Anita was raised by her mother, a strong-willed and competent women who ran her own beauty salon and was financially successful enough to send her daughter to an excellent private college. Anita, who has always been tall and robust, gained about twenty unwanted pounds during those four years, the result of too many late-night pizza parties and study-break snacks. When she graduated, she vowed to lose the extra weight and over about a year succeeded, following a program of healthy eating and exercise. She had a goal, to wear a bikini and feel good about herself when she did, and she met it. Anita's outgoing, self-confident personality rests in part on her comfort with herself. She will never be mistaken for a fashion model, but that doesn't bother her at all.

The fact that the majority of women are not tall, swizzle-stick thin, and forever young has created a multibillion-dollar beauty industry to sell cosmetics, vitamins, face creams, plastic surgery, and high-heeled shoes. Worse than emptying your pocketbook, the Barbie-doll standard put forward by the beauty industry (among others) has made millions of women psychologically miserable. Poor body image can influence a woman's sense of self-worth and well-being, as well as her sense of sexual attractiveness. Eating disorders, including anorexia nervosa and bulimia, are certainly linked to dissatisfaction with body size, shape, or weight.

It is not surprising that teenagers are insecure and self-conscious about how they look. Their bodies are changing rapidly and at this time of life being "average" is the most desirable state. Girls who have their growth spurts and menstrual periods later or earlier than their friends are likely to feel awkward. It is at this time of life that negative body images are most likely to develop. During their reproductive years, many women suffer body-image problems during pregnancy, though some women who enjoy being pregnant take pleasure in the capacity of their bodies to reproduce. Others, who have put emotional energy into controlling their weight, feel anxiety as they see their waistlines spread, notice the appearance of stretch marks, and watch the scales creep upward.

Because our culture glorifies youth, women also suffer from negative body image and the consequent loss of self-esteem as they grow older, even though they may have fit comfortably into the stereotypes of beauty when they were younger.

Many women have found help through counseling. Your internist or family-practice physician can help—as can dietitians, mental health counselors, and some university health and counseling centers.

The goal, to accept ourselves as we are throughout life, is not easy when society imposes such narrow limits, but recognition of the problem is the first step. Perhaps the best solution, from adolescence on, is to strive for health through balanced nutrition and enjoyable exercise.

Afterword

MANY women compare their relationships with their mothers to their relationships with their daughters. We must always take care of ourselves for our own primary health, but we must also understand that we are role models for our daughters as our mothers were for us.

Although my mother was a wonderful role model intellectually and professionally, she was hardly a healthy role model. I grew up assuming that all women wore size 18 dresses (after all, when we shopped at Loehmann's, that was where we looked for hers), smoked a pack of Chesterfields a day, and never exercised. And even though her father's entire family were diabetics, it wasn't until I made the diagnosis for her when she was 52 (she never went to the doctor) that she decided that in order to avoid the insulin I suggested, maybe she ought to lose the fifty extra pounds she carried.

I was also actively discouraged from athletic participation. Sports were for dummies, my mother would say. So I remained my somewhat chubby self, and only after I insisted that I needed to learn how to ride a bike at age 10 was I allowed one for my birthday. I pursued this sedentary existence until I had the good fortune to attend a medical school where athletics were glorified (we had a squash court in the library and tennis courts behind it). I realized then that attendance at the Payne Whitney Cathedral of Sports (which is how we referred to our gym) was a blast.

Unfortunately, my mother is now paying heavily for her unhealthy lifestyle as a younger woman. Last year she became severely demented with what we presume is a vascular disease, secondary to years of obesity, smoking, and inactivity on top of her diabetes. She really cannot enjoy her grandchildren and cannot travel, which she used to relish. And although I obviously know that I have a genetic predisposition to diabetes, I will do my best to avoid its potentially devastating consequences by not smoking, keeping my weight under control so that I can continue to wear a size 12 dress, and running 15–20 miles a week.

Most important, my daughter sees me doing these things. She is upset that she cannot have a normal conversation with her grandmother and would be devastated if she could not communicate with me in a few years. I am trying to keep my daughter healthy in other ways too, besides living a healthy life. For example, at the request of the health teachers, I went to the middle school in our town to lecture the eighth graders on the consequences of sexual promiscuity as teenagers, including the ubiquity of the human papilloma virus and the fact that it can lead to cervical cancer years later (proving of course that sex can cause cancer).

Since my daughter has heard me talk in a general way of the sadness of older patients who have infertility woes, she has decided that she is going to get married at age 30 and have her first child at 32. Of course she doesn't fully understand some of the social issues, but she is certainly being exposed to the medical situations.

I hope that I can influence other women too by providing medical information. I encourage all of you to lead healthy, happy lives, and to serve as excellent role models for those around you.

M.J.M.

My mother was quite the opposite of Mary Jane's in terms of lifestyle. She was small (peaking at about 5′1″ and 110 pounds, but shrinking as she aged), and she had an iron will plus a huge amount of physical energy. A hard worker and a housekeeper of impeccable standards, she scrubbed the bathroom floors every day until my sister was born (slacking off thereafter to once or twice a week), washed the windows (inside and out), raked the leaves, waxed the car. She also performed an annual spring cleaning that left no surface inside our house untouched. She finished off the project by washing, starching, and ironing all the curtains and turning the mattresses. If that wasn't enough physical activity, she took up golf when she was in her 50s or early 60s and continued to play until she was 90, walking the course and pulling her cart behind her. She made friends with a group of women who shared her interest in the sport, but finally had to give up because the heat in Southern California got to be too much for her. Still, she could climb three flights of stairs when she was 94.

My mother was diligent about her weight. After a period of plumpness in her teens (which, of course, I never saw), she controlled her fondness for desserts and stayed at 110 pounds for her entire life. It really struck her as unfair during her last years that her waist got bigger even though her weight remained the same. Although I'm sure that genes had something to do with her long, healthy life, I believe that much had to do with her lifestyle. The only thing she did "wrong," in terms of health activities, was avoid milk, which she never liked. In her later years she managed to down a cup of cocoa every morning, but by then she was stooped by osteoporosis.

My own daughter is now an adult, and any role modeling I could have done for her has been accomplished. As far as establishing and maintaining healthy habits, she and I both struggle against weight gain and inactivity, and we learn from each other. She has become a regular at the gym and finds it mentally and physically rewarding. We both look up to my mother, her grandmother, for her high standards, work ethic, and determination.

C.V.W.

▶ GLOSSARY

amenorrhea The condition of not having menstrual periods. Primary amenorrhea meaning never having menstruated; secondary amenorrhea, having started but then stopped.

ablation The destruction of the tissue, usually the lining, of the uterus by freezing, heating, or laser technology.

abortion The ending of a pregnancy. Can be spontaneous, happening on its own, or induced by medical intervention.

abruption In pregnancy, the premature separation of the placenta from the wall of the uterus.

ACE inhibitors Angiotensin-converting enzyme inhibitors; medications that lower the blood pressure by hindering production of a protein that makes the blood vessels constrict.

adenomatous Glandular.

adenomyosis A condition in which the glands that line the uterus penetrate its internal muscle walls. Sometimes called internal endometriosis. Often associated with painful and heavy periods.

adhesions Scar tissue that causes one structure or organ to stick to another to which it should not be attached.

agonist A chemical that acts in a similar fashion to another chemical.

AID Artificial insemination with donor sperm.

AIDS Acquired immune deficiency syndrome; the final stage of infection with the human immunodeficiency virus.

AIH Artificial insemination with husband's sperm.

AIS Androgen insensitivity syndrome; a condition in which a person produces testosterone and is genetically male (has a Y chromosome) but looks and behaves like a female. Also called testicular feminization syndrome.

amniocentesis Sampling the fluid around the fetus by inserting a needle into the abdomen. The procedure is used for genetic testing or to check whether there is infection around the fetus.

androgenic Producing or leading to male characteristics.

anencephaly A congenital birth defect in which brain tissue does not develop.

angina Chest pain associated with lack of oxygen to the heart, usually caused by narrowed coronary arteries.

anorexia nervosa An eating disorder whereby people starve themselves.

anteverted Tilted forward.

antifungal Referring to substances that act against yeast and other fungi, and are often used to fight yeast infections.

anti-inflammatory Referring to substances that act against inflammation and sometimes to combat menstrual cramps. Frequently applied to drugs used to treat arthritis (for example, Motrin or Anaprox).

areola The pigmented area of the breast around the nipple.

ASCUS Atypical squamous cells of undetermined significance; a category of Pap test classification.

Asherman's syndrome Scarring of the lining of the uterus resulting in loss of periods and infertility.

atherosclerosis A thickening of the walls of arteries, primarily composed of fat. Also known as arteriosclerosis.

atypia Referring to cells with unusual characteristics; sometimes associated with inflammation, sometimes with precancerous changes.

autoimmune A reaction in which the immune system attacks the body's own cells or tissues, as in rheumatoid arthritis and lupus.

AZT Azidothymidine; one of the antiviral drugs most commonly used in treating HIV infections. Also known as zidovudine.

bacterial vaginosis Bacterial infection of the vagina.

basal body temperature Temperature taken first thing in the morning before arising. Drops at about the time of ovulation and then goes up about half a degree.

basement membrane A thin layer that divides the superficial cells of an organ from its deeper cells; the "skin" of an organ.

beta-blockers A family of drugs that block the activity of adrenaline. Used primarily to slow the heart rate and lower the blood pressure.

Bethesda system A system for evaluating Pap smears, devised by the National Institutes of Health, located in Bethesda, Maryland.

Billings method Natural family-planning method based on predicting the time of ovulation.

biopsy A sample; or (as a verb) to take a sample of tissue.

birth control pills Oral contraceptive pills. Contain estrogen and progesterone, which suppress the release of an egg by the ovary, thus preventing pregnancy.

bisphasic Referring to oral contraceptive pills with two levels of progestin.

BRCA1, BRCA2 Genes that are markers for increased risk of breast cancer and ovarian cancer.

breakthrough bleeding Bleeding between periods. Usually associated with usage of low-dose birth control pills. Also called dysfunctional uterine bleeding or metrorrhagia.

CAD Coronary artery disease; thickening of the walls of blood vessels to the heart, with obstruction to blood flow. Also known as atherosclerosis. Often leads to angina.

canavan disease A genetic disorder that involves metabolism of complex sugars in the body; it has a higher incidence in Jews than in the rest of the population.

candidiasis A yeast infection.

cannula A narrow tube.

carcinogenic Causing cancer.

carcinoma A cancer that begins in the lining layer of an organ.

carcinoma in situ Cancerous changes within cells, but without invasion of nearby cells.

cardiac disease Heart problems. Usually either CAD or disease of the valves that control the blood in the chambers of the heart.

catamenial Occurring with or at the same time as a menstrual period.

cauterize Destroy tissue by freezing or burning (with electricity), or by using chemicals.

cerebral cortex The outer part of the brain, where the bulk of thinking occurs.

cervical cap A contraceptive device that sits on the cervix and prevents sperm from passing into the uterus and beyond.

cervical mucus Secretions made by the cells of the cervix, primarily to provide lubrication.

cervix The neck of or entrance to the uterus; opens in labor to expel the fetus.

cesarean section Surgical delivery of a fetus through an incision in the mother's abdomen and uterus.

chancre An ulceration of the skin, usually in the genital area; painless ones can be associated with syphilis.

chlamydia A sexually transmitted disease, caused by a virus-like bacterium.

"chocolate" cyst Another name for an endometrioma. An endometrial cyst filled with dark blood, so called because it resembles chocolate syrup.

cholesterol The organic molecule and building block for all steroid hormones. HDL (high-density lipoprotein) is "good" cholesterol and helps prevent heart disease. LDL (low-density lipoprotein) is "bad" cholesterol and promotes heart disease.

CIN Cervical intraepithelial neoplasia; abnormal growth of the tissue on the surface of the cervix.

clinical trials Experiments to check the effectiveness of a new medication; some people are given a drug to be tested and others are given a placebo.

clitoris The female equivalent of the penis; sits at the top of the labia and is involved in sexual response.

Clomid Clomiphene citrate; a drug that induces ovulation.

collagen A substance that acts like glue and holds many cells together. Softer than bone; supports the skin and other structures.

colostomy A surgical incision into the colon, which is then brought out to the surface of the body for drainage; often temporary.

colposcope A giant microscope used to examine and magnify the cervix and vulva. Used to aid in the diagnosis of precancerous and cancerous conditions of the cervix, vagina, and vulva. Can also be used to examine the penis.

conception The fertilization of an egg by a sperm.

condom A device of rubber or natural skin that mechanically covers the penis or vagina and prevents sperm from reaching the cervix. Made for both men and women.

condyloma lata Flat warts associated with syphilis infection; different from genital warts.

condyloma virus A sexually transmitted virus that can cause genital warts. Also associated with increased risk of cervical cancer.

cone biopsy A surgical procedure in which a cone-shaped wedge of tissue is removed from the cervix. Used to diagnose and treat precancerous and cancerous conditions of the cervix.

contraindicated A term for something that is a poor idea—say, a medication or treatment that is absolutely wrong for a certain condition and will make it get worse.

copper T-380 A A type of IUD that is coated with copper as the spermicidal agent.

corpus luteum Literally, "yellow body." The cyst that forms after an egg is released by the ovary. Secretes progesterone and thus readies the lining of the uterus to receive a fertilized egg.

cryoablation The destruction of the lining of the uterus by freezing.

cryosurgery Freezing. Usually used in gynecology to treat genital warts and precancerous conditions of the cervix. Also known as cryotherapy.

CT scan, also called CAT scan Computerized axial tomography; an x-ray technique that focuses in at different levels of an organ or body cavity. Allows a three-dimensional visualization; usually fairly expensive.

cul-de-sac End of the abdominal cavity behind the uterus and cervix, and in front of the rectum.

culdocentesis Insertion of a needle through the vaginal wall into the cul-de-sac; used to check for blood or pus.

curette A surgical device used to remove cells from the wall of the uterus.

cyst A sac containing fluid.

cystic fibrosis A genetic disease associated with production of thick mucus in the lungs and pancreas.

cystitis A bladder infection.

cystocele A bulging out of the bladder into the vagina.

danazol Danocrine, a hormone used to treat endometriosis.

D&C Dilation and curettage; a procedure in which the cervix is stretched so that the lining of the uterus can be scraped.

D&E Dilation and evacuation; a procedure used to terminate a pregnancy that has continued beyond the first trimester.

dental dam An oral condom for prevention of sexually transmitted diseases.

Depo-Provera An injected form of medroxyprogesterone, used as a contraceptive and also for endometriosis therapy.

DES Diethylstilbestrol; a synthetic estrogen used in the 1950s and 1960s in the mistaken belief that it prevented miscarriage.

diabetes A medical condition characterized by abnormally large amounts of sugar in the blood.

diaphragm A small rubber cup that fits over the top of the vagina and covers the cervix; used for contraception.

diuretic A medication that pushes the kidney to excrete water, thereby increasing urine output.

diverticulum An abnormal outpouching of the lining of a hollow organ (for example, of the bowel or bladder).

DNA Deoxyribonucleic acid; the basic genetic material of all cellular organisms.

douching Rinsing out the vagina with a solution of vinegar, baking soda, or other product; intended as a means of personal hygiene, not effective as contraception.

dysmenorrhea Painful menstrual cramps.

dysplasia Abnormal development of cells.

ectocervix The outer part of the cervix; covered with flat (squamous) cells.

ectopic pregnancy A pregnancy outside the uterus, most commonly in one of the fallopian tubes.

ejaculation Emission of sperm from the penis.

electrocautery The use of electric current to stop bleeding or to cut tissue.

embolus Blood clot.

endocervix The inner part of the cervix; covered with glandular (columnar) cells.

endometrial ablation Electrical or laser destruction of the lining of the uterus; a treatment for heavy bleeding.

endometrial cancer Cancer of the lining of the uterus.

endometrioma A cyst of endometriosis, usually on an ovary.

endometriosis A condition in which endometrial-type tissue is found in locations outside the uterus. It can be anywhere in the pelvis, possibly near the bladder or bowel; rarely, as far away as in the lungs.

endometrium The innermost lining of the uterus, composed of glandular tissue.

endorphins Chemicals released in the brain that give a sense of well-being; commonly released with exercise.

epithelium The outermost layer of many organs. Skin is one kind of epithelium.

erectile dysfunction Formerly called impotence; the inability to maintain an erection.

ERT Estrogen replacement therapy; the giving of supplemental estrogen to replace that not made by the body. Women who have had hysterectomies often take ERT (estrogen only). Sometimes used as a synonym for HRT (hormone replacement therapy).

estrogen One of the primary female hormones.

ethinyl estradiol A synthetic derivative of the natural female hormone estradiol, used in birth control pills.

exotoxins Chemicals secreted by bacteria that can act like poisons.

exuberant Very heavy in growth.

fallopian tubes Narrow tubular structures attached to the uterus and extending toward the ovaries; conduits for eggs to go from the ovaries into the uterus. Fertilization occurs in the fallopian tubes.

false negative A test result saying that a condition is not present when it actually is.

false positive A test result saying that a condition is present when it is not.

FDA Food and Drug Administration; the agency of the federal government responsible for testing the safety of medications before they can be marketed to the public.

fertilization Penetration of an egg by a sperm.

fetal alcohol syndrome A condition affecting infants in utero if pregnant mothers drink two or more glasses of alcohol daily. May lead to mental retardation.

fibrocystic breast disease Lumpy breast tissue, often associated with discomfort.

fibroid A benign excess growth of the smooth muscle wall of the uterus. Also called a myoma, fibromyoma, or leiomyoma.

fibroma A collection of dense collagen-like tissue; sometimes seen on the ovary.

fimbriae The ends of the fallopian tubes; have fingerlike projections.

fimbrioplasty An infertility operation to fix scarred fimbriae.

Fitz-Hugh-Curtis syndrome Inflammation around the liver, associated with gonorrhea or chlamydial infection.

follicle A collection of cells in the ovary that surround the developing egg.

follicular phase The first portion of the menstrual cycle, the part before ovulation while the follicles are developing.

FSH Follicle-stimulating hormone; a peptide chemical made by the pituitary gland that stimulates egg development and estrogen production.

FTA-ABS Fluorescent treponemal antibody absorption test; a blood test for syphilis. Used in conjunction with the VDRL test.

gamete A reproductive cell, either an egg or a sperm.

genital warts Benign growths of tissue in the genital area, usually caused by the condyloma or papilloma virus.

gestational age In pregnancy, the number of weeks that have elapsed since the beginning of the last menstrual period.

GIFT Gamete intrafallopian transfer; an infertility procedure in which sperm and eggs are mixed outside the body, then deposited through a laparoscope into the fimbriated end of one of the fallopian tubes.

GLA Gammalinoleic acid; an essential fatty acid.

GnRH Gonadotropin-releasing hormone; a chemical produced by the hypothalamus that makes the pituitary gland secrete FSH and LH.

gonadotropins Hormones involved in reproduction. The pituitary secretes FSH and LH; the placenta secretes hCG.

gonorrhea A sexually transmitted disease caused by the gonococcus bacterium; can cause pelvic inflammatory disease and later infertility in women.

granulosa cells Cells that surround the maturing egg in the ovarian follicles.

gumma A wad of tissue infected with syphilis.

hCG or HCG Human chorionic gonadotropin; a hormone secreted by the placenta to keep the uterus hospitable to the fetus during pregnancy.

HDL High-density lipoprotein; "good" cholesterol.

hematocrit A measurement of red blood cells; the percentage of red blood cells in a known volume of blood.

hematoma A swelling filled with blood; a bruise.

hemoglobin The iron and protein compound in red blood cells that transports oxygen; a test measuring the number of red blood cells in the bloodstream.

hepatitis Inflammation of the liver.

herpes A family of viruses whose members cause genital herpes, fever blisters, chicken pox, shingles, and other diseases. Genital herpes, caused by the herpes simplex virus, is sexually transmitted.

HIV Human immunodeficiency virus, the virus that causes AIDS; weakens the body's ability to fight infections and cancers.

HMO A health maintenance organization.

hormone A chemical messenger used by cells to communicate with other cells and their targets.

HPV Human papilloma virus, the virus that causes genital warts.

HRT Hormone replacement therapy, usually includes progestin as well as estrogen; supplemental hormones given to replace those not made by the body.

HSV Herpes simplex virus.

hymen The plate of tissue covering the vaginal opening. Can be stretched or broken by sexual intercourse, exercise, or tampon use.

hyperplasia Benign but excessive growth of tissue, which if left unchecked can occasionally turn malignant.

hypertension High blood pressure.

hyperthyroidism Overactivity of the thyroid gland.

hypothalamus A portion of the brain that sits on top of the pituitary gland and governs much of the hormonal activity of the body.

hypothyroidism Underactivity of the thyroid gland.

hysterectomy Surgical removal of the uterus.

hysterogram An infertility test in which dye is injected into the uterus in order to visualize it on an x-ray. When the dye spills into the fallopian tubes and shows whether or not the tubes are open, the test is called a hysterosalpingogram.

hysteroscope A narrow tube containing a light that is passed through the cervix and used to look inside the uterus.

ICSI Intracytoplasmic sperm injection; used with in vitro fertilization when the sperm do not function well.

immunoglobulin A protein in the blood that fights infections.

implantation Attachment of the embryo to the lining of the uterus, where it then develops.

incompetent cervix A weakened neck of the uterus (cervix), which allows the cervix to dilate during pregnancy long before it is supposed to. Often associated with loss of pregnancy in the second trimester. The term is inept and inappropriate.

inflammatory response The action of the body that mounts its defenses to fight off infection.

in situ In place; refers to cancerous changes that "stay put" and do not invade nearby cells.

interferon An antiviral protein normally produced by the body in response to a viral infection. Can be manufactured genetically by pharmaceutical companies to give to people with viral infections.

intramural In the wall; for example, an intramural fibroid is located in the wall of the uterus.

IUD An intrauterine device; a small plastic device placed in the uterus to prevent pregnancy.

IVF In vitro fertilization; the technique whereby sperm and eggs are mixed in a test tube and then introduced into the uterus.

IVP Intravenous pyelogram; a kidney x-ray.

keloid Excessive scar formation, usually raised and thick. More common in black people than in Caucasians.

labia majora The outer lips of the vagina.

labia minora The smaller inner lips of the vagina.

laminaria Seaweed, strips of which are inserted into the cervix to help it stretch.

laparoscope A narrow metal tube, inserted into the abdominal cavity, that allows a look at the inside of the abdomen. Can be used to operate without making a large incision.

laparoscopy A technique for looking around inside the body using a laparoscope.

laparotomy An incision to look into the abdomen.

laser A highly focused light that delivers enough energy to actually cut tissue.

LDL Low-density lipoprotein, "bad" cholesterol; high levels can lead to heart disease.

LEEP Loop electrical excision procedure; a surgical technique for removing a piece of tissue, usually of the cervix, using an electrically heated wire.

leiomyosarcoma A cancer arising in the muscular tissue of a fibroid; very rare.

levonorgestrel A type of synthetic progestin used in birth control pills.

LH Luteinizing hormone; a chemical produced by the pituitary gland that leads to egg maturation and release by the ovary.

lipoproteins Fat molecules in the blood.

lithotripsy A procedure to dissolve kidney stones or sometimes gall stones.

lobule A little lobe; one of the glands in the breast where milk is produced.

local anesthesia A drug that temporarily deadens nerve endings; injected into the area to be numbed.

lumpectomy The surgical removal of a lump of tissue; usually refers to breast tissue.

Lunelle An injectable monthly hormonal contraceptive.

Lupron A drug that simulates menopause; used in therapy for endometriosis or fibroids.

luteal phase The second half of the menstrual cycle after ovulation, during which the corpus luteum secretes progesterone and readies the lining of the uterus to receive a fertilized egg.

Lyme disease An infection transmitted by ticks infected with the bacterium *Borrelia burgdorferi*.

lymph A clear fluid derived from body tissues that contains white blood cells.

lymphatics The circulatory vessels of the lymphatic system, which fights infection.

mammogram A breast x-ray.

marker A chemical that can be measured and may indicate the presence of some condition. For example, CA-125 can be used as a marker for ovarian cancer.

mastitis An infection of the breast.

menarche The onset of menstrual periods at puberty.

menopause The final cessation of menstrual periods.

menorrhagia Heavy loss of blood with menstrual periods.

menstrual extraction A suctioning out of the lining of the uterus; often used as an early form of abortion. Also called miniabortion or minisuction.

menstruation The monthly shedding of the lining of the uterus.

mestranol A synthetic estrogen used in birth control pills.

methotrexate A drug used in chemotherapy to kill cancer cells.

microinvasion Minimal spread of cancer cells beyond the border of the tumor itself.

mifepristone RU-486, a drug long used in Europe for abortion; acts by lowering progesterone levels. FDA approved in 2000 for use in the United States, but rarely utilized.

migraine A headache caused by changes in the blood vessels.

minilaparotomy A small incision made in the abdomen to operate in the pelvis.

minipill A birth control pill that contains only progesterone.

Mirena A recently developed IUD with progestin.

mittelschmerz Midcycle pain associated with ovulation.

monophasic A birth control pill containing a constant dose of progestin.

mons pubis The top of the vulva; a pad of fat over the pubic bone.

morcellator A device for cutting into little pieces. Used for fibroids.

MRI Magnetic resonance imaging; a diagnostic technique that can make thin-section images from any angle of any area within the body; can be used to assess soft tissue as well as bone. Its great advantage over x-rays or CT scans is that it does not subject the patient to radiation or require that contrast dyes be injected into the body. Especially valuable for looking at soft tissue and, although expensive, used for diagnosing back pain, stroke, brain tumors, heart, circulatory, and other problems.

mucinous Containing a jelly-like substance.

mucosa The inner lining of the uterus or another organ.

myomectomy Surgical removal of a fibroid or fibroids, leaving the uterus intact.

myometrium The muscular lining of the uterus.

neural tube A term in embryology for the tissue from which the brain and spinal column develop.

nonoxynol-9 The spermicidal agent used in most contraceptive creams, foams, or jellies.

norethindrone A synthetic progesterone used in birth control pills.

norgestrel Another synthetic progesterone used in birth control pills.

Norplant A long-lasting contraceptive containing progestin, no longer on the market in the United States; placed under the skin, it provided contraceptive protection for about five years.

NSAID A nonsteroidal anti-inflammatory medication; for example, aspirin or ibuprofen.

omentum The fatty apron of tissues that surrounds the intestines.

orgasm Sexual climax.

osteoporosis Loss or softening of bone, associated with increased risk of bone breakage; weakening of bone through loss of its hard inner structure. A frequent problem for women after menopause.

ovaries The female sex organs where eggs are matured, stored, and then released; the primary source of estrogen in the body.

ovulation The ripening, maturation, and release of an egg by the ovary.

Pap test, or Pap smear Often used as a test for cervical cancer; involves scraping superficial cells of the cervix and examining them for changes.

paracervical block Injection of a local anesthetic such as novocaine next to the cervix to relieve pain from an endometrial biopsy or D&C.

pathological Abnormal, associated with disease.

pathologist A doctor trained to look at tissue samples for diagnostic purposes.

PCOS Polycystic ovarian syndrome; a condition associated with multiple small cysts in the ovary. Leads to problems with ovulation.

pedicle The supporting tissue for an organ or, in surgery, the tissue from which a structure is released. (The stem of a mushroom could be considered its pedicle.)

pelvic exam Physical examination of the female reproductive organs, including the external female genitalia, the cervix, and, by palpation (feeling), the internal female organs.

Perganol An injectable medication made of gonadotropins, used to induce ovulation.

perimenopause The time "around menopause." Describes the period before menopause when ovarian function and hormone production are declining but have not yet totally stopped.

perineum Area between the vaginal opening and the anus.

PID Pelvic inflammatory disease; infection of the cervix, uterus, fallopian tubes, and/or ovaries.

pipelle A small plastic tube used to take samplings of the lining of the uterus.

pituitary gland The part of the brain immediately behind the bridge of the nose. Secretes hormones that regulate the activity of most of the glands in the body.

placebo A sugar pill, a "dummy" pill without effective ingredients. Often used in drug trials to see whether a patient is just thinking herself better or is actually receiving benefits from the specific drug being tested.

PMDD Premenstrual dysphoric disorder; severe PMS.

PMS Premenstrual syndrome; the symptoms can be emotional, including mood swings, or physical, including headaches and breast pain.

podophyllin A plant-derived chemical used to treat genital warts.

polyp An outgrowth of normal tissue, usually benign, attached to a mucuous membrane by a stem or stalk. Can occur in many body sites, singly or in groups. Polyps in the lining of the uterus may be associated with bleeding.

Progestasert An IUD with progestin; one of two basic types of IUD presently marketed in the United States.

progesterone A steroid hormone made by the corpus luteum in the ovary during the second half of the menstrual cycle; stabilizes the lining of the uterus and prepares it for implantation of a fertilized egg.

progestin Any of several synthetic forms of progesterone made in the laboratory.

prolactin A hormone made by the pituitary gland, which stimulates the secretion of breast milk. Elevated levels in nonpregnant women may be associated with irregular menstruation or infertility.

prolapsed uterus A uterus that is hanging down into the vagina, occasionally extending out of the vagina.

prophylactic Preventing or defending against something; a device, such as a condom, that prevents something (such as pregnancy or the spread of disease).

prostaglandins A family of hormones, made by the uterus and many other bodily organs, that stimulate the activity of smooth muscle, including the uterine wall.

psammona bodies A term from pathology; clumps of tissues often associated with ovarian cancer.

psoriasis An inflammatory skin disease.

pyelonephritis Bacterial infection of the kidney.

quants The abbreviation for quantitative human chorionic gonadotropin levels; measured to assess the well-being of an early pregnancy.

rape trauma syndrome The psychological aftermath of a sexual assault.

regional anesthesia A method of pain relief that involves placing a local anesthetic into the spinal canal (spinal anesthesia) or into the space around the spinal canal (epidural anesthesia).

retroverted Tilted backward.

Rhogam An immune globulin shot; prevents sensitization of Rh-negative women to subsequent Rh-positive pregnancies.

rhythm method A contraceptive practice based on timing intercourse to avoid the days surrounding ovulation.

risk factor Something that increases your chances of getting a disease. Smoking is a risk factor for lung cancer, among other diseases.

Risperdal A drug used to treat schizophrenia.

salpingostomy A surgical procedure in which the fallopian tube is opened; often used to treat ectopic pregnancy.

sarcoma A kind of cancer arising from connective or supportive tissue; for example, from bone or cartilage.

serosa The inner lining of the uterus.

serotonin A brain chemical responsible for mood; a serotonin deficiency may cause depression.

sickle-cell anemia, or sickle-cell disease A disorder of red blood cells. More common in blacks than in whites; can cause clumping of the cells in the blood vessels.

SIDS Sudden infant death syndrome.

SIL Squamous intraepithelial lesion; also known as cervical intraepithelial neoplasia.

sonography The process of using ultrasound technology for diagnostic or other purposes.

speculum An instrument used to look into the vagina; holds the vaginal walls apart so that the cervix is visible.

spermicide Something that kills sperm; the most common active ingredient is nonoxynol-9.

spina bifida A birth defect associated with an opening in the spinal canal.

spironolactone A diuretic that pushes the kidneys to excrete urine.

SSRI Selective serotonin re-uptake inhibitor; a medication that increases serotonin levels in the brain (Prozac was the first).

stat Immediately, at once; a stat dose of medication works in one use.

STD A sexually transmitted disease.

stereotactic A procedure that uses needles in conjunction with x-ray technology to locate an area of tissue that needs to be biopsied.

sterilization Permanent contraception of either men or women; a surgical procedure done in women cutting or blocking the fallopian tubes; in men, by cutting the vas deferens.

stromal Pertaining to the supporting tissue; the stromal tissue in the ovaries supports the egg-making apparatus.

submucosal Under the lining of an organ.

systemic Affecting the entire body (as opposed to "topical," which refers to a specific area).

tamoxifen A selective estrogen receptor modulator that blocks estrogen activity at the breast. Used to treat and prevent breast cancer.

Tay-Sachs disease A genetic disorder that leads to severe neurological impairment and early childhood death. More common in Jews and French Canadians than in others.

teratoma A tumor of the ovary, usually benign, which contains tissue that resembles tissue from other parts of the body (for example, teeth or hair). Also called a dermoid cyst.

testosterone The "male" steroid hormone. Also made by women, but in much smaller amounts.

thermogram A type of x-ray that picks up heat from tissue; occasionally used for detecting breast cancer.

thrombophlebitis Inflammation of the veins.

topical Applied to the surface of the body (as opposed to systemic).

totipotent A term describing a cell, for example an egg cell, that can turn into anything. Possible because all cells contain the same DNA.

toxic shock syndrome A general body reaction to poisonous substances released by staphylococcus infections.

triage Medically, sorting patients into groups so that those who are sickest get attention first.

trichomoniasis A vaginal infection produced by an amoeba-like organism; usually sexually transmitted.

triphasic When referring to oral contraceptives, pills with three levels of progestin.

tubal ligation A surgical procedure that severs the fallopian tubes.

tuboplasty An operation to repair scarred fallopian tubes.

tumor A swelling due to abnormal growth of cells.

Turner syndrome A genetic condition characterized by the presence of one X chromosome instead of two; individuals with this condition are women but cannot reproduce. Also called gonadal dysgenesis.

ultrasound A diagnostic tool that uses sound waves to examine the inside of the body. Often used to determine if a mass is solid or filled with fluid (cystic). Ultrasound procedures are basically risk free, as they do not involve exposure to radiation.

ureters The tubes that connect the kidneys to the bladder.

urethra The opening of the bladder to the outside of the body.

urethritis An inflammation of the urethra.

urinary tract infection Infection of the bladder and urethra.

urologist A physician who deals with the bladder, urethra, and kidneys and with problems of male infertility.

uterus The womb; the central part of the female reproductive tract, which houses the developing fetus.

vagina The tube leading from the uterus to the outside of the body.

vaginal flora The normal bacteria that live in the vagina.

vaginitis Inflammation of the vagina.

vagus nerve The "wandering" nerve; goes from the brain to distant organs such as the cervix and the diaphragm.

variocele A cluster of varicose veins in the scrotum near the testes.

vascular Referring to blood vessels.

vas deferens The tube that connects the penis and the testes.

vasectomy The surgical cutting of the vas deferens; a procedure for male sterilization.

vasovagal reaction Stimulation of the vagus nerve, for gynecological reasons, by manipulating the cervix; rarely, can cause the patient to pass out.

VDRL Venereal Disease Research Laboratory; a blood test for syphilis.

viability Ability to live, specifically outside the uterus.

von Willebrand's disease A bleeding disorder.

vulva The female external genitalia, the tissue surrounding the opening of the vagina.

ZIFT Zygote intrafallopian transfer; an infertility procedure in which the egg is fertilized outside the body, then the fertilized egg (the zygote) is introduced into one of the fallopian tubes.

▶ RESOURCES

This section contains ideas for additional reading, suggested Web sites, and the names and addresses of organizations that may provide information and support for you. In recent years the Internet has become a major source of information about health and disease. A word of warning: all Internet information is not equal. Unlike the articles in medical journals, which are reviewed by experts in the field before they are published, or printed books, which also are subjected to early editorial scrutiny, information on the Net has not necessarily been carefully examined. Many sites are sponsored by companies with an interest in selling their products: pharmaceuticals, herbals, vitamins, and other remedies. Other sites are hosted by people interested in the subject matter, who may or may not have accurate knowledge.

So if you are browsing the Net, be alert for bias, outdated material, and misinformation. Be aware of the source of the information and evaluate its objectivity. Discuss Web-based material with your physician before you follow its recommendations. Above all, use your common sense.

GENERAL SOURCES

ORGANIZATION

National Women's Health Resource Center, Inc.

120 Albany Street, Suite 820

New Brunswick, NJ 08901

Tel.: toll free (877) 98-NWHRC or (877) 986-9472

Web site: *www.healthywomen.org*

A nonprofit clearinghouse of information and resources about women's health. The organization publishes *National Women's Health Report,* a bimonthly newsletter; maintains a database on local hospitals, services, and other resources; and offers books and publications.

FURTHER READING

Berkow, Robert, editor. *The Merck Manual of Medical Information: Home Edition.* Whitehouse Station, NJ: Merck Research Laboratories, 1997.

An all-purpose, encyclopedic reference to medical problems and procedures from abdominal abscesses to zygote intrafallopian transfer. It offers the insights of two hundred medical experts and contains a useful glossary of medical terms, information on legal issues, a section on generic and brand-name pharmaceuticals, and a list of organizations offering information and support for a number of diseases and conditions.

Scialli, Anthony R., editor. *The National Women's Health Resource Center Book of Women's Health: Your Comprehensive Guide to Health and Well-Being.* New York: William Morrow, 1999.

This straightforward, basic discussion of health issues that affect women includes sections on nutrition, exercise, mental health, and cosmetic surgery as well as information on contraception, pregnancy, labor and delivery, and other clinical topics.

WEB SITES

Healthfinder

www.healthfinder.gov

This gateway site sponsored by the federal government provides links to more than fourteen hundred other sites, including on-line journals, libraries, and medical dictionaries.

The site gives advice about evaluating and choosing health care information offered on the Internet.

JAMA Women's Health Information Center

www.ama-assn.org/special/womh/womh.htm

Sponsored by the *Journal of the American Medical Association* and directed at physicians and health care professionals, the site contains information on topics of interest to women (eating disorders, STDs, osteoarthritis), and a library of articles from peer-reviewed medical journals.

Mayo Clinic

www.mayohealth.org

The site offers information on a wide range of topics, including women's health. It includes guides to making medical decisions and a section on healthy living.

Medhunt

www.hon.ch

Another gateway with links to a broad range of organizations, this site is sponsored by Health On the Net Foundation (HON), a not-for-profit organization headquartered in Geneva, Switzerland, dedicated to realizing the benefits of the Internet in the fields of health and medicine. One resource is a set of links to medical articles from daily news sources, sorted by topic.

National Institutes of Health (NIH)

www.nih.gov

The NIH is the focus for government-sponsored biomedical research in the United States. The site gives access to its prodigious health resources, including consumer health publications, information about clinical trials, health hotlines, MEDLINE (a catalog of articles published in medical journals), the NIH Information Index (a subject-word guide to diseases and conditions under investigation at NIH). Particularly useful is MEDLINEplus, a database of information for the general public: *www.nlm.nih.gov/medlineplus*.

National Women's Health Information Center

Toll-free hotline: (800) 994-9662 or (800) 994-WOMAN

www.4woman.gov

This site, a service of the Office on Women's Health in the U.S. Department of Health and Human Services, is a gateway to the vast women's health information resources of the federal government. The toll-free information line is available Monday through Friday, 9:00–6:00, eastern time.

ABORTION

ORGANIZATION

National Abortion Federation (NAF)
1755 Massachusetts Avenue, N.W., Suite 600
Washington, DC 20036
Tel.: (202) 667-5881; hotline: (800) 772-9100; in Canada: (800) 424-2280
Web site: *www.prochoice.org*
The NAF is an association of providers of abortion in the United States and Canada; it was founded to make high-quality abortion services accessible to all women. It has developed professional standards on medical, nursing, counseling, administrative, and ethical aspects of abortion services and has established evaluation systems based on these standards. The Web site includes a guide to choosing abortion facilities, information on the legal and political aspects of abortion, fact sheets, and statistics on abortion in the United States. The hotline will provide referrals to qualified providers as well as help in navigating abortion restrictions in various states.

FURTHER READING

Adler, N. E., H. P. David, B. N. Major, S. H. Roth, N. F. Russo, and G. E. Wyatt. Psychological factors in abortion: A review. *American Psychologist* 47(10): 1194–1204 (Oct. 1992).
A classic paper on the psychological aspects of abortion and the feelings of women after the procedure.

Kaufmann, K. *The Abortion Resource Handbook.* New York: Fireside, 1997.
Explains how to find a safe prochoice clinic, examines parental consent laws, suggests questions to ask doctors, lists prochoice organizations by state.

Schneider, Karen A., editor. *Choices: Women Speak Out About Abortion.* Seattle: Seal Press, NARAL Foundation, 1998.
In observation of the 25th anniversary of the *Roe* v. *Wade* decision, the NARAL Founda-

tion (an arm of the National Abortion and Reproductive Rights Action League) published this book, which includes a dozen accounts by women of their abortion experiences.

WEB SITE

NARAL (National Abortion and Reproductive Rights Action League)
www.naral.org
The Web site of this activist organization includes information about the political struggle to keep abortion legal.

AFRICAN AMERICAN WOMEN'S HEALTH CONCERNS

ORGANIZATION

Celebrating Life Foundation
P.O. Box 224076
Dallas, TX 75222-4076
Tel.: (800) 207-0992
Web site: *www.celebratinglife.org/*
The Celebrating Life Foundation was established in 1995 to promote breast cancer awareness among women of color. The Web site has information about breast cancer as related to African American women, interviews with cancer survivors, answers to frequently asked questions, lists of support groups, and links to other major sites.

FURTHER READING

Villarosa, Linda, editor. *Body and Soul: The Black Woman's Guide to Physical Health and Emotional Well-Being.* New York: Harper Perennial Library, 1994.
Sponsored by the National Black Women's Health Project, this guide speaks to the physical and emotional issues surrounding good health.

White, Evelyn C., editor. *The Black Women's Health Book: Speaking for Ourselves.* Seattle: Seal Press, 1994.
These collected essays by African American women about health issues that affect them, their families, and their communities cover menopause, breast-feeding, holistic healing, fibroids, diet, skin color issues, teenage sexuality, and HIV. Contributors include Marian Wright Edelman, Toni Morrison, Alice Walker, and Faye Wattleton. Though the book is out of print, you may find it at your library.

AIS (ANDROGEN INSENSITIVITY SYNDROME, OR TESTICULAR FEMINIZATION)

ORGANIZATION

Androgen Insensitivity Syndrome Support Group
www.medhelp.org/www/ais/
This support group was started in Great Britain by the mother of an AIS infant and formalized in 1993. The Web site offers information about AIS, a newsletter, personal stories, a bibliography listing both scientific papers and popular works, and links to sites focused on infertility and adoption, social issues, and other relevant topics.

FURTHER READING

Kessler, Suzanne J. *Lessons from the Intersexed.* New Brunswick, NJ: Rutgers University Press, 1998.
The book discusses AIS and the lives of people with this syndrome; it is recommended by the AIS Support Group.

ALTERNATIVE THERAPIES AND COMPLEMENTARY MEDICINE

ORGANIZATION

National Center for Complementary and Alternative Medicine (NCCAM)
Tel. (clearinghouse), toll free: (888) 644-6226
Web site: *nccam.nih.gov*
NCCAM was established in 1998 by the federal government to evaluate and support complementary and alternative medicine. Although it facilitates and conducts research, it is not a referral service. The Web site provides access to the Complementary and Alternative Medicine (CAM) Citation Index (CCI) of more than 180,000 bibliographic citations dating back to 1963, as well as fact sheets about dietary supplements and alternative treatments.

FURTHER READING

Cassileth, Barrie R. *The Alternative Medicine Handbook.* New York: W. W. Norton, 1998.
A well-balanced and thorough look at alternative and complementary treatments from acupuncture to yoga, this book is by a founding member of the advisory council to the NIH Office of Alternative Medicine.

Moyers, Bill. *Healing and the Mind.* New York: Doubleday, 1993.
This intelligent exploration of mind-body interactions was written as a companion to the series on public television.

Sifton, David W., editor. *The PDR Family Guide to Natural Medicines and Healing Therapies.* New York: Three Rivers Press, 1999.
A comprehensive and useful book, this guide includes information about herbal remedies, alternative approaches, and nutritional supplements. For each treatment the guide mentions possible side effects, drug interactions, and precautions during pregnancy or breast-feeding. It further describes alternative therapies and their goals, and suggests when to consult a conventional physician.

BODY IMAGE

FURTHER READING

Cash, Thomas F. *The Body Image Workbook: An 8-Step Program for Learning to Like Your Looks.* Oakland, CA: New Harbinger Press, 1997.
This workbook, written by a clinical psychologist who has also published scholarly work, contains a self-help program on overcoming unhealthy attitudes toward physical appearance.

BREAST CANCER

ORGANIZATIONS

National Alliance of Breast Cancer Organizations (NABCO)
9 East 37th Street, 10th floor
New York, NY 10016
Tel.: for information (888) 80-NABCO; for administrative offices (212) 889-0606
Web site: *www.nabco.org*
A source of timely information for media, medical organizations, professionals, patients, and their families, NABCO is also a political organization advocating regulatory change and legislation that benefits women with breast cancer and women at risk. The Web site has general information about breast cancer, news of clinical trials, and listing of support groups.

Susan G. Komen Breast Cancer Foundation

5005 LBJ Freeway, Suite 370

Dallas, TX 75244

Tel.: (972) 855-1600 or (800) I'M AWARE (462-9273)

Web site: *www.komen.org/*

The foundation, started by the sister of Susan G. Komen who died of breast cancer, offers information and support to women who have the disease. It promotes medical research with the goal of eradicating breast cancer; the Race for the Cure is one of its projects. The help line has information to assist women in making decisions about treatment. The site has a forum where survivors and their families and friends can share their thoughts, and a list of relevant articles on developments in the field including research updates.

Y-ME National Breast Cancer Organization

212 W. Van Buren Street, Suite 500

Chicago IL 60607-3908

Tel.: (312) 986-8338 or toll free: (800) 221-2141

Web site: *www.y-me.org*

Y-ME National Breast Cancer Organization is committed to providing information and support to anyone who has been touched by breast cancer. The site includes information on screening and detection, and a profiler for finding treatment options.

FURTHER READING

Hirshaut, Yashar, Peter I. Pressman, and Amy S. Langer. *Breast Cancer: The Complete Guide,* rev. ed. New York: Bantam Books, 1997.

This book, written by a surgeon and an oncologist, discusses diagnosis, treatment, recovery, and life after cancer. It explores factors such as heredity, race, diet, alcohol and caffeine use, smoking, radiation exposure and other environmental causes, as well as hormones, birth control pills, and hormone replacement therapy.

Kaye, Ronnie. *Spinning Straw into Gold: Your Emotional Recovery from Breast Cancer.* New York: Fireside, 1991.

Written by a psychotherapist who was diagnosed with breast cancer, the book suggests the possibility of transforming a devastating crisis into an opportunity for growth.

LaTour, Kathy. *The Breast Cancer Companion.* New York: Avon Books, 1994.
Written by a breast cancer survivor, the book addresses both medical and emotional issues surrounding the disease.

BREAST IMPLANTS AND RECONSTRUCTION

FURTHER READING

Berger, Karen, and John Bostwick III. *A Woman's Decision: Breast Care, Treatment and Reconstruction.* St. Louis: Quality Medical Publishing, 1998.
Along with information on breast cancer and treatment options including breast reconstruction, the book offers personal stories, information about communicating with your doctor, and the effect of breast cancer on relationships.

Bruning, Nancy Pauline. *Breast Implants: Everything You Need to Know,* rev. ed. Alameda, CA: Hunter House, 1995.
Written by a breast cancer survivor, the book covers the controversial history of silicone gel implants and explains how to evaluate the issues and risks of implant surgery and implant removal.

CANCER: GENERAL RESOURCES

ORGANIZATIONS

American Cancer Society
1599 Clifton Road NE
Atlanta, GA 30329
Tel.: (800) 227-2345
Web site: *www.cancer.org*
Founded in 1913, the American Cancer Society has programs in research, patient services, and advocacy and offers education for prevention, detection, and treatment. The Web site has general cancer information, as well as articles about alternative and complementary medicine and new scientific developments.

Cancer Care
275 Seventh Avenue
New York, NY 10001

Tel.: (212) 712-8080; hotline: (800) 813-HOPE (4673)

Web site: *www.cancercare.org*

This national social service agency is dedicated to providing free emotional support, information, and practical help to people with cancer, their loved ones, and caregivers. Founded in 1944, Cancer Care focuses on helping people cope with the emotional, social, and financial burdens of cancer.

National Cancer Institute

9000 Rockville Pike

Bethesda, MD 20892

Tel.: (800) 4-CANCER (422-6237)

To write for information:

NCI Public Inquiries Office

Building 31, Room 10A31

31 Center Drive, MSC 2580

Bethesda, MD 20892-2580

Web site: *www.cancer.gov/cancer_information*

Part of the NIH, the Cancer Institute's Web site offers a wealth of information from peer-reviewed scientific papers to information on clinical trials. There are also links (for both the public and health care professionals) to sites focused on specific types of cancer.

CONTRACEPTION

ORGANIZATIONS

Planned Parenthood of America

810 Seventh Avenue

New York, NY 10019

Tel.: (212) 541-7800; toll-free help line: (800) 230-PLAN (230-7526)

Web site: *www.plannedparenthood.org*

Founded by Margaret Sanger, Planned Parenthood offers affordable reproductive health care. Services include family planning counseling, birth control, pregnancy testing and counseling, emergency contraception, Pap tests, breast exams, HIV testing and counseling, screening for STDs, age-appropriate sex education, abortion or abortion referrals, and other services. The Web site will find a clinic near you.

Population Council
One Dag Hammarskjold Plaza
New York, NY 10017
Tel.: (212) 339-0500
Web site: *www.popcouncil.org*
The Population Council is a nonprofit research organization focusing on reproductive health and population control around the world, to find a balance between population and resources. It analyzes population issues and trends, conducts research in the social and reproductive sciences, develops new contraceptives, and works with public and private agencies to improve the quality of family planning and reproductive health services. The Web site includes information on emergency contraception, long-term contraception, and news about contraceptives under development.

DOMESTIC VIOLENCE / ABUSE

ORGANIZATIONS

National Coalition Against Domestic Violence
P.O. Box 18749
Denver, CO 80218
Tel.: (303) 839-1852
Web site: *www.ncadv.org/*
The site has information about personal safety, phone numbers of state organizations, and links to other relevant Web sites.

National Domestic Violence Hotline
(800) 799-SAFE (7233) or (800) 787-3224 (TTY). For emergencies call 911.
Web site: *www.ndvh.org*
The hotline is a project of the Texas Council on Family Violence and provides counseling for women in troubling and possibly dangerous relationships.

FURTHER READING

Herman, Judith Lewis. *Trauma and Recovery,* rev. ed. New York: Basic Books, 1997.
Written by a faculty member of Harvard Medical School, this book examines post-traumatic stress disorder and draws parallels between domestic violence, the experience of combat, and political terrorism.

Jones, Anne, and Susan Schechter. *When Love Goes Wrong: What to Do When You Can't Do Anything Right.* New York: Harper Perennial Library, 1993.

This "how-to" book, written by two women who have worked for many years with victims of domestic violence, contains advice for victims, social workers, counselors, and concerned friends.

Miller, Mary Susan. *No Visible Wounds: Identifying Nonphysical Abuse of Women by Their Men.* Chicago: Contemporary Books, 1995. Reprinted by Fawcett Books, 1996.

Miller discusses psychological abuse, including social and economic manipulation, and other forms of emotional battering, offering the experiences of women who have escaped abusive relationships and providing guidelines to women who are considering leaving such a relationship.

WEB SITE

American Bar Association Commission on Domestic Violence
www.abanet.org/domviol/home.html
Directed primarily at lawyers who deal professionally with the problem of domestic abuse, this site has safety tips, information about getting legal aid, statistics, and educational material.

DRUGS AND MEDICATIONS

FURTHER READING

Donjon, Richard P. *Mosby's Over-the-Counter Medicine Cabinet Medicines.* St. Louis: Mosby Lifeline, 1996.

This book lists more than five hundred over-the-counter medications, describes symptoms of common problems, and suggests over-the-counter drugs for specific conditions. In addition, it describes possible drug interactions and side effects.

Graedon, Joe, and Teresa Graedon. *The People's Pharmacy,* rev. ed. New York: St. Martin's Press, 1998.

This book is an authoritative and popular reference guide to prescription drugs, over-the-counter medications, and home remedies. Includes information on drug interactions and side effects.

Graedon, Joe, and Teresa Graedon. *Deadly Drug Interactions: The People's Pharmacy Guide: How to Protect Yourself from Harmful Drug/Drug, Drug/Food, Drug/Vitamin Combinations.* New York: St. Martin's Press, 1997.

The Physicians' Desk Reference, 56th ed. Montvale, NJ: Medical Economics Company, 2002.
This volume is the standard reference to prescription medications, known in the profession as the *PDR.* Published annually, it is directed at physicians and written in technical language.

Sifton, David, ed. *The PDR Family Guide to Over-the-Counter Drugs.* New York: Ballantine Books, 1998.

EMERGENCY CONTRACEPTION

WEB SITE

Not-2-Late.com
ec.princeton.edu
Operated by the Office of Population Research at Princeton University and by the Association of Reproductive Health Professionals, this site offers information about emergency contraception.

ENDOMETRIOSIS

FURTHER READING

Ballweg, Mary Lou, editor, and the Endometriosis Association. *The Endometriosis Sourcebook: The Definitive Guide to Current Treatment Options, the Latest Research, Common Myths About the Disease and Coping Strategies.* New York: McGraw Hill, 1995.
This guide to current treatment options, research, and coping strategies was compiled by the Endometriosis Association and its president, who lived with the disease for years. It examines the connections between endometriosis and autoimmune diseases and looks at treatments based on Chinese medicine and those of modern medical technology. Included are letters from women detailing their experiences.

HIV/AIDS

ORGANIZATIONS

Body Health Resources Corporation
250 West 57th Street, Suite 415
New York, NY 10107
Tel.: (212) 541-8500
Web site: *www.thebody.com*
Body Health Resources maintains this excellent Web site for nonprofit organizations. It offers information by and for women living with HIV/AIDS, a section on the basics of prevention for women, chat rooms, bulletin boards, and forums on diet, nutrition, exercise, and treatment.

CDC National Prevention Information Network
P.O. Box 6003
Rockville, MD 20849-6003
Tel.: (800) 458-5231; AIDS hotline: (800) 342-AIDS (2437) (24 hours a day, 7 days a week)
Web site: *www.cdc.gov/hiv/dhap.htm*
Topics on the Web site include vaccine research, prevention tools, treatment, and statistics documenting the epidemic, and answers to frequently asked questions. Some of the information is technical, some directed at the public. The site is a useful source for recent information and updates.

FURTHER READING

Bartlett, John G., and Ann K. Finkbeiner. *The Guide to Living with HIV Infection: Developed at the Johns Hopkins AIDS Clinic,* 4th ed. Baltimore: Johns Hopkins University Press, 1998.
This updated edition of a comprehensive book contains new information on HIV treatment strategies; it discusses the effectiveness, availability, and side effects of new drugs, coping with the emotional effects of the infection, financial and legal concerns, and special problems of women.

Ward, Darrell E. *The AmFAR AIDS Handbook: The Complete Guide to Understanding HIV and AIDS.* New York: W. W. Norton, 1998.
Compiled by AmFAR, the nonprofit American Foundation for AIDS Research, this com-

prehensive guide offers information on combination therapy and other treatment options.

WEB SITE

HIV InSite

hivinsite.ucsf.edu/InSite

Hosted by the University of California at San Francisco, the site provides a gateway to all kinds of HIV/AIDS information. It includes clinical information from textbooks as well as discussions, case studies, and down-to-earth insights into what works and what does not for preventing HIV infection. There are also discussions of social and legal issues and links to the latest available national and global statistics.

INFERTILITY

ORGANIZATIONS

American Society for Reproductive Medicine

1209 Montgomery Highway

Birmingham, AL 35216-2809

Tel.: (205) 978-5000

Web site: *www.asrm.org*

The American Society for Reproductive Medicine (formerly the American Infertility Society) is the professional organization for physicians working in this field. The Web site has answers to frequently asked questions, links to other professional organizations, fact sheets and booklets, information about state infertility insurance laws, and updates on current research.

RESOLVE, Inc.

1310 Broadway

Somerville, MA 02144-1731

Tel.: (617) 623-1156; help line: (617) 623-0744

Web site: *www.resolve.org*

RESOLVE, the national support organization for couples coping with infertility, offers a membership network, information about physicians, and a newsletter. Visitors to the Web site can access its services and follow links to Centers for Disease Control (CDC) statistical reports on the success of assisted reproductive technologies.

FURTHER READING

Berger, Gary S., Marc Goldstein, and Mark Fuerst. *The Couple's Guide to Infertility,* rev. ed. New York: Doubleday, 1994.

Carter, Jean W., and Michael P. Carter. *Sweet Grapes: How to Stop Being Infertile and Start Living Again,* rev. ed. Indianapolis: Perspectives Press, 1998.
Written by a doctor and her husband who have experienced infertility, this guide offers suggestions on making positive choices and reordering priorities that may have become skewed during the quest for a biological child.

Peoples, Debby, and Harriette Rovner Ferguson. *What to Expect When You're Experiencing Infertility.* New York: W. W. Norton, 1998.
Written with compassion and respect for those undergoing the ordeal, this book deals in depth with the emotional, medical, and financial issues surrounding infertility.

WEB SITE

National Center for Chronic Disease Prevention and Health Promotion
www.cdc.gov/nccdphp/drh/art.htm
The center, part of the CDC, posts annual statistical reports on the success of assisted reproductive technologies.

MISCARRIAGE

ORGANIZATIONS

Compassionate Friends
P.O. Box 3696
Oak Brook, IL 60522-3696
Tel.: (630) 990-0010
Web site: *www.compassionatefriends.org*
This organization, founded in England in 1969, now has branches in the United States and serves as a support group offering friendship and understanding to families who are grieving the death of a child of any age, from any cause. The Web site has a chapter locator, links to recent relevant newspaper stories and articles, and publications on coping with loss and grief.

SHARE
St. Joseph Health Center
300 First Capitol Drive
St. Charles, MO 63302-2893
Tel.: (314) 947-6164 or (800) 821-6819
Web site: *www.nationalshareoffice.com*
Founded in 1977, SHARE now has 130 chapters here and abroad. Its Web site offers links to
the chapters and other organizations, chat rooms, and news.

OVARIAN CANCER

ORGANIZATION

Gilda Radner Familial Ovarian Cancer Registry
Roswell Park Cancer Institute
Elm and Carlton Streets
Buffalo, NY 14263-0001
Tel.: (800) 682-7426 (800-OVARIAN)
Web site: *www.overiancancer.com*
The site contains basic information about ovarian cancer and a newsletter detailing devel-
opments in research, as well as the familial registry itself.

FURTHER READING

Piver, M. Steven, with Gene Wilder. *Gilda's Disease: Sharing Personal Experiences and a
Medical Perspective on Ovarian Cancer.* New York: Broadway Books, 1998.

PMS

FURTHER READING

Dalton, Katharina, and Wendy Holton. *Once a Month: Understanding and Treating PMS.*
Alameda, CA: Hunter House, 1999.
A reissue of a classic work, updated with new information on PMS and osteoporosis, the
book describes common symptoms and self-help strategies.

Hahn, Linaya. *PMS—Solving the Puzzle: Sixteen Causes of PMS and What to Do About It.*
Evanston, IL: Chicago Spectrum Press, 1995.
A self-help guide based on personal experience by a worker in holistic medicine, this dis-

cussion suggests causes and offers recommendations, including dietary changes, exposure to full-spectrum light, and improving quality of sleep.

SEX EDUCATION: RESOURCES FOR PARENT-CHILD DISCUSSION OF SEX

ORGANIZATIONS

Kaiser Family Foundation
2400 Sand Hill Road
Menlo Park, CA 94025
Tel.: (650) 854-9400
Web site: *www.kff.org/*
This independent health care philanthropy focuses on major national health care issues. The site offers guidelines for talking with children about difficult issues, including sex, violence among young people, and drugs and alcohol.
Web site: *www.talkingwithkids.org*

National Campaign to Prevent Teen Pregnancy
1776 Massachusetts Avenue, N.W., Suite 200
Washington, DC 20036
Tel.: (202) 478-8500
Web site: *www.teenpregnancy.org*
This organization places great value on communication between parents and children. The site gives parents tips on talking to their children about sex in a meaningful and intelligent way. It has links to other organizations with a similar mission, as well as a list of publications, including free materials.

FURTHER READING

Moglia, Ronald Filiberti, and Jon Knowles, editors. *All About Sex: A Family Resource on Sex and Sexuality.* New York: Crown Books, 1997.
Endorsed by Planned Parenthood, this guide provides information about all aspects of human sexuality and includes clear explanations of human reproduction and sexual pleasure, as well as entries on the psychology of sex and laws affecting our sexuality. It is directed at open-minded families with teenagers and preteens.

SEXUAL IDENTITY

FURTHER READING

White, Jocelyn C., and Marissa C. Martinez. *The Lesbian Health Book: Caring for Ourselves.* Seattle: Seal Press, 1997.
The essays in this book, written from the perspective of doctors, patients, researchers, and health care advocates, deal with physical and mental health, including discussions of parenting, menopause, aging, and death.

WEB SITE

www.pridenet.com/
The PrideNet site, with links for every state, has information about support groups, hotlines and information services, physicians, and other professional services.

SEXUAL PERFORMANCE AND RESPONSE

FURTHER READING

Barbach, Lonnie Garfield. *For Yourself: The Fulfillment of Female Sexuality,* Reissue. New York: Anchor Books, 1990.
This classic book, originally published in 1976, provides support and reassurance and a practical course in freeing up sexuality.

Comfort, Alex. *The New Joy of Sex: A Gourmet Guide to Lovemaking in the Nineties.* New York: Crown Publishers, 1994.
Comfort's sex manual, first published in 1972, became a classic, selling millions of copies. Its frank words and explicit line drawings captured the spirit of the sexual revolution. It has been updated to include information on sex in the age of HIV and other health concerns, as well as "how-to" information.

Westheimer, Dr. Ruth K. *Sex for Dummies: A Reference Guide for the Rest of Us.* Foster City, CA: IDG Books, 1995.
Despite its unfortunate title, the book contains the warmth and wisdom of Dr. Ruth, the well-known sex therapist, and includes discussion of the psychological aspects of sex. Like the outspoken doctor herself, it does not shy away from sensitive topics such as impotence, physical disabilities, and "coming out" for people who have been married and have children. It is a useful resource for parents talking to young people.

TURNER SYNDROME

ORGANIZATION

Turner Syndrome Society of the United States
14450 TC Jester, Suite 260
Houston, TX 77014
Tel.: (800) 365-9944
Web site: *www.turner-syndrome-us.org*
The site has answers to frequently asked questions, fact sheets, and a list of support groups.

► INDEX